Emerging Technologies in Biomedical Imaging

Emerging Technologies in Biomedical Imaging

Editor: Ricky Collier

hayle medical
New York

Hayle Medical,
750 Third Avenue, 9th Floor,
New York, NY 10017, USA

Visit us on the World Wide Web at:
www.haylemedical.com

ISBN 978-1-64647-558-2 (Hardback)

Cataloging-in-Publication Data

Emerging technologies in biomedical imaging / edited by Ricky Collier.
p. cm.
Includes bibliographical references and index.
ISBN 978-1-64647-558-2
1. Imaging systems in medicine. 2. Diagnostic imaging.
3. Imaging systems in medicine--Technological innovations.
4. Medical radiology. I. Collier, Ricky.
R857.O6 E44 2023
616.075 4--dc23

Contents

Preface

In my initial years as a student, I used to run to the library at every possible instance to grab a book and learn something new. Books were my primary source of knowledge and I would not have come such a long way without all that I learnt from them. Thus, when I was approached to edit this book; I became understandably nostalgic. It was an absolute honor to be considered worthy of guiding the current generation as well as those to come. I put all my knowledge and hard work into making this book most beneficial for its readers.

Biomedical imaging is a field that deals with capturing the images of the internal organs of the body for diagnostic and therapeutic purposes. It helps create informative images of the organs and structures of the body for clinical purposes. Micro-electro-mechanical systems (MEMS) technology has demonstrated enormous potential in biomedical imaging applications due to its outstanding advantages such as miniaturization, high speed, higher resolution, and convenience of batch fabrication. Emerging technologies in biomedical imaging include artificial intelligence (AI), augmented reality (AR), and cinematic rendering and digital twin technology. AI can be used to guide the radiologists on positioning the machine and preparing the optimum settings for the scan. These settings can be based on age, gender, area or disease of focus. This book unravels the recent studies in the field of biomedical imaging, focusing on the emerging technologies and applications. It will prove to be immensely beneficial to students and researchers in this field.

I wish to thank my publisher for supporting me at every step. I would also like to thank all the authors who have contributed their researches in this book. I hope this book will be a valuable contribution to the progress of the field.

Editor

1

Wide Field-of-View Fluorescence Imaging with Optical-Quality Curved Microfluidic Chamber for Absolute Cell Counting

Mohiuddin Khan Shourav [1], Kyunghoon Kim [2,3], Subin Kim [1] and Jung Kyung Kim [1,2,*]

[1] Department of Mechanical Engineering, Graduate School, Kookmin University, 77 Jeongneung-ro, Seongbuk-gu, Seoul 02707, Korea; khan@kookmin.ac.kr (M.K.S.); subinkim@kookmin.ac.kr (S.K.)

[2] School of Mechanical Systems Engineering, Kookmin University, 77 Jeongneung-ro, Seongbuk-gu, Seoul 02707, Korea

[3] Department of Mechanical and Aerospace Engineering, North Carolina State University, Raleigh, NC 27695, USA; kkim15@ncsu.edu

* Correspondence: jkkim@kookmin.ac.kr

Academic Editors: Shih-Chi Chen and Wei-Chuan Shih

Abstract: Field curvature and other aberrations are encountered inevitably when designing a compact fluorescence imaging system with a simple lens. Although multiple lens elements can be used to correct most such aberrations, doing so increases system cost and complexity. Herein, we propose a wide field-of-view (FOV) fluorescence imaging method with an unconventional optical-quality curved sample chamber that corrects the field curvature caused by a simple lens. Our optics simulations and proof-of-concept experiments demonstrate that a curved substrate with lens-dependent curvature can reduce greatly the distortion in an image taken with a conventional planar detector. Following the validation study, we designed a curved sample chamber that can contain a known amount of sample volume and fabricated it at reasonable cost using plastic injection molding. At a magnification factor of approximately 0.6, the curved chamber provides a clear view of approximately 119 mm^2, which is approximately two times larger than the aberration-free area of a planar chamber. Remarkably, a fluorescence image of microbeads in the curved chamber exhibits almost uniform intensity over the entire field even with a simple lens imaging system, whereas the distorted boundary region has much lower brightness than the central area in the planar chamber. The absolute count of white blood cells stained with a fluorescence dye was in good agreement with that obtained by a commercially available conventional microscopy system. Hence, a wide FOV imaging system with the proposed curved sample chamber would enable us to acquire an undistorted image of a large sample volume without requiring a time-consuming scanning process in point-of-care diagnostic applications.

Keywords: curved chamber; fluorescence imaging; aberration; field curvature; field of view; cell counting

1. Introduction

The term "aberration" is generally used to describe errors in optical images. Aberrations are caused by different focus positions on the image plane. Field curvature is one among the various types of monochromatic aberrations. For a flat detector surface, Petzval and field curvature must be corrected by balancing positive and negative power surfaces [1]. To overcome this problem, conventional microscope objectives are designed with multiple lenses. Although this usually corrects all aberrations, it is quite expensive to implement. The resulting system cost, size, and complexity limit accessibility of the device to well-funded laboratories with the required space and personnel trained in device operation and maintenance. Although unconventional solutions are becoming more popular for some applications, balancing performance and cost is challenging [2]. Smith et al. [3] proposed two common biomedical devices, a microscope and a spectrometer, as simple and inexpensive add-ons to a commercial cell phone camera. Although other researchers have previously demonstrated similar devices, such as mobile phone-based clinical microscope [4] that has both bright field and fluorescence imaging modes, the phone attachments proposed by Smith et al. are considerably smaller, simpler, and low in cost while still maintaining acceptable levels of performance. With increasing demand for fluorescence imaging in diagnostics, many imaging techniques have been developed. A cytometry platform [5] was designed and installed on a cell phone for blood cell analysis in field settings, enabling cost-effective and rapid measurement of the density of blood cells and hemoglobin concentration. Choi et al. [6] proposed and developed a fast-scanning method for fluorescence detection in three-dimensional (3D) cell culture by introducing a digital micromirror device (DMD), and Benjamin et al. proposed adaptive scanning optical microscopy (ASOM) [7], a unique wide-field imaging system designed with inexpensive techniques compared to conventional microscopy. However, the design of the latter is complex and might warrant careful handling.

Field curvature is a type of monochromatic aberration. Although all aberrations encountered with a conventional microscopic objective can be corrected using multiple lens elements, doing so is quite expensive. The advantages of a curved image plane have been described [8,9]. A curved imager provides a large degree of freedom in camera system design. It affords better resolution and brightness, in addition to reducing primary aberrations. Curved focal plane arrays (FPAs) have been proposed to remove spherical aberrations caused by spherical mirrors. Moreover, large field-of-view (FOV) cameras, spherical imagers, artificial retinas, and biomimetic optical sensors, equipped with curved FPAs have been proposed [10,11]. Jung et al. [12] recently made progress toward the realization of an eyeball camera. Realistic images can be collected by functional silicon devices. Despite the fact that these systems have advantages over a conventional planar detector, their curved detector with fixed curvature leads to discrepant variable zoom when using simple lenses.

A few lens-free approaches to point-of-care (POC) diagnosis have been proposed and advanced [13–17]. These may make the system more compact and easier to use for personnel. A giga-pixel fluorescent imaging system has been developed by modifying a commercially available scanner, which can analyze 2.2 mL of sample volume [18]. For lens-free imaging, samples are to be placed over the image sensor before image capture. Sample image does not have the optical aberration that may occur with lens imaging. However, the area of these images depends on the sensor size, and to place the sample over the sensor, a custom-fabricated chamber is required. Conventional imaging systems employ several lenses to eliminate primary aberration, because of which, designing systems for remote and on-site applications becomes expensive and complicated. These challenges can be overcome using a curved imaging surface to reduce the number of lenses in the imaging system and eliminate primary aberration and field curvature. However, sophisticated engineering skills are required to fabricate the designed system, and the curved imaging sensor might not be affordable to people from resource-confined areas. A curved refractive mirror was introduced as a substitute for correcting objective lens to compensate for field curvature or the Petzval effect [19]. The proposed system leads transmitted rays to a flat image plane and ensures uniform focus on the flat image plane for flat objects.

Herein, we describe a simple optical imaging system for large-field absolute counting of white blood cells (WBCs). An alternative approach is developed to correct field curvature in a flat image plane by replacing the conventional planar sample chamber with a curved one while using a single lens. The Petzval theory was revisited, and an optical simulation was conducted to determine the lens-specific curvature of the curved sample substrate that reduces field curvature in a compact single-lens fluorescence imaging system. The proposed method was validated further by experimental studies conducted using a custom-made curved sample substrate and an optical-quality curved sample chamber with fluorescent microbeads and white blood cells.

2. Materials and Methods

2.1. Theory

Petzval field curvature can be determined as below [20]:

$$\frac{1}{r_k} = -n_k \sum_{i=1}^{k} \frac{K_i}{n_{i-1} n_i} \tag{1}$$

where n_i is the refractive index of the i-th material, r_i is the radius of curvature of the i-th material, and K_i is the power of the i-th lens, defined as $K_i = (n_i - n_{i-1})/R_i$, where R_i is the radius of the i-th lens. The field curvature or Petzval radius of a single lens can be calculated as follows:

$$\frac{1}{n_0 r_0} - \frac{1}{n_2 r_2} = \frac{K_1}{n_0 n_1} + \frac{K_2}{n_1 n_2} \tag{2}$$

where r_0 and r_2 are the radii of curvature of the object and the image surfaces, respectively. Because light is projected through a single lens, n_0, n_1, and n_2 are the refractive indices after refraction in the three-media system. We found that r_0 and r_2 are symmetric to each other, and assuming the image surface is flat ($r_2 \rightarrow \infty$), Equation (2) reduces to:

$$\frac{1}{n_0 r_0} = \frac{K_1}{n_0 n_1} + \frac{K_2}{n_1 n_2} \tag{3}$$

2.2. Imaging Setup

We used Zemax (ZEMAX LLC, Kirkland, WA, USA), a ray-tracing simulation tool that helps model, analyze, and design optical systems, to optimize the design for minimal field curvature and reduced aberrations. Our model included one single biconvex lens, and the refractive material was N-BK7. At the start of the optimization process, the variables were sample object radius and fixed FOV to be imaged. The practicality of model assembly was kept by setting the object at a position beyond the focal length of the lens.

In our optics setup, a fluorescence imaging platform and fluorescent micro-objects located within a large-area curved substrate were designed as shown in Figure 1a. The working distance increases because of the large FOV target, which ensures that sample handling is comfortable.

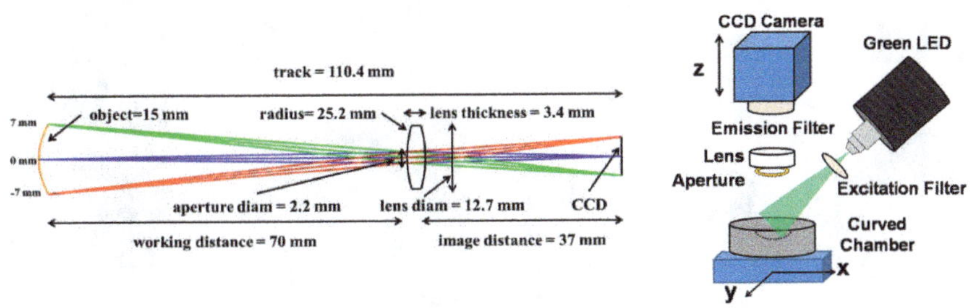

(a) (b)

Figure 1. (**a**) Optical prescription for prototype curved-substrate imaging system, designed for a wavelength of 560 nm. A single commercial lens was used for imaging. All dimensions are in millimeters. (**b**) Schematic of experimental setup.

A commercial CCD camera sensor (DMK 51BUC02, ImagingSource, Bremen, Germany) with a resolution of 1600 × 1200 pixels and a pixel size of 4.4 μm was used. We used a biconvex lens

(LB1014, Thorlabs, Newton, NJ, USA), the focal length and refractive index of which were 25 mm and 1.517, respectively. The lens, an emission filter (XF3083, Omega Optical, Brattleboro, VT, USA) and the camera were aligned with a C-mount extension tube (25 mm length, #58-736, Edmund Optics, Barrington, NJ, USA) and a C-mount lens mount (12.5 mm diameter, #55-246, Edmund Optics) was then fixed with a dovetail stage (22 mm travel, #03-682, Edmund Optics). These integrated parts of optics enable the system to move along the *z*-axis to adjust the focus. An *x*-*y* positioning stage was attached with the integrated part to keep a rigid distance between the lens and the sample chamber as illustrated in Figure 1b. The light source was fixed separately, as shown in the schematic. This structure makes the system robust and not too sensitive.

2.3. Fabrication of Curved Sample Chamber

Images produced by the two optical systems were simulated in an accurate model by using Zemax software and considering relative illumination, geometric aberration, and point spread functions (PSFs) at various heights on the sample substrate. Following the proof-of-concept simulation with the curved sample substrate, we designed a curved sample chamber consisting of two parts, an upper window and a lower substrate. Both parts have spherical dome shapes with lens-dependent curvatures and can be snapped together manually with a gap of 50–500 μm to hold a fixed sample volume. A sample solution can be loaded into the chamber through a hole made in the lower substrate. The volume of the sample filled in the chamber is proportional to the gap thickness between the window and the substrate. Figure 2a shows a 3D model of the curved sample chamber. To fabricate the disposable optical-quality curved chambers, we used a transparent acrylic material for the upper window which was prepared using a plastic injection molding technique. The lower substrate was colored black to reduce a reflective light at the surface. The cost for making a mold for the sample chamber is about 4000 USD and we have produced 200 pieces for our study. The cost per piece is reduced exponentially with the number of pieces in a batch produced by injection molding process. Large FOV fluorescence imaging is enabled by a simple lens (~20 USD) and a curved sample chamber without using a sample scanning mechanism, which reduces the system cost greatly. Figure 2b shows various views of the fabricated curved sample chamber. For comparing the fluorescent particle images taken in the curved chamber with those taken in the planar chamber, we used the central part of a glass bottom culture dish (P35G-0-14-C, MatTek, Ashland, MA, USA) covered with a circular coverslip as a planar sample chamber.

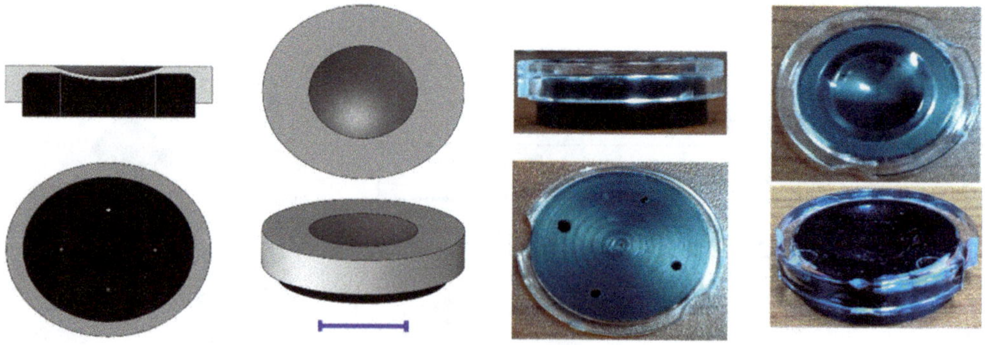

(a) (b)

Figure 2. (**a**) 3D model of curved sample chamber composed of an upper window (gray color) and a lower substrate (black color). A sample solution is introduced into the gap of 100-μm thickness between those two separable parts through one of the holes in the lower substrate. The other three holes are air vents. (Scale bar = 10 mm). (**b**) Curved sample chamber fabricated by plastic injection molding technique. The upper window is optically clear for image acquisition and the lower substrate is colored black to minimize light reflection at the surface.

A schematic of the cross-sectional view of the sample chamber with the distribution of the cells is depicted in Figure 3a. Cells are distributed across the gap rather than deposited at the curved bottom part. A large field-of-view image of the cells is taken immediately after loading the sample into the chamber, and thus even those cells with a high density are not deposited on the bottom during image acquisition. As the field of view of our imaging system is large and the depth of focus is greater than the gap thickness, cells are imaged sharply regardless of their positions inside the chamber. It is quite easy to load a cell suspension into the sample chamber by a micropipette as shown in Figure 3b, as there are air vents in the lower substrate. No leakage is observed through the air vents.

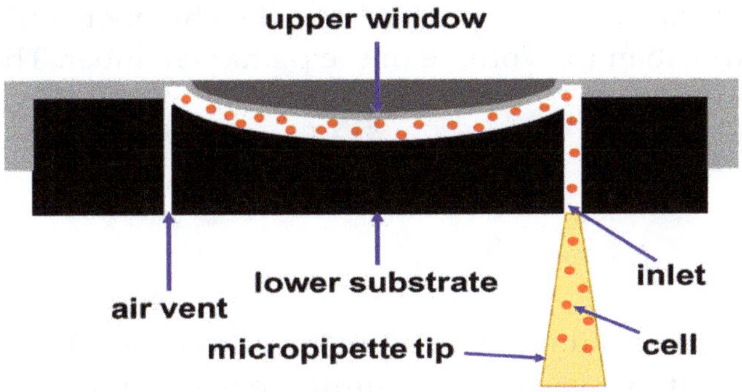

(a)

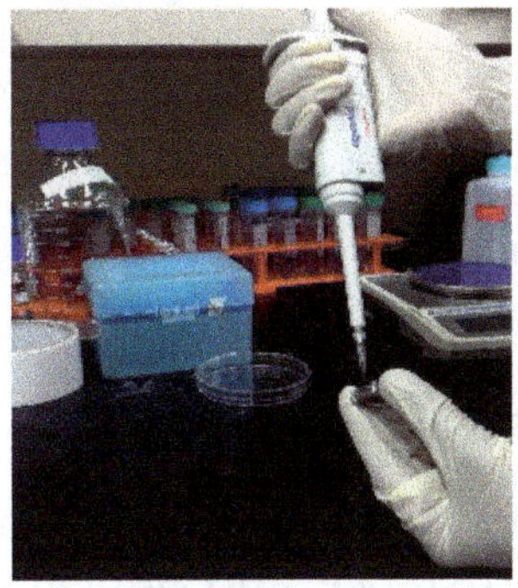

(b)

Figure 3. (**a**) A schematic of the cross-sectional view of the curved sample chamber and suspended cells in the gap between upper window and lower substrate; and (**b**) loading of cell suspension with a micropipette is facilitated by air vent holes made through the lower substrate as shown in (**a**).

Our curved chamber was designed to be used as a disposable one to prevent infection. If there is no concern about infection, it can be reused after separating the upper window and the lower substrate and cleaning each part with a distilled water or a diluted ethanol solution. It does not take long or require a tedious process for cleaning as, cells are not adhered to the bottom substrate.

2.4. Sample Preparation

A small amount of whole blood was donated by members of our laboratory. We used 1× RBC (red blood cell) lysis buffer by diluting the original 10× RBC lysis buffer to 1× working concentration with deionized water (DW). A 10:1 ratio was maintained to form 1× RBC lysis buffer. Before using, we keep the buffer at room temperature for 10 min. Then, we added 2 mL of 1× RBC lysis buffer to each e-tube containing up to 100 μL of whole blood. For mixing, we gently vortexed each tube immediately after adding the lysed solution. We maintained the vortexed tubes at room temperature for 10–15 min. We centrifuged the sample at 500 G for 5 min. Then, we pulled out carefully the upper part of the sample without disturbing the pellet. Then, we washed the sample by adding 1× PBS (phosphate buffered saline) + 2 mM EDTA (ethylenediaminetetraacetic acid) + 0.2% BSA (bovine serum albumin) and suspending the cell pellet with 4 mL PBS. Then, we centrifuged the samples for 5 min and collected the supernatant.

We prepared 8 different samples with different WBC concentrations. After extracting WBCs from whole blood, we mixed it with different quantities of PBS buffer. The prepared samples had WBC concentrations of 100%, and 10%–70% with an interval of 10%. The WBC samples were then stained with a fluorescence dye. We added 20 μL of 1 mM SYTO82 orange fluorescent nucleic acid stain (Thermo Fisher Scientific, Waltham, MA, USA) to 200 μL of each sample solution.

2.5. Image Acquisition and Cell Counting

We imaged WBCs with conventional microscopy using a 4× magnification lens with an exposure time of 30 ms in a handmade slide glass chamber, which covers a FOV of 2.2 mm × 1.65 mm, and the volume enclosed by this area is 0.8 μL. Chamber height is 220 μm, and the total area is 180 mm^2 (15 mm × 12 mm), which makes the total volume 40 μL. ImageJ software was used to binarize the image to count WBC manually. The raw images were then processed using a FFT bandpass filter, which subtracts the background from the image. Images of large structures over 40 pixels and small debris less than 3 pixels were removed. With the single-lens imaging system, we imaged the same chamber and our designed curved chamber with an exposure time of 30 ms to directly compare WBC counts. The size of the image is 10.66 mm × 8 mm and the enclosed sample volume is 18.76 μL for flat chamber. Likewise a curved chamber was also imaged in the single lens imaging system with the same area covered but the volume was 8.51 μL. The height of the curved chamber between the cover and the base was 100 μm and chamber diameter was 12.7 mm, which means the chamber could hold 12.67 μL of sample. This is around three times lower than the volume of the planar chamber. The magnification factor of the single-lens imaging system was 0.66.

3. Results and Discussion

3.1. Simulation Study

Zemax software was used to model the imaging system to determine the aperture radius, lens-to-camera distance, and optical resolution, as well as to simulate the image on the image plane. However, the aperture radius was optimized independently.

The model included one single biconvex lens (LB1450, Thorlabs) made of refractive material N-BK7, an aperture, object at a fixed distance to achieve a certain FOV, and a flat image plane. The lens diameter was 12.7 mm, thickness 3.9 mm, focal length 20 mm, and radius of curvature 19.9 mm, and it was placed 50 mm from the sample substrate. An aperture stop of 2 mm was mounted toward the front surface of the lens. The optics simulation began with the flat substrate and a preset FOV, as shown in Figure 4a. The software was initially allowed to optimize the image by viewing a dot grid model. Then, the calculated substrate curvature was simulated, as shown in Figure 4c, and the dot grid was analyzed. The dot grid was simulated at three different heights on the flat and calculated curved substrates, as shown in Figure 4b,d, respectively. Optimally focused images were obtained when the radius of curvature of the substrate was kept within the sagittal value of the lens, as shown in Figure 4b. Figure 4e,f shows a quantitative analysis consisting of field curvature graphs for flat and curved substrates, respectively. The red and blue lines represent the sagittal and tangential surfaces, respectively. The on-axis position (H = 0 mm) in this graph is considered the center of the 12 mm substrate. The focus points are deviated from the image plane with increasing height. However, in Figure 4f, the sagittal surface becomes more flat and aligned with the image plane. Thus, the curved substrate can focus the rays to a point in the flat plane.

The sagittal surface was calculated by first determining mathematically the Petzval surface, a natural characteristic that exists in every optical system. The ratio of the distance between the Petzval surface and the tangential and sagittal surfaces is 3:1. The sagittal surface can thus be calculated as follows:

$$\frac{1}{R_s} = \frac{1}{R_p} - \frac{1}{f} = \frac{1+n}{nf} \tag{4}$$

where R_s and R_p are the radii of the sagittal and the Petzval surface curvatures, respectively; n is the refractive index of the medium; and f is the focal length. From Equations (3) and (4), for the lens used in this study, the Petzval sagittal radii are −29.19 mm and 12 mm, respectively.

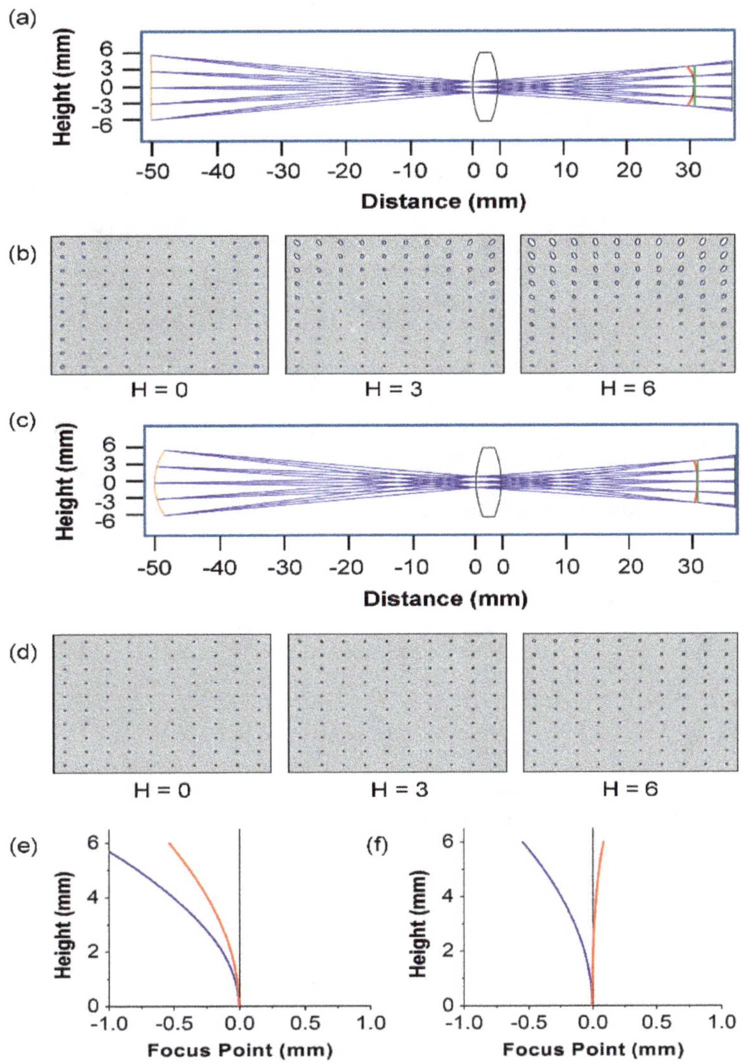

Figure 4. Ray tracing simulation of astigmatism field curvature. Ray tracing of a simple biconvex lens for: (**a**) flat substrate; and (**c**) curved substrate. The grayscale images in (**b**,**d**) were acquired using the flat and the curved substrates, where the image plane was kept flat. The images in (**b**,**d**) represent 0, 3, and 6 mm sample substrate height. The field curvature graphs for the flat and the curved substrates are shown in (**e**,**f**), respectively, where the blue and red lines denote tangential and sagittal surfaces.

The designed optical system was simulated by a ray-tracing numerical model using Zemax software. Zemax helps confirm the results of the analytical model and evaluate optical performance over the FOV. The spot diagram, modulation transfer function (MTF), and point spread function (PSF) of the curved substrate show considerably better agreement (Figure 5) than those of the flat substrate. The radius of the Airy disk was 9.87 μm for both the flat and the curved substrates in the optical system. The RMS radius of the spot diagram in Figure 5a diverges with increasing field height for the flat substrate, but it remains in the Airy disk radius for the curved substrate, as shown in Figure 5d. Numerical modeling results obtained across the FOV are shown in Figure 5b,e, where the optimal FOV was used to calculate the MTF. The MTF of this system is plotted for a field point on the optical axis and another point at the edge of the FOV. The field point on the optical axis shows a nearly diffraction-limited response at a spatial frequency of about 120 cycles/mm for the curved substrate in comparison with that for the flat substrate [21].

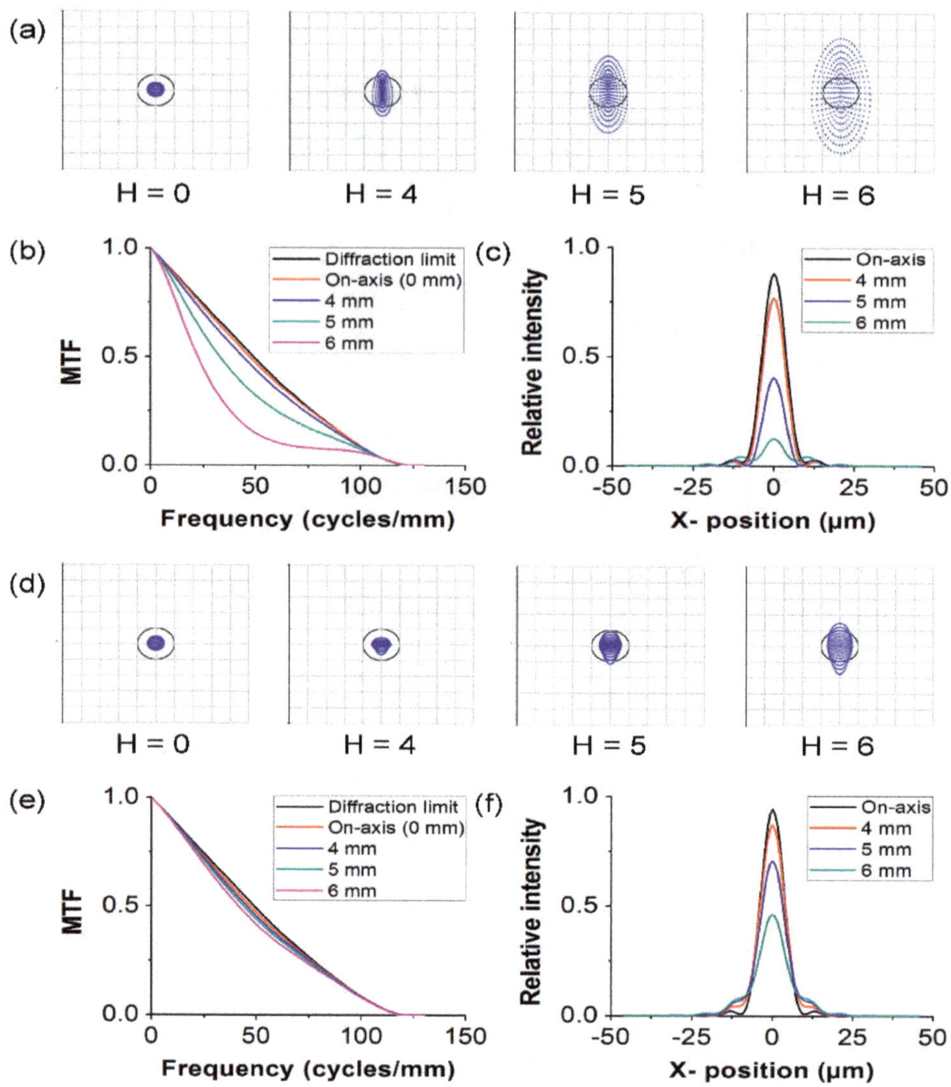

Figure 5. Analytical characterization of simple imaging system for flat and curved substrates. The spot size diagrams include a circle showing the Airy disk (9.87 μm in radius) for the flat and the curved substrates in (**a**,**d**), respectively. (**b**,**e**) MTF and (**c**,**f**) PSF of flat and curved substrates, respectively. In the MTFs, the black line shows the diffraction limit, and the red and pink lines represent the on- and off-axis image fields, respectively.

The PSFs on the image plane at 560 nm are shown in Figure 5c,f. The advantage of a curved substrate is clear on the image plane. This PSF represents light intensity over the entire FOV on the imaging surface. The on-axis image intensities are similar to each other but vary with the field height. The off-axis PSF of the curved substrate exhibits a higher peak than that of the flat substrate, and it is more uniform with respect to the wavelength and image height, thus resulting in better image formation.

3.2. Validation Study

The curvature radii of objects used in this experiment were calculated for different lenses considering their field curvature radii. Curved objects were fabricated as described in the Materials and Method Section. Figure 6 shows the change in object radii with a change in lens radius. The Petzval radii of the biconvex and the plano-convex lenses used in our experiment were calculated.

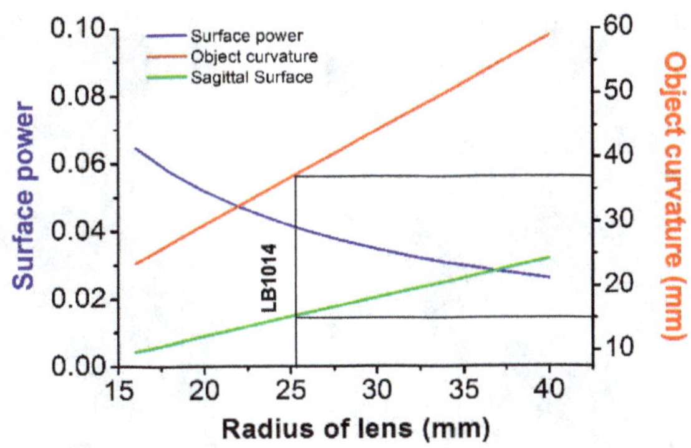

Figure 6. Change in surface power and object curvature with change in curvature radius of lens. These radii of the lens consider both sides of biconvex lens, and have the same focal length as the radius.

We determined the object curvature using Equation (2), while the image surface was kept infinity. Finally, we calculated the power of the lens surface as follows:

$$\frac{n_1 - n_0}{R_1} = K_1 \tag{5}$$

By using the above formulas, we found the Petzval radius and the surface power of the lens. Here we used a commercial lens LB1014 for designing the chamber. Table 1 below lists the specifications of lenses with different curvature and because the FOV is fixed, the volume varies.

Table 1. Specification of imaging system for simulation.

Lens	Inner Surface of Sphere			Outer Surface of Sphere		
	Radius (mm)	Height (mm)	Volume (mm^3)	Radius (mm)	Height (mm)	Volume (mm^3)
LB1014	15.06	1.25	71.88	15.56	1.75	144.09
LB1258	18.08	1.03	59.114	18.58	1.53	132.89
LB1378	24.12	0.8	47.96	24.62	1.3	128.41
LB1844	30.135	0.605	34.42	30.635	1.105	116.10

Figure 6 shows plots for a certain FOV, and it can be seen that upon increasing the FOV, system length increases. Thus, choosing a short focal length lens can reduce the size of the imaging system.

A validation study was conducted with the planar and curved sample chambers, in which a fluorescent microbead suspension was loaded. The imaging setup is discussed in the Methods Section, and a schematic diagram is shown in Figure 1b. As shown in Figure 7a,b, the fluorescent microbeads were distributed uniformly over the entire FOV. The brightest circular region in the center of the image shown in Figure 7b is attributed to the fluorescent microbeads aggregated at the inlet hole. It can be removed by changing the position of the hole in the lower substrate. In our curved sample chamber, the well-focused area is approximately 119 mm^2, which is twice as large as the approximately 64 mm^2 aberration-free area of the planar chamber. Furthermore, the image in the curved chamber also exhibits almost uniform brightness over the FOV (Figure 7d), while, in the case of the planar chamber, the distorted portion at the edge has much lower intensity than the central region (Figure 7c). The fluorescent microbeads positioned at the edge part of the curved chamber exhibit a small distortion, which is attributed to other type of optical aberration such as coma. As mentioned earlier, our curved sample chamber with a single-lens imaging system can reduce the field curvature only and enlarge the focused area of the image.

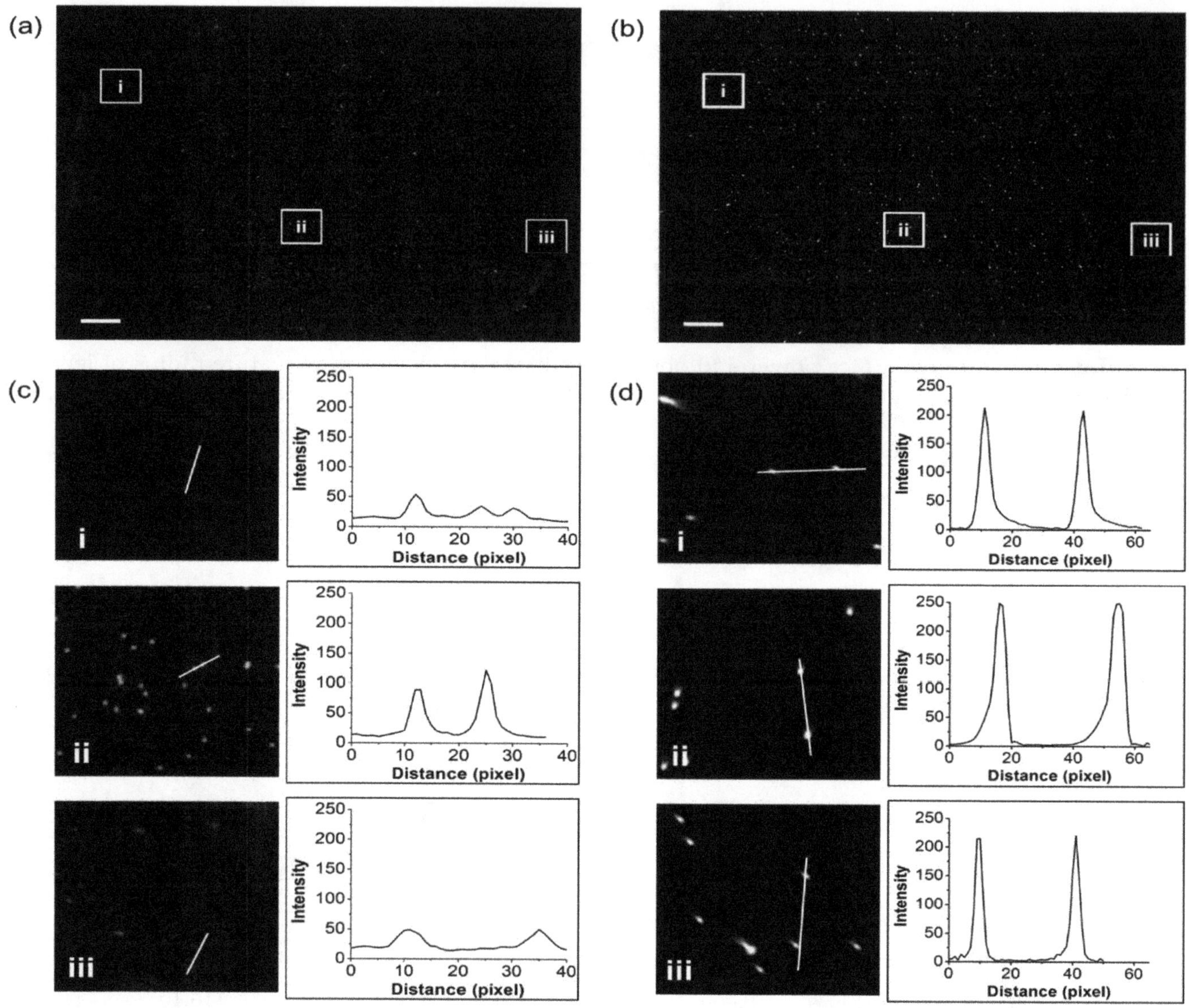

Figure 7. Imaging performance of single-lens fluorescence microscopy with curved sample chamber. Fluorescence images taken for beads of diameter 10 μm for: (**a**) planar; and (**b**) curved sample chambers. The fluorescent microbeads are distributed uniformly over the entire FOV. The intensity profiles of the bead images are shown in (**c**,**d**). As observed for the curved substrate, a wider area of the bead image is more focused in (**b**), and the aberration is lower than that in (**a**). (Scale bar = 1 mm).

3.3. *Absolute Counting of WBC*

We investigated the feasibility of our curved chamber platform by analyzing SYTO82 stained WBCs at different locations within the chambers. The image shown in Figure 8a has an area of 2.2 mm × 1.65 mm of flat chamber achieved using 4× magnification and Figure 8b,c show images of the flat and the curved chambers taken over a large field with an area of 10.66 mm × 8 mm. Portions corresponding to the 4× magnification area were digitally cropped from the whole images of the flat chambers as shown in Figure 8d. For comparison purpose, the same regions of the sample were also cropped from the curved chamber as shown in Figure 8e. For the flat chamber, the area cropped from the edge part shows the presence of few cells, which decreases the average number of cells in total. However, the cropped image of the curved chamber shows uniform number of cells throughout, and the average cell count deviates negligibly across the image. WBC detection at the edges of both the flat and the curved chambers showed a significant difference. The cell count at the edge of the flat chamber was very low, as shown in Figure 8d (i and iii), and, as expected from our validation study, the cell count at the edge of the curved chamber was higher (Figure 8e (i and iii)), which attributes to the uniform fluorescence intensity in the curved chamber image. As some monochromatic aberrations still exist in our single-lens imaging system, there are limited applications such as cell counting. However, our approach serves wide FOV absolute cell counting by reducing the field curvature effect.

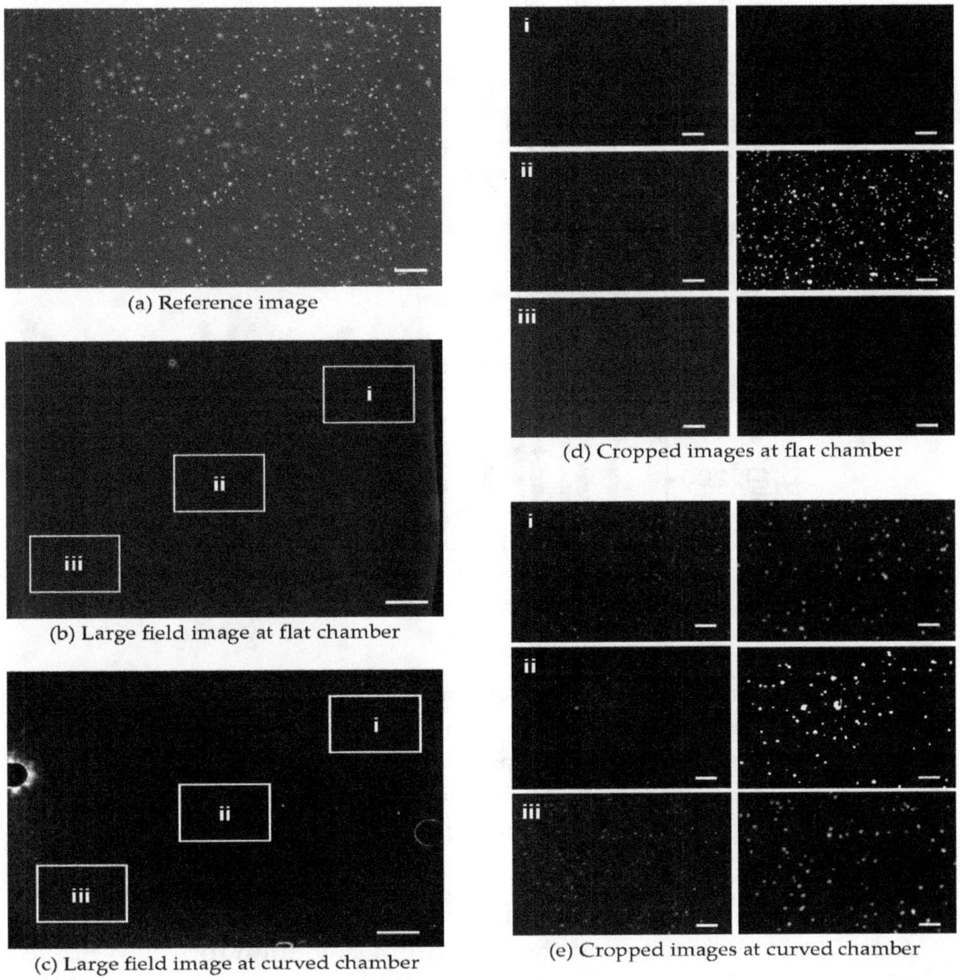

Figure 8. Fluorescence images of stained white blood cells in small and large field imaging. (**a**) Microscopic image of flat chamber. The inset white boxes in (**b**,**c**) are of the same size in the microscopy images of the flat and curved chambers. (**d**,**e**) Cropped areas of the flat and curved chamber images, where (ii) denotes the center part of an image. All cropped images are of the same size. The cell counts in the center (ii) were similar for both chambers. The bars in (**b**,**c**) represent a scale of 1 mm, while those in the other figures represent a scale of 200 μm.

The main purpose of this research is to determine the absolute count of WBCs, defined as the total number of WBCs in a microliter of blood, in the designed chamber. By considering the microscopy result as the reference, we analyzed the flat and curved chamber images for WBC counts obtained from samples with eight different dilution levels. As shown in Figure 9a, a very good agreement is found between the counts using the reference microscopic images and the curved chamber images. However, the results obtained with the large flat chamber and those obtained with the curved chamber are considerably different from those obtained using conventional microscopy. The slope between the reference and the flat chamber is 0.25, while that between the reference and the curved chamber is 0.97.

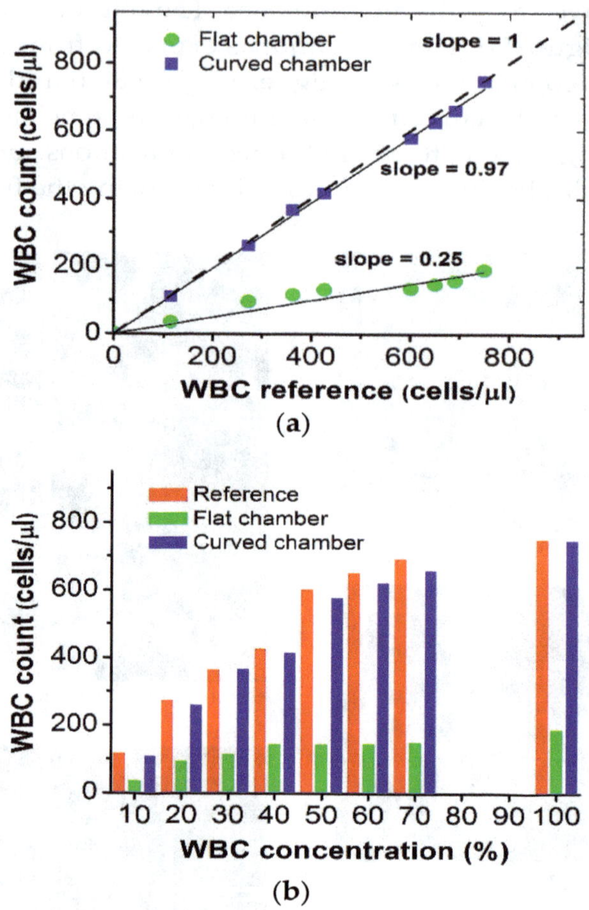

Figure 9. (**a**) WBC count obtained using planar chamber is remarkably different from the reference cell count obtained with conventional microscopy; and (**b**) WBC concentrations of 10%–70% with an interval of 10% and 100% were compared for absolute counting obtained by microscopic, flat, and curved chamber imaging. The count obtained with the curved chamber is close to that obtained with conventional microscopy. However, the corresponding result with the flat chamber differs considerably for large fields.

In Figure 9b, the bar chart shows the average cell counts for the microscopic, flat and curved chamber imaging. Among the eight samples, the maximum deviation for the WBC counts from whole images obtained using the single-lens imaging system is found to be 5.12% at WBC concentration of 70%.

We measured WBC size in two imaging methods to optimize our count results. This validation study confirms the same particle counting inside the chamber. Same size of the microscopic image is cropped at the center part from the large field of view image. To justify the WBC size obtained with both imaging systems, we measured the number of pixels occupied by the fluorescent dye. In Figure 10, the bottom panel shows the normalized intensity profiles of fluorescently-labeled WBCs. However, fluorescence covers an area greater than the particle size owing to the emission of light. We analyzed the full width at half maximum (FWHM) to measure WBC size, which is shown with red line in Figure 10d–f. The average number of pixels in the microscopic image is 11, and because 1376 pixels span a length of 2.2 mm, the size of an individual WBC cell is 17.58 μm. In the single-lens images, each fluorescence signal covers 2.5 pixels, and 1600 pixels span 10.66 mm; hence, the size of an individual WBC cell is 16.65 μm. It should be noted that those three images have different noise levels and signal-to-noise ratios as we compared our single lens imaging system with a conventional microscopy. In addition, for the single lens imaging system, difference in signal-to-noise ratio (SNR) can be seen because of different material properties of the sample chambers.

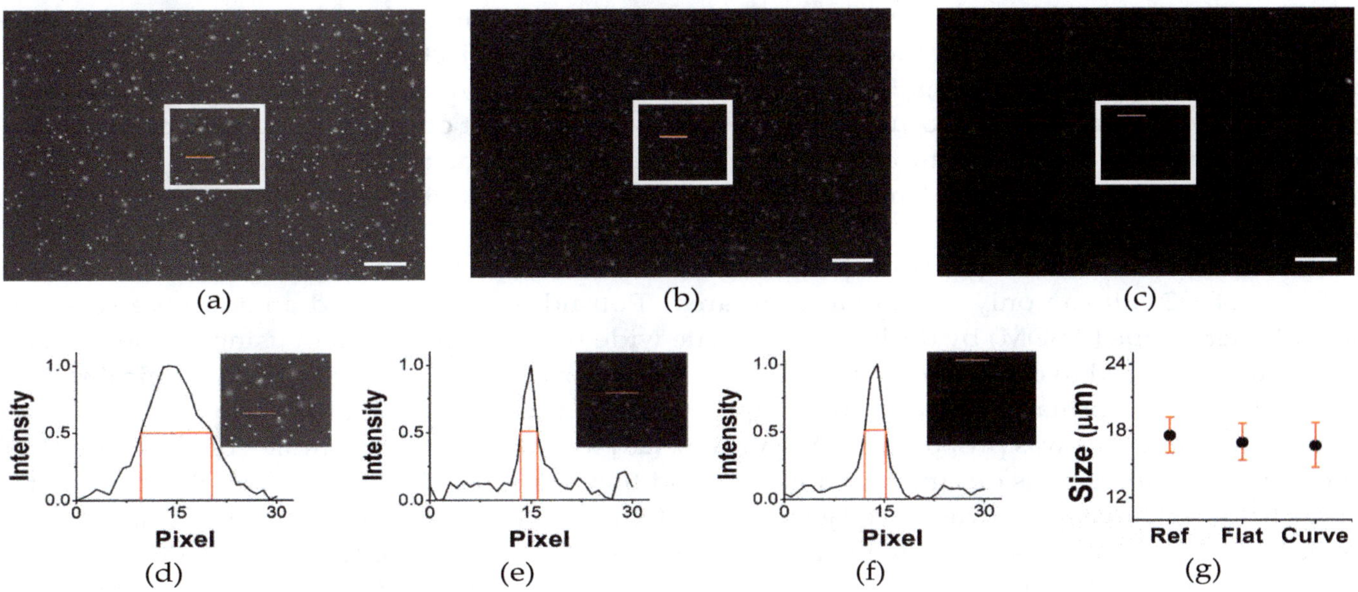

Figure 10. (**a–c**) The reference, flat, and curved chamber images with 500 μm^2 white boxes inside, respectively (scale bar = 0.5 mm); (**d–f**) the normalized intensity profiles of a fluorescently-labeled WBC in those three images; and (**g**) the size of the fluorescent WBCs measured with microscopy, and flat and curved imaging, represented by Ref, Flat, and Curved on the x-axis of the graph, respectively. The range of WBC size is 16–20 μm. The normalized intensity profile of the fluorescence shows the size of the SYTO-stained WBC in pixels, and the inset images are cropped from the center part of the processed image.

3.4. Advantages of Large FOV Imaging with Curved Sample Chamber

Using an eight-megapixel cell phone camera, Zhu et al. [22] achieved a FOV of approximately 81 mm^2 in the central region of an approximately 162 mm^2 image with a magnification factor (MF) of 0.3. The curved substrate enables us to enlarge the FOV by approximately 50% at an even higher MF of approximately 0.6. The FOV can be widened further if we use a lens with a longer focal length, while maintaining the MF within a reasonable range. Owing to this large FOV, an imaging system incorporating a curved sample chamber can image a large sample volume without a time-consuming scanning process, which is particularly important for rapid screening of samples such as blood, water, and urine. We demonstrated that an optical-quality curved sample chamber can be fabricated by the plastic injection molding process, which is beneficial from the viewpoint of lowering the cost of mass-producing disposable curved sample chambers. For laboratory-scale research, 3D printing with a transparent polymer resin can be employed as an alternative method for fabricating the curved sample chamber [23].

Rogers' group developed an electronic eye, in which the image sensor was designed by considering the Petzval surface. Although other groups have reported the advantage of a curved focal image plane, meticulous engineering is required for fabrication. As we aimed to make a simple imaging system, we used a curved chamber instead of a curved image sensor. Despite the substantial reduction in field curvature, other aberrations still exist in the fluorescence image taken in the curved chamber because we use a single-lens imaging system and do not use any lens- or image-processing scheme to enhance image quality. The Petzval surface works only when the imaging system is corrected for astigmatism [24]. Note that the constant distance between the sagittal and the tangential surfaces in Figure 4e,f is attributed to the slightly deformed object (astigmatism) at the periphery of the image shown in Figure 7d. Nevertheless, those regions with aberrations are available for particle counting in the fluorescence imaging mode.

The aberration field curvature is related to astigmatism, but it might exist in a system that does not suffer from astigmatism. In the case of field curvature, an object is imaged on a curved surface rather than on a plane. The image is not blurred by this aberration, but it is simply projected onto a curved surface. This cannot be focused on with a flat sensor for flat object imaging. Our experimental and computational analyses demonstrate that the image can be focused on to a greater extent so no particles in the sample are lost. This is useful from the viewpoint of counting particles or cells in a large sample volume.

A traditional microscope can achieve high resolution over the entire image field. However, in terms of FOV, it can only capture a small area. Potsaid et al. proposed an adaptive scanning optical microscope (ASOM) by designing a unique wide field imaging system using an inexpensive technique compared to conventional microscopy. They introduced a microelectromechanical system (MEMS)-based deformable mirror with complex design of lens array. A high-throughput imaging system without a lens was proposed by Arpali et al. [25] for imaging large sample volumes. A special microfluidic chamber was designed in this case, and they system achieved good resolution over the image field. As the chamber was placed just over the CCD image sensor, it did not show the aberrations in the imaging system caused by a regular lens. However, a large CCD sensor was used, and it required sophisticated expertise in optics design. Previously, we developed a dual-mode high-throughput microscopy system to scan a wide field of asbestos slide sample [26]. Two translational stages of this system move along the x- and y-directions to acquire a series of small images over a large area of the sample slide. One of the drawbacks of this system is a limited FOV.

The design of a simple imaging system with a curved chamber has not received much attention, partly because calculation of the curvature varies with lens specifications, and there is no practical, low-cost technique for large-scale diagnostic imaging. Large FOV images have a number of advantages, and we can reduce the standard deviation of cell count by using large sample volume, which would allow us to count all cells in a single image. Different image areas from a single sample can have different amount of cells, which can be confusing for sample analysis. The proposed curved sample chamber and practical diagnostic imaging tool can be applied to point-of-care diagnosis such as absolute cell counting and detection of parasites in resource-constrained areas.

High precision in cell counting is vital for reliable diagnosis. A statistical term, coefficient of variation (CV), is used for the measurement of precision and calculated as

$$CV(\%) = \frac{100}{\sqrt{n}} \tag{6}$$

where, n represents the number of cells counted in a sample [27]. In our study, the sample of lowest concentration contains 92 cells per 0.8 μL and 747 cells per 6.8 μL for 4× and 0.66× magnified images, respectively, and CVs are given as 10.4 and 3.65, respectively. For the sample of highest concentration at both magnifications, counts are 600 cells per 0.8 μL and 5077 cells per 6.8 μL, where CVs decrease to 4.08 and 1.40, respectively. Higher number of cells counted in a sample gives less variation and higher precision in absolute cell counting. Thus, a single image containing a large sample volume can decrease CV greatly, which is a strong advantage of large FOV imaging with our curved sample chamber.

4. Conclusions

We proposed an optical-quality curved sample chamber to reduce the field curvature, which is inherently unavoidable in optical imaging of a flat substrate with a simple lens system. Ray tracing simulations and experiments demonstrated that the optical distortion at the planar camera sensor could be corrected by using a curved sample chamber with a lens-dependent curvature. An application to absolute cell counting for the fluorescently-labeled white blood cells confirmed that a large field-of-view imaging with our curved sample chamber can reduce the variation in counting cells while increasing the precision of measurement. The present study supports the use of an unconventional curved sample chamber for designing a compact and cost-effective single-lens fluorescence imaging system.

Acknowledgments: This research was supported by the National Research Foundation (NRF) of Korea grant funded by the Ministry of Education (NRF-2013R1A1A2059539) and the Human Resources Development Program (20134010200580) of the Korea Institute of Energy Technology Evaluation and Planning (KETEP) funded by the Ministry of Trade, Industry and Energy, Republic of Korea. Mohiuddin K. Shourav was funded by the Global Scholarship Program for Foreign Graduate Students at Kookmin University in Korea.

Author Contributions: J.K.K. conceived and designed the experiments; M.K.S. and K.K. performed the experiments; M.K.S. and J.K.K. analyzed the data; S.K. prepared samples; and M.K.S. and J.K.K wrote the paper.

References

1. Jenkins, F.A.; White, H.E. *Fundamentals of Optics*, 4th ed.; Shirley, G., Ed.; McGraw-Hill: New York, NY, USA, 2001.
2. Cybulski, J.S.; Clements, J.; Prakash, M. Foldscope: Origami-based paper microscopy. *PLoS ONE* **2014**, *9*, e98781. [CrossRef] [PubMed]
3. Smith, Z.J.; Chu, K.; Espenson, A.R.; Rahimzadeh, M.; Gryshuk, A.; Molinaro, M.; Dwyr, D.M.; Lane, S.; Matthews, D.; Wachsmann-Hogiu, S. Cell-phone-based platform for biomedical device development and education application. *PLoS ONE* **2011**, *6*, e17150. [CrossRef] [PubMed]
4. Breslauer, D.N.; Maamari, R.N.; Switz, N.A.; Lam, W.A.; Fletcher, D.A. Mobile phone based clinical microscopy for global health applications. *PLoS ONE* **2009**, *4*, e6320. [CrossRef] [PubMed]
5. Zhu, H.; Sencan, I.; Wong, J.; Dimitrov, S.; Tseng, D.; Nagashima, K.; Ozcan, A. Cost-effective and rapid blood analysis on a cell-phone. *Lab Chip* **2013**, *13*, 1282–1288. [CrossRef] [PubMed]
6. Choi, J.R.; Kim, K.J.; Kim, D.H. In situ fluorescence optical detection using a digital micromirror device (DMD) for 3D cell-based assays. *J. Opt. Soc. Korea* **2012**, *16*, 42–46. [CrossRef]
7. Potsaid, B.; Finger, F.P.; Wen, J.T. Automation of challenging spatial-temporal biomedical observations with the adaptive scanning optical microscope (ASOM). *IEEE Trans. Autom. Sci. Eng.* **2009**, *6*, 525–535. [CrossRef]
8. Hecht, E. *Optics*, 4th ed.; Addison Wesley: San Francisco, CA, USA, 2002; p. 226.
9. Rim, S.B.; Catrysse, P.B.; Dinyari, R.; Huang, K.; Peumans, P. The optical advantages of curved focal plane arrays. *Opt. Exp.* **2008**, *16*, 4965–4971. [CrossRef]
10. Jin, H.; Abelson, J.R.; Erhardt, M.K.; Nuzzo, R.G. Soft lithographic fabrication of an image sensor array on a curved substrate. *J. Vac. Sci. Technol. B* **2004**, *22*, 2548–2551. [CrossRef]
11. Malyarchuk, V.; Jung, I.; Rogers, J.A.; Shin, G.; Ha, J.S. Experimental and modeling studies of imaging with curvilinear electronic eye cameras. *Opt. Exp.* **2010**, *18*, 27346–27358. [CrossRef] [PubMed]
12. Jung, I.; Xiao, J.; Malyarchuk, V.; Lu, C.; Li, M.; Liu, Z.; Rogers, J.A. Dynamically tunable hemispherical electronic eye camera system with adjustable zoom capability. *Proc. Natl. Acad. Sci. USA* **2011**, *108*, 1788–1793. [CrossRef] [PubMed]
13. Ozcan, A.; Demirci, U. Ultra wide-field lens-free monitoring of cells on-chip. *Lab Chip* **2008**, *8*, 98–106. [CrossRef] [PubMed]
14. Greenbaum, A.; Luo, W.; Su, T.W.; Göröcs, Z.; Xue, L.; Isikman, S.O.; Coskun, A.F.; Mudanyali, O.; Ozcan, A. Imaging without lenses: Achievements and remaining challenges of wide-field on-chip microscopy. *Nat. Methods* **2012**, *9*, 889–895. [CrossRef] [PubMed]
15. Seo, S.; Isikman, O.S.; Sencan, I.; Mudanyali, O.; Su, T.W.; Bishara, W.; Erlinger, A.; Ozcan, A. High-throughput lens-free blood analysis on a chip. *Anal. Chem.* **2010**, *82*, 4621–4627. [CrossRef] [PubMed]
16. Su, T.W.; Erlinger, A.; Tseng, D.; Ozcan, A. Compact and light-weight automated semen analysis platform using lensfree on-chip microscopy. *Anal. Chem.* **2010**, *82*, 8307–8312. [CrossRef] [PubMed]
17. Mudanyali, O.; Oztoprak, C.; Tseng, D.; Erlinger, A.; Ozcan, A. Detection of waterborne parasites using field-portable and cost-effective lensfree microscopy. *Lab Chip* **2010**, *10*, 2419–2423. [CrossRef] [PubMed]
18. Göröcs, Z.; Ling, Y.; Yu, M.D.; Karahalios, D.; Mogharabi, K.; Lu, K.; Wei, Q.; Ozcan, A. Giga-pixel fluorescent imaging over an ultra-large field-of-view using a flatbed scanner. *Lab Chip* **2013**, *13*, 4460–4466. [CrossRef] [PubMed]
19. Ulrich, W.; Shafer, D.; Bader, D.; Epple, A. Refractive Optical Imaging System, in Particular Projection Objective for Microlithography. U.S. Patent 7,511,890, 31 March 2006.
20. Malacara, D.; Malacara, Z. *Handbook of Optical Design*, 2nd ed.; Marcel Dekker: New York, NY, USA, 2004.
21. Hagen, N.; Tkaczyk, T. Foveated endoscopic lens. *J. Biomed. Opt.* **2012**. [CrossRef] [PubMed]

22. Zhu, H.; Yaglidere, O.; Su, T.; Tseng, D.; Ozcan, A. Cost-effective and compact wide-field fluorescence imaging on a cell-phone. *Lab Chip* **2010**, *11*, 315–322. [CrossRef] [PubMed]
23. Lee, W.; Kwon, D.; Choi, W.; Jung, G.Y.; Jeon, S. 3D-printed microfluidic device for the detection of pathogenic bacteria using size-based separation in helical channel with trapezoid cross-section. *Sci. Rep.* **2015**. [CrossRef] [PubMed]
24. Smith, W.J. *Modern Optical Engineering*, 4th ed.; McGraw-Hill: New York, NY, USA, 2007; p. 90.
25. Arpali, S.A.; Arpali, C.; Coskun, A.F.; Chiang, H.H.; Ozcan, A. High-throughput screening of large volumes of whole blood using structured illumination and fluorescent on-chip imaging. *Lab Chip* **2012**, *12*, 4968–4971. [CrossRef] [PubMed]
26. Cho, M.O.; Chang, H.M.; Lee, D.; Yu, Y.G.; Han, H.; Kim, J.K. Selective detection and automated counting of fluorescently-labeled chrysotile asbestos using a dual-mode high-throughput microscopy (DM-HTM) method. *Sensors* **2013**, *9*, 5686–5699. [CrossRef] [PubMed]
27. Shapiro, M.H. *Practical Flow Cytometry*, 4th ed.; Wiley-Liss: Hoboken, NJ, USA, 2003; pp. 18–20.

2

Enhanced Axial Resolution of Wide-Field Two-Photon Excitation Microscopy by Line Scanning Using a Digital Micromirror Device

Jong Kang Park [1], Christopher J. Rowlands [2] and Peter T. C. So [1,3,*]

1 Department of Biological Engineering, Massachusetts Institute of Technology, Cambridge, MA 02139, USA; jongpark@mit.edu
2 Department of Chemical Engineering and Biotechnology, Cambridge University, Cambridge CB2 1TN, UK; cjr52@cam.ac.uk
3 Laser Biomedical Research Center (LBRC), Massachusetts Institute of Technology, Cambridge, MA 02139, USA
* Correspondence: ptso@mit.edu

Academic Editors: Shih-Chi Chen and Wei-Chuan Shih

Abstract: Temporal focusing multiphoton microscopy is a technique for performing highly parallelized multiphoton microscopy while still maintaining depth discrimination. While the conventional wide-field configuration for temporal focusing suffers from sub-optimal axial resolution, line scanning temporal focusing, implemented here using a digital micromirror device (DMD), can provide substantial improvement. The DMD-based line scanning temporal focusing technique dynamically trades off the degree of parallelization, and hence imaging speed, for axial resolution, allowing performance parameters to be adapted to the experimental requirements. We demonstrate this new instrument in calibration specimens and in biological specimens, including a mouse kidney slice.

Keywords: multiphoton microscopy; temporal focusing; digital micromirror device

---

1. Introduction

Multiphoton-excited fluorescence microscopy is a technique that can obtain axially resolved fluorescence images of various specimens, and is often employed in biomedical applications on account of its high resolution, intrinsic optical sectioning capability, and biocompatibility [1]. Since its invention, and with the aid of recent advances in femtosecond pulsed lasers, it has now become one of the standard microscopic tools in the field of biology [2–5]. Despite its utility for structural and functional studies on biological systems, conventional multiphoton microscopy is slow, based as it is on conventional raster-scanning of a tightly focused laser beam; the maximum imaging speed is often limited by the physical speed of a scanning mirror. This mechanical limitation hampers studies of the high-speed dynamics of a system of interest. To illuminate large areas at high speeds, new methods are needed [6].

Temporal focusing, a highly parallelized excitation technique, was proposed independently by Oron et al. and Zhu et al. [7,8]. This technique achieves parallelization of the excitation process by reflecting a high-peak-power femtosecond optical pulse off of a diffraction grating, and imaging the light from the grating onto the sample of interest using a high-resolution microscope. By spatially dispersing the optical pulse with the grating, the laser's pulse width is broadened temporally, and the peak power is reduced everywhere apart from at the focal plane of the microscope, thus ensuring that multiphoton excitation is confined to this plane. This technique has been successfully implemented in various applications including cellular dynamic imaging [9], depth-resolved lifetime imaging [10,11], optogenetics [12,13], and microfabrication [14–16]. Although this approach gives rise to wide-field multiphoton excitation, conventional wide-field temporal focusing does not achieve axial resolution comparable to point-scanning multiphoton microscopy, instead achieving axial resolution similar to that of a line-scanning multiphoton microscope [7,17].

Nevertheless, by patterning the temporal focusing excitation plane, the axial resolution can be improved. Line scanning temporal focusing is one example of patterning the excitation plane by focusing the light into a line, as demonstrated by Tal et al. [18]. In their paper, a cylindrical lens was used to generate a line pattern at the grating, and the resulting line shape at the sample plane had a ~1.5 μm axial extent, resulting in axial resolution close to that of conventional point-scanning multiphoton microscopy. This improved axial resolution does not come for free though; it requires the user to raster this excitation line along the orthogonal dimension using a galvo-mirror.

In this paper, we demonstrate a simple and programmable implementation of the line scanning temporal focusing technique, by employing a digital micromirror device (DMD). Using the DMD, a number of lines can be illuminated simultaneously, and swept across the sample at high speed. Unlike in a conventional line-scanning temporal focusing system [18,19], this approach enables trivial modification of the number of lines and the line thickness, allowing the tradeoff between the illuminated area and the axial resolution to be explored. The number of simultaneously swept lines can be also increased arbitrarily, helping to increase the photon efficiency, since fewer photons will be lost as the fraction of "on" pixels on the DMD is increased. In this study, particular attention is paid to the axial resolution of this system as a function of line thickness and the number of lines, and to demonstrate that the technique is not limited to test samples, a sectioned mouse kidney slice was imaged to highlight the superior axial resolution of DMD-based line scanning temporal focusing compared to wide-field temporal focusing. The experimental results clearly show that the DMD-based line scanning temporal focusing technique, with its ability to control the parameters of the projected line patterns, provides improved axial resolution in biological microscopy while maintaining high pixel throughput.

2. Materials and Methods

2.1. Digital Micromirror Device (DMD)-Based Line Scanning Temporal Focusing Multi-Photon Microscope

Figure 1 shows the schematic diagram of the DMD-based line temporal focusing multiphoton microscope. An ultrafast pulsed laser beam (120 fs pulse width, 10 kHz repetition rate, ~8 mm beam diameter ($1/e^2$)) from a regenerative amplifier (Legend Elite, Coherent, Santa Clara, CA, USA) was demagnified to ~6 mm and diffracted from a reflective ruled grating with a grating period of 1200 lines/mm (53033BK02-530R, Richardson Gratings, Rochester, NY, USA). The grating was followed by a 4f-lens system consisting of two planoconvex lenses (f = 300 mm; LA1256, Thorlabs and f = 750 mm; LA1727, Thorlabs, Newton, NJ, USA), which served to project and magnify the image of the grating onto the DMD (V-7000, Vialux, Chemnitz, Germany). The beam diameter of ~15 mm slightly overfilled the active area of the DMD. Arbitrary patterns could be uploaded onto the DMD using a control program (EasyProj) provided by Vialux. The light from the DMD was then allowed to pass through a tube lens (f = 750 mm; LA1227, Thorlabs), reflected off a dichroic filter (FF750-SDi02, Semrock, Rochester, NY, USA) and into an objective (water immersion 20×/1.0 numerical aperture; 421452-9880-000, Zeiss) to focus the image of the DMD into the sample. The geometric dispersion of the system ensured that the pulse width was broad enough to minimize multiphoton excitation except for at the sample plane. For wide-field temporal focusing, that is to say, when all 256 × 256 pixels of the DMD were on a field of view of ~60 μm × 60 μm was generated at the sample plane. The two-photon excited fluorescence from the sample was collected by the same objective lens and imaged by another tube lens (f = 200 mm; PAC064, Newport, Irvine, CA, USA) on to a CMOS camera (GS3-U3-32S4M-C,

FLIR, Wilsonville, OR, USA). Residual excitation light was filtered out by the dichroic filter and a short pass filter (ET680SP-2PS, Chroma, Bellows Falls, VT, USA).

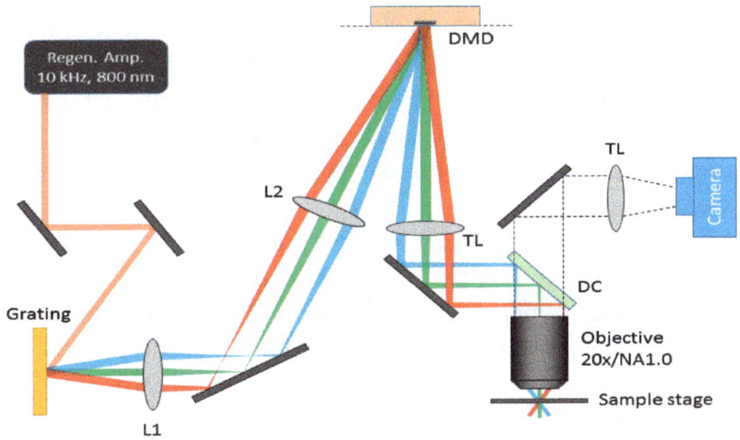

Figure 1. Schematic diagram of digital micromirror device (DMD)-based temporal focusing two-photon excited fluorescence microscope. L: lens; DMD: digital micromirror device; TL: tube lens; DC: dichroic mirror. L1: f = 300 mm, L2: f = 750 mm, TL (excitation): f = 750 mm.

For all experiments, fluorescence signals were collected in epi-fluorescence mode. Data from the camera were transferred using control software written using LabVIEW 2015 (National Instruments, Austin, TX, USA), which also controlled an objective piezo positioner (MIPOS-500, Piezosystem Jena, Jena, Germany) in order to obtain focal stacks.

Because a DMD can also act as a diffraction grating, there exists a remote possibility that this dispersion will affect the system. The effect of the DMD's dispersion is unlikely to have a major effect, since the "grating period" of the DMD in our configuration is high compared to that of the grating. Nevertheless, since the DMD is imaged onto the sample through an achromatic lens system, any additional dispersion from the DMD is actually likely to *improve* the axial resolution slightly, since this dispersion will lead to additional separation of the spectral components at the back aperture of the microscope objective.

2.2. Preparation of Calibration and Biological Samples

A thin, fluorescent layer of green quantum dots (supplied by QDVision, Lexington, MA, USA) was used to characterize the axial resolution of the system. Quantum dots dispersed in hexane (10 μL) were dropped onto a coverslip (thickness 170 μm) and allowed to dry. The coverslip was affixed to a glass slide and sealed. Another, more disperse quantum dot sample was prepared by diluting the quantum dot solution by a factor of 400 and repeating the procedure. A pollen grain slide (Carolina Biological Supply Inc., Burlington, NC, USA) was used to visually compare the optical sectioning capability of wide-field vs. line scanning two-photon temporal focusing. We further used a prepared slide of sectioned mouse kidney (F24630, Invitrogen, Carlsbad, CA, USA) to demonstrate the utility of DMD-based line scanning two-photon temporal focusing. For all line scanning measurements, each line pattern was illuminated for 2 ms, and total imaging time per frame was 1–2 s. For the line scanning modes, the generated lines swept the imaged area multiple times per frame. For example, a 1-pixel-thick line would sweep an area 128 pixels thick in 256 ms. Therefore, for an integration time of two seconds, the entire area was swept approximately eight times. For wide-field mode, square patterns were illuminated for less than 40 ms per frame. Excitation powers were adjusted to avoid saturation of the camera.

3. Results and Discussion

3.1. Axial Resolution Comparison Between Wide-Field and Line-Scanning Temporal Focusing

A thin layer of green fluorescent quantum dots (QD) was used to compare the axial resolution of wide-field temporal focusing and DMD-based line scanning temporal focusing techniques. Four measurements were performed for each imaging mode, and the integrated fluorescence intensity profile in the z-axis ($I_{p,z}$) was fitted using a Lorentzian function. The full-width half maximum (FWHM) of the fitted Lorentzian functions were averaged and used as a quantitative indicator of the axial resolution throughout this work.

For the wide-field temporal focusing, 128 × 128 pixels at the center of the DMD were set to an "on" state during the illumination time. The rest of the micromirrors outside the selected area remained "off" at all times. A line pattern was generated using 128 × 3 "on" micromirror pixels, and subsequent lines of the same thickness were scanned on the DMD to sweep the same area as the 128 × 128 pixel wide-field mode. Excitation powers were adjusted so as not to saturate the fluorescence signals from the thin quantum dot layer.

Wide-field (128 × 128 "on" pixels) illumination resulted in an axial FWHM of 9.03 ± 0.38 μm (mean ± SEM, $N = 4$) from $I_{p,z}$ (Figure 2). This value is close to the FWHM 7.6 μm obtained from our previous work (the literature value was obtained with an oil immersion 40×/1.3 NA objective) [17] but slightly broader, possibly due to underfilling of the back aperture of the objective. Although the initial microscope design deliberately did not overfill the back aperture of the objective lens in order to maximize illumination intensity at the sample plane, this reduction in axial resolution relative to the literature should affect both the wide-field and line-scanning modalities equally; hence, relative comparisons of the two different modalities is still valid. The FWHM of the line pattern illumination (128 × 3 "on" pixels) was determined to be 3.55 ± 0.02 μm, which is significantly reduced compared to the wide-field illumination. This result clearly demonstrates the improved axial resolution of line scanning over that of wide-field illumination.

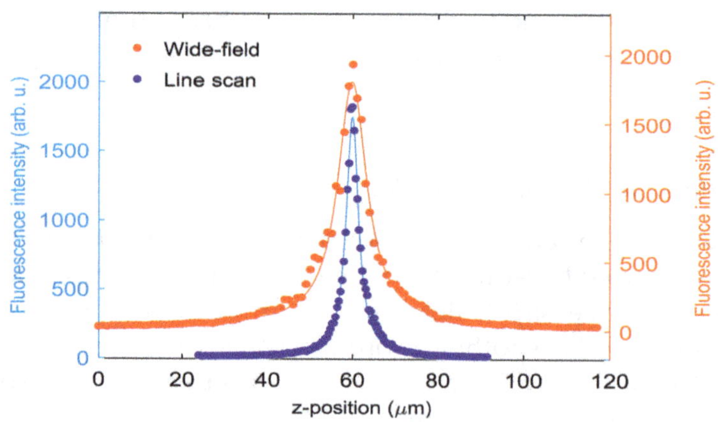

Figure 2. The comparison of z-axis integrated fluorescence intensity profile from wide-field temporal focusing excitation (red dots) and line scan temporal focusing excitation (blue dots). Pixels of the DMD with dimensions of 128 × 128 were "on" for the wide-field measurement, and a sequence of 128 × 3 pixels were "on" for the line scan mode. The data were fitted with Lorentzian function (solid lines).

3.2. Axial Resolution Dependence on the Line Thickness and the Number of Lines

We further studied the effect of pixel thickness on $I_{p,z}$ FWHM. The thickness of the lines (each of which had a length of 128 pixels at the DMD) was changed from 128 (wide-field), to 31, 15, 11, 7, 3, 2, and 1 pixels. As an illustration of the scanning process, a line of thickness of 1 was composed of 128 sequentially projected patterns of 128 × 1 "on" pixels, in order to illuminate the same area as the 128 × 128 wide-field illumination. Individual line patterns were illuminated for 2 ms and camera exposure times were kept to 1–2 s to maximize the image signal-to-noise ratio. For each pixel thickness, four z-stacks were obtained. $I_{p,z}$ plots were obtained from each z-stack measurement and fitted with a Lorentzian function. The averaged Lorentzian fit result is summarized in Figure 3 and Table 1. Interestingly, the $I_{p,z}$ FWHM exhibited a threshold-like response, rapidly transitioning from a wide-field like FWHM to a single-pixel line-like FHWM with a line thickness of 11 pixels, which corresponds to a thickness of ~106 μm immediately after the DMD, or ~1.17 μm at the sample once it has been imaged by the tube lens (f = 750 mm) and the objective lens (f_{eff} = 8.25 mm). The FWHM of $I_{p,z}$ continued to drop as the line thickness decreased, but not to as great a degree. The minimum FWHM 3.07 ± 0.15 μm was obtained when the line was 1 pixel thick. This FWHM (3.07 μm) is significantly reduced compared to that (9.03 μm) of the wide-field illumination of the same illumination width. However, it is still broader than the theoretical diffraction limit of point scanning, which is ~1.1 μm ($\left(0.886\lambda/\sqrt{2}\right)\left(1/\left(n-\sqrt{n^2-NA^2}\right)\right)$, where λ = 800 nm, n = 1.3, and NA = 1.0, equivalent to our experimental conditions) [20,21], as well as the FWHM (~1.5 μm) of line temporal focusing achieved using a cylindrical lens [18]. The broader FHWM is possibly due to the underfilled back aperture of the objective as mentioned above. To exclude the possibility of a thick QD layer broadening the FWHM, we prepared another QD slide after diluting the QD solution by a factor of 400, and observed a similar $I_{p,z}$ FWHM of 3.57 ± 0.20 μm from 3-pixel-thick line illumination, confirming that the QD slide that was used was sufficiently thin.

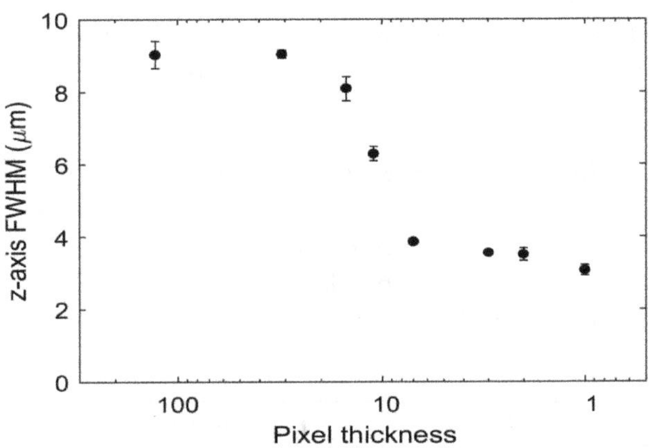

Figure 3. The dependence of $I_{p,z}$ full-width half maximum (FWHM) of a thin quantum dot layer upon illumination with pixel thicknesses of line (128 × T) excitation, generated by DMD. Four measurements (N = 4) were performed for each pixel thickness and fitted with Lorentzian function. Pixel thicknesses corresponded to T = 128, 31, 15, 11, 7, 3, 2, and 1.

Table 1. FWHM of a thin quantum dot slide varying the thickness of line pattern on the DMD. Four measurements (N = 4) were performed and averaged for each pixel thickness (pixel size of 128 × T).

Pixel Thickness (128 × T)	FWHM (μm)	Standard Error (μm)
128 (wide-field)	9.03	0.38
31	9.04	0.10
15	8.10	0.33
11	6.29	0.20
7	3.87	0.05
3	3.55	0.02
2	3.51	0.18
1	3.07	0.15

To explain the threshold-like response, we propose a "two-regime" model in which the axial resolution is constrained by two different phenomena—the temporal focusing and the geometric focusing effects. In the first regime, with a wide thickness, the dominant effect is temporal focusing—out-of-plane excitation is suppressed by the temporal focusing dispersion, so no matter how wide the excitation, there is a limiting axial resolution. As the line thickness becomes thinner, geometric focusing also contributes—as one focuses the line tighter and tighter, axial resolution is improved in exactly the same way as a normal multiphoton microscope. Finally, the resolution plateaus as the diffraction limit and residual optical aberrations in the system start to constrain how narrow the projected lines can be.

The most salient benefit of using a DMD-based microscope is to generate arbitrarily patterned illumination; multiple lines of various thicknesses can be generated by a DMD, while conventional line temporal focusing using a cylindrical lens [18] can only produce one. We generated multiple 3-pixel-thick lines with the DMD and measured $I_{p,z}$ FWHM of the thin QD slide (Table 2). FWHMs of $I_{p,z}$ remained in the region of 3.4–3.5 μm, from a single line up to 16 lines (duty cycles, or the ratio of on and off pixels, were 0.023, 0.094, 0.19, and 0.38 for 1, 4, 8, and 16 lines, respectively); thus, each individual line behaved in an isolated manner, not affecting the other projected lines. With 32 lines, however, corresponding to duty cycle of 0.73, the FWHM of 7.75 μm became worse by a factor of 2 compared to 1, 4, 8, and 16 lines. The upper limit of multiple lines illumination is wide-field illumination, in which the FWHM is 9.03 μm (Table 1). Knowing the limit of the number of lines that can be exposed while maintaining a minimum level of axial resolution is important to maximize imaging speed; the exposure time is inversely proportional to the number of identical lines. As a guide, illuminating multiple lines with a duty cycle below ~0.4 is a safe estimate in order to reduce the image acquisition time while maintaining the axial resolution of the system.

Table 2. Axial FWHMs of a thin quantum dot layer, varying the number of illuminating lines when single or multiple 128 × 3-pixel-thick lines were used. Line patterns were spaced equally so that the total number of patterns decreased as the number of lines increased, in order to illuminate the same sample area, corresponding to 128 × 128 "on" pixels. Four measurements ($N = 4$) were performed, and fitted FHWMs were averaged for each pixel thickness.

Number of Lines ($L \times (128 \times 3)$)	FWHM (μm)	Standard Error (μm)
1	3.55	0.02
4	3.40	0.12
8	3.38	0.17
16	3.40	0.23
32	7.75	0.43

3.3. Imaging of a Pollen Grain and Biological Sample

We collected two-photon temporal focusing fluorescence images of a pollen grain in order to demonstrate the utility of DMD-based line temporal focusing (Figure 4). The pollen grain was imaged at 1 μm steps along the *z*-axis, both with equally spaced 8 lines (128 × 3 "on" pixels) and with wide-field (128 × 128 "on" pixels) temporal focusing. Clearly, DMD-generated line scanning displayed a sharper axial fluorescence intensity profile than wide-field illumination on the same pollen grain (Figure 4c). In addition to better axial optical sectioning, line scanning removes the "ghost" interference pattern that appears in the wide-field mode (Figure 4a); the striped pattern on the pollen grain is not a real feature. The ghost pattern potentially originates from interference among multiple spectral components or between multiply reflected beams passing through the many optical components in the system.

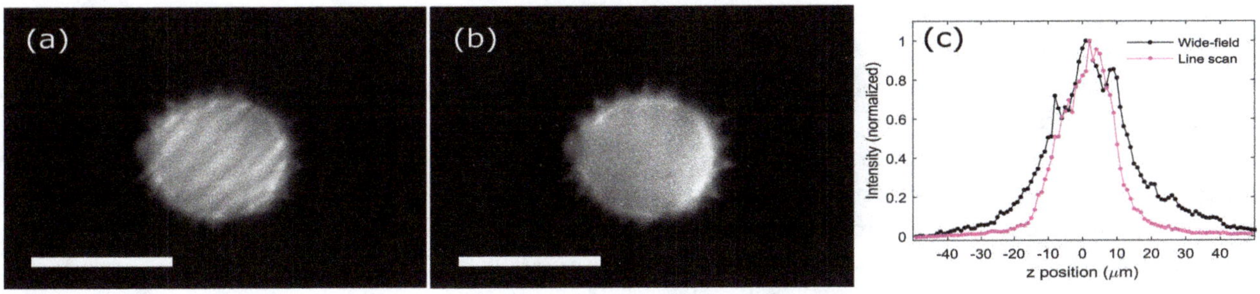

Figure 4. Two-photon temporal focusing fluorescence images of a pollen grain. The pollen grain was imaged with wide-field, 128 × 128 "on" pixels and 8 lines of 128 × 3 "on" pixels. The images of the pollen grain at maximum fluorescence intensity by the wide-field and the line scan modes are shown (**a**,**b**), respectively. (**c**) Normalized fluorescence z-profile of the wide-field (black) and the line scan (magenta) modes on the pollen grain. Scale bar is 30 μm in (**a**,**b**).

We next imaged a prepared slide of sectioned mouse kidney (F24630, Invitrogen). The sample was imaged at a 0.5 μm step size with a 40 μm axial scanning range to ensure that no sample features were missed. Both line scanning (16 lines of 256 × 3 "on" pixels corresponding to duty cycle of 0.19) and wide-field (256 × 256 "on" pixels) illumination were used. While convoluted tubule structures in a mouse kidney can be identified by both the line scanning (Figure 5a–c) and wide-field (Figure 5d) temporal focusing, fine structures are more discernible by line scanning mode.

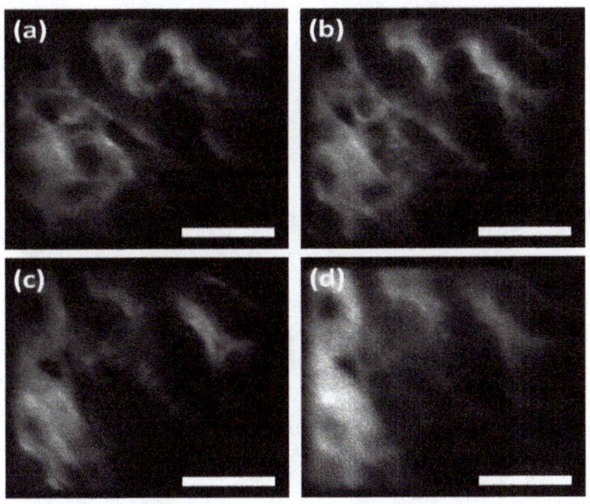

Figure 5. Line scanning temporal focusing two-photon excited fluorescence images of an excised mouse kidney slice. Three of the line scanning (16 lines of 256 × 3 "on" pixels) z-stack images taken at 2 μm intervals are shown in (**a**–**c**). Scale bar; 20 μm. Wide-field (256 × 256 "on" pixels) temporal focusing image at the same z-position with (**b**) is shown for comparison in (**d**).

4. Conclusions

We have demonstrated a line-scanning temporal focusing two-photon excited fluorescence microscope using a digital micromirror device. While wide-field temporal focusing can only achieve a broad axial resolution of 9.03 μm measured using a thin fluorescent quantum dot layer, line-scanning temporal focusing generated by a DMD shows an enhanced axial resolution of up to 3.07 μm, which is an improvement of a factor of three over that of the wide-field mode. We were also able to determine that, by illuminating the sample with lines of different thicknesses, the transition between wide-field-like and single-line-like axial resolutions occurs very rapidly. This observation leads us to recommend the use of multi-pixel thick line scans for a better signal-to-noise ratio without sacrificing axial resolution. Equally spaced multiple lines were also examined, confirming that multiple lines do not degrade the axial resolution until a certain duty cycle is reached, which was ~0.4 for our experimental conditions.

We also have visually compared the axial resolution by wide-field and multiple line scanning temporal focusing microscopy of the autofluorescence of a pollen grain. The fluorescence trace from the pollen grain as a function of focal position clearly demonstrated that line scanning temporal focusing has better optical sectioning capability than the wide-field mode. We also observed that the line scanning mode can remove interference patterns that appeared in the wide-field mode; patterns which might mislead the user under some circumstances. A mouse kidney slice was imaged using the line-scanning mode, which produced a sharper transition from the background to fluorescence signal at the boundary between the kidney tissue and the coverslip. This result demonstrates the utility of DMD-based line scanning temporal focusing two-photon excited fluorescence in the field of biomedical imaging.

Acknowledgments: We acknowledge support from the National Institute of Health 5-P41-EB015871-28, 2R01EY017656-06, R21-NS091982-01, 1-U01-NS090438-01, 1U01CA202177-01, and 1R01HL121386-01A1, Singapore-MIT Alliance for Science and Technology, Connecticut Children's Medical Center, Hamamatsu Corp., and Samsung Advanced Institute of Technology. C.J.R. further acknowledges support from the Wellcome Trust 093831/Z/10/Z.

Author Contributions: J.K.P., C.J.R., and P.T.C.S. conceived and designed the experiments; J.K.P. performed the experiments; J.K.P. analyzed the data; J.K.P. and C.J.R. contributed reagents/materials/analysis tools; J.K.P., C.J.R., and P.T.C.S. wrote the paper.

References

1. Denk, W.; Strickler, J.H.; Webb, W.W. Two-photon laser scanning fluorescence microscopy. *Science* **1990**, *248*, 73–76. [CrossRef] [PubMed]
2. Helmchen, F.; Denk, W. Deep tissue two-photon microscopy. *Nat. Methods* **2005**, *2*, 932–940. [CrossRef] [PubMed]
3. Mertz, J. Nonlinear microscopy: New techniques and applications. *Curr. Opin. Neurobiol.* **2004**, *14*, 610–616. [CrossRef] [PubMed]
4. So, P.T.C.; Dong, C.Y.; Masters, B.R.; Berland, K.M. Two-Photon excitation fluorescence microscopy. *Annu. Rev. Biomed. Eng.* **2000**, *2*, 399–429. [CrossRef] [PubMed]
5. Hoover, E.E.; Squier, J.A. Advances in multiphoton microscopy technology. *Nat. Photon.* **2013**, *7*, 93–101. [CrossRef] [PubMed]
6. So, P.T.C.; Yew, E.Y.S.; Rowlands, C. High-throughput nonlinear optical microscopy. *Biophys. J.* **2013**, *105*, 2641–2654. [CrossRef] [PubMed]
7. Oron, D.; Tal, E.; Silberberg, Y. Scanningless depth-resolved microscopy. *Opt. Express* **2005**, *13*, 1468–1476. [CrossRef] [PubMed]
8. Zhu, G.; van Howe, J.; Durst, M.; Zipfel, W.; Xu, C. Simultaneous spatial and temporal focusing of femtosecond pulses. *Opt. Express* **2005**, *13*, 2153–2159. [CrossRef] [PubMed]
9. Therrien, O.D.; Aubé, B.; Pagès, S.; Koninck, P.D.; Côté, D. Wide-field multiphoton imaging of cellular dynamics in thick tissue by temporal focusing and patterned illumination. *Biomed. Opt. Express* **2011**, *2*, 696–704. [CrossRef] [PubMed]
10. Choi, H.; Tzeranis, D.S.; Cha, J.W.; Clémenceau, P.; de Jong, S.J.G.; van Geest, L.K.; Moon, J.H.; Yannas, I.V; So, P.T.C. 3D-resolved fluorescence and phosphorescence lifetime imaging using temporal focusing wide-field two-photon excitation. *Opt. Express* **2012**, *20*, 26219–26235. [CrossRef] [PubMed]
11. Choi, H.; Yew, E.Y.S.; Hallacoglu, B.; Fantini, S.; Sheppard, C.J.R.; So, P.T.C. Improvement of axial resolution and contrast in temporally focused widefield two-photon microscopy with structured light illumination. *Biomed. Opt. Express* **2013**, *4*, 995–1005. [CrossRef] [PubMed]
12. Andrasfalvy, B.K.; Zemelman, B.V.; Tang, J.; Vaziri, A. Two-photon single-cell optogenetic control of neuronal activity by sculpted light. *Proc. Natl. Acad. Sci. USA* **2010**, *107*, 11981–11986. [CrossRef] [PubMed]
13. Papagiakoumou, E.; Anselmi, F.; Begue, A.; de Sars, V.; Gluckstad, J.; Isacoff, E.Y.; Emiliani, V. Scanless two-photon excitation of channelrhodopsin-2. *Nat. Methods* **2010**, *7*, 848–854. [CrossRef] [PubMed]

14. Kim, D.; So, P.T.C. High-throughput three-dimensional lithographic microfabrication. *Opt. Lett.* **2010**, *35*, 1602–1604. [CrossRef] [PubMed]
15. Li, Y.-C.; Cheng, L.-C.; Chang, C.-Y.; Lien, C.-H.; Campagnola, P.J.; Chen, S.-J. Fast multiphoton microfabrication of freeform polymer microstructures by spatiotemporal focusing and patterned excitation. *Opt. Express* **2012**, *20*, 19030–19038. [CrossRef] [PubMed]
16. Li, Y.-C.; Yeh, T.-F.; Huang, H.-C.; Chang, H.-Y.; Lin, C.-Y.; Cheng, L.-C.; Chang, C.-Y.; Teng, H.; Chen, S.-J. Graphene oxide-based micropatterns via high-throughput multiphoton-induced reduction and ablation. *Opt. Express* **2014**, *22*, 19726–19734. [CrossRef] [PubMed]
17. Yew, E.Y.S.; Sheppard, C.J.R.; So, P.T.C. Temporally focused wide-field two-photon microscopy: Paraxial to vectorial. *Opt. Express* **2013**, *21*, 12951–12963. [CrossRef] [PubMed]
18. Tal, E.; Oron, D.; Silberberg, Y. Improved depth resolution in video-rate line-scanning multiphoton microscopy using temporal focusing. *Opt. Lett.* **2005**, *30*, 1686–1688. [CrossRef] [PubMed]
19. Dana, H.; Kruger, N.; Ellman, A.; Shoham, S. Line temporal focusing characteristics in transparent and scattering media. *Opt. Express* **2013**, *21*, 5677–5687. [CrossRef] [PubMed]
20. Kim, D. Ultrashort optical pulse delivery for nolinear optical microscopy. In *Handbook of Biomedical Nonlinear Optical Microscopy*; Masters, B.R., So, P.T.C., Eds.; Oxford University Press: New York, NY, USA, 2008; p. 239.
21. Zipfel, W.R.; Williams, R.M.; Webb, W.W. Nonlinear magic: Multiphoton microscopy in the biosciences. *Nat. Biotechnol.* **2003**, *21*, 1369–1377. [CrossRef] [PubMed]

3

Single-Pixel MEMS Imaging Systems

Guangcan Zhou [1], Zi Heng Lim [1], Yi Qi [1] and Guangya Zhou [1,*]

Micro and Nano Systems Initiative, Department of Mechanical Engineering, National University of Singapore, Singapore 117575, Singapore; E0115906@u.nus.edu (G.Z.); limziheng@nus.edu.sg (Z.H.L.); mpeqiyi@nus.edu.sg (Y.Q.)

* Correspondence: mpezgy@nus.edu.sg

Abstract: Single-pixel imaging technology is an attractive technology considering the increasing demand of imagers that can operate in wavelengths where traditional cameras have limited efficiency. Meanwhile, the miniaturization of imaging systems is also desired to build affordable and portable devices for field applications. Therefore, single-pixel imaging systems based on microelectromechanical systems (MEMS) is an effective solution to develop truly miniaturized imagers, owing to their ability to integrate multiple functionalities within a small device. MEMS-based single-pixel imaging systems have mainly been explored in two research directions, namely the encoding-based approach and the scanning-based approach. The scanning method utilizes a variety of MEMS scanners to scan the target scenery and has potential applications in the biological imaging field. The encoding-based system typically employs MEMS modulators and a single-pixel detector to encode the light intensities of the scenery, and the images are constructed by harvesting the power of computational technology. This has the capability to capture non-visible images and 3D images. Thus, this review discusses the two approaches in detail, and their applications are also reviewed to evaluate the efficiency and advantages in various fields.

Keywords: single-pixel imaging; microelectromechanical systems (MEMS); computational technology; MEMS scanners; MEMS modulators

---

1. Introduction

In conventional imaging systems, the scenery is usually focused by camera lenses onto a focal plane where it is captured by a pixel array detector. Current cameras can obtain an image with millions of pixels using a silicon-based sensor chip, owing to the mature technology of complementary metal-oxide-semiconductor (CMOS) and charge-coupled devices (CCDs). The number of pixels on the sensor chip is usually adopted to evaluate its performance and marketing value, but this type of sensor only works efficiently at the specified wavelength range. It is noticed that there is increasing demand for imaging systems that can operate at wavelengths unavailable for silicon-based sensors to meet different sensing applications, such as far-infrared and deep ultraviolet sensing. Sensor arrays in these operating ranges are either expensive or unavailable; thus, single-pixel imaging (SPI) technology provides an alternative method to construct an imager with just one single-pixel detector in these cases. Based on the general architectures, the SPI systems can be divided into two main research subcategories, namely the scanning-based approach and the encoding-based approach.

The scanning-based method originates from the reported televisor in 1929 [1], which employs a light sensitive detector and a spiral-perforated disc, the Nipkow disk [2], to raster-scan the target scenery at different positions. Modern scanning imagers are typically established with various scanning devices to direct the light from the scenery onto a single-pixel photodetector, and each pixel of the scenery is separately scanned and recorded at each scanning step. This type of imager is commonly applied in imaging where the operating wavelengths cannot be sensed efficiently by silicon-based sensor arrays, where its performance may be affected when the light intensity from each pixel is too weak to be efficiently detected, for example in long-range imaging. The performance of such mechanism is highly related to the mechanical properties of the applied scanners, and its pixel resolution is decided by the achievable number of measurements (scanning points) employing specific scanners. With the encoding-based approach, the scenery is usually encoded with time-varying patterns generated by a spatial light modulator (SLM), while the encoded light is synchronously collected with a single-pixel detector. In this case, the image is recovered through specified algorithms, and thus the efficiency of this method mainly relies on the power of computational technology instead of hardware. The encoding system is generally performing a sampling process to sense the light from multiple pixels at each sampling step, thus benefiting from the improved detected efficiency and low dark count. In addition, some well-established mathematical theories allow us to compress the signal during the acquisition process to reduce sampling time and data storage requirement [3], which is significant in real-time imaging systems [4] or hyperspectral imaging systems [5]. However, the computational overhead is still an important consideration when constructing an encoding-based SPI system.

Over the past few decades, the miniaturization of imagers has drawn the attention and interest of researchers to meet the increasing demand of portable devices for field applications. Considering that microelectromechanical systems (MEMS) technologies are capable of integrating multiple functionalities within small devices, this technology has been explored to develop various compact SPI systems by miniaturizing the scanners and modulators in the two approaches mentioned. Until now, many MEMS scanners have been widely explored in truly miniaturized imaging systems, such as endoscopes. In addition, there also exist many demonstrations of the encoding-based SPI systems using MEMS technology for these imaging areas where traditional cameras get limited efficiency. This paper reviews these single-pixel MEMS imaging systems with the purpose of providing useful information to anyone planning to construct a compact imager for a specific application. The operating principles of the two methods will be briefly introduced in this paper, followed by a review of the typical system architectures. This paper also focuses on the applications of single-pixel MEMS imaging systems to evaluate its efficiency and advantages in various industrial fields. The potential of this technology is also described in this paper considering its latest imaging applications, such as 3D imaging.

2. Scanning-Based Approach

After the first scanning mirror was reported in 1980 [6], MEMS scanners have become an important research topic in the MEMS area and also drive the development of portable and truly miniaturized imaging systems. Compared with traditional scanning optical devices, such as galvanometric scanners, MEMS scanners are preferable in field applications, considering their capability of miniaturization, lower power consumption and high performance at resonant driving conditions. Figure 1 depicts two general approaches to build an SPI system using MEMS scanners. In the first approach, a scanning imager can be implemented by a single dual-axis scanning mirror, which scans the target scenery and directs the scanned light intensity onto a single-pixel detector. In the second approach, two orthogonal single-axis scanning mirrors are employed to scan the scenery instead, thereby increasing the system complexity. When designing such imagers, scan angles and scan speed should be designed properly to ensure the appropriate field-of-view and framerates. In addition, it is also noticed that some scanners have been developed with the ability of additional axial scan to achieve 3D images, which are desired in imaging applications.

The inset of Figure 1a schematically gives the scanning trajectories of three commonly applied strategies in MEMS scanning imagers. Raster scan was the first sampling strategy used for SPI systems and consists of slow scanning and fast scanning in two orthogonal directions. The acquisition time of this imager is mainly determined by the lower scanning frequency, which should be increased to acceptable levels for real-imaging applications. Such a scanning mechanism can be easily obtained with torsional MEMS scanners or fiber scanners, and thus it is widely applied in MEMS imaging systems. Flexible micro-springs are desired in the architecture of torsional scanners for slow motion to ensure the scanning range (field-of-view) [7–9], while high driving voltage is required for fiber scanners. Another solution to scan the scenery is to utilize the Lissajous scan, which can conduct simultaneous biaxial high frequency scans. Its scanning range and framerate can be ensured by operating it at resonant mode, and thus this strategy benefits from the mechanical stability and low power consumption [10]. It is noticed that spiral scanning is also employed in some scenarios [11] using a bare-fiber scanner, which allows for miniaturization. To achieve the shown trajectory in the inset, two separate signals with the same frequency are set with a 90° phase-shift to drive the scanner along two orthogonal axes, while the amplitude along the radius is modulated during the scanning process. However, it should be noted that the scanning speed and illumination density distribution condition may affect the performance of this scanning approach [12,13]. One can choose the proper sampling strategy according to the application requirements, and some selection rules can be found in [14].

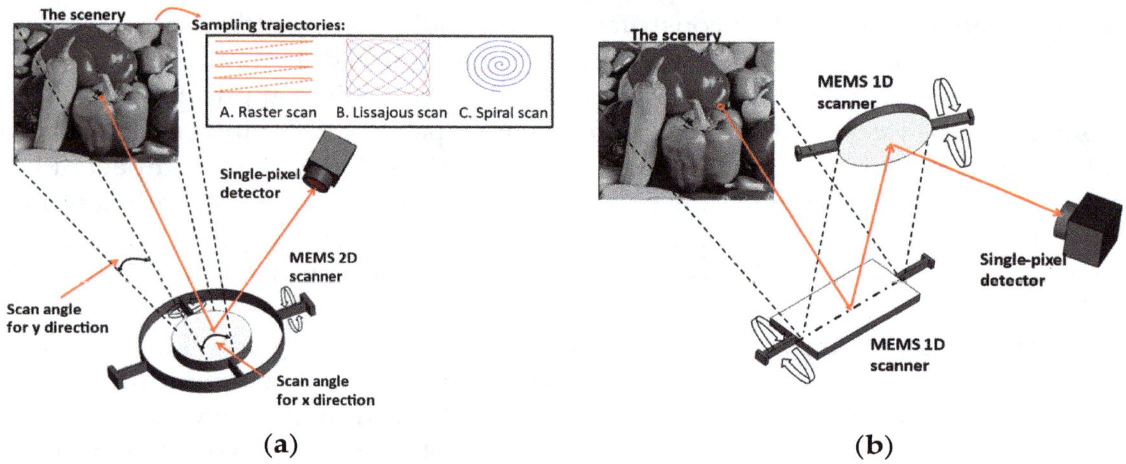

Figure 1. Schematic of two scanning strategies to build a single-pixel imaging system: (**a**) using a single dual-axis scanner; (**b**) using two orthogonal single-axis scanners.

2.1. Microelectromechanical Systems (MEMS) Scanners Technologies

There are four predominant driving mechanisms commonly applied in the construction of MEMS scanners, namely electrostatic, electromagnetic, piezoelectric and electrothermal actuation. Each actuation approach has its potential applications as well as limitations in image capture, and it should be noted that a variety of MEMS scanning mirrors have also been reported in other fields, such as MEMS displays and optical communication. This paper will focus on the application of MEMS scanners to construct SPI systems, and thus much attention is focused on these parameters, which affect the performance of imagers. More specifically, a large field of view is typically achieved with large scan angles, while a higher scan frequency can increase the framerate. It should be noted that mirror smoothness is also an important parameter in imaging applications considering that the deformation of the mirror may distort the images. In this section, a brief introduction is given on the basic working principles of the four actuation mechanisms, followed by some imaging applications of each technology.

2.1.1. Electrostatic Actuation

Considering the fabrication complexity and the ease of integration, electrostatic actuation is an attractive actuation method for the MEMS scanner. This actuation mechanism utilizes the electrostatic force generated between two oppositely charged components to tilt the micromirrors. There are two architectures, comb-drive actuation and parallel plate actuation, to be explored for the driving of MEMS scanners in imaging applications. In comb-drive architectures, the movable comb structures are typically offset from the fixed comb structures at the initial condition, and the electrostatic force can be generated to move the movable fingers up and down with a supplied voltage. The micromirror connected with the movable comb structures can then be titled to the specified scan angles. Figure 2a shows a MEMS scanner actuated by an angular vertical-comb (AVC) actuator [15]. The device was constructed through surface and bulk micromachining processes and can achieve a scan angle of ±6° under non-resonant operation, while the resonant frequencies were measured to be 463 and 140 Hz for the inner and outer axis, respectively. In addition to providing 2D images, various efforts have also been devoted to building 3D scanning architecture, which can capture the side view as well through specific optical configurations or scanner design. In this case, the micromirror was integrated within an optical coherence tomography (OCT) catheter of 5 mm diameter and can provide a side view with 2 mm working distance by mounting the mirror tilted to the optical path at ±45°. This system can achieve a 1.8 mm × 1 mm × 1.3 mm field of view with 500 × 500 × 1000 pixels for in vivo imaging applications, and the frame rate was reported to be 4 frames/s. In reference [16], a 2D scanner was demonstrated with gimbal-less electrostatic actuators. Separate fabrication processes were conducted to form the actuators and the mirror with a size of 1 mm × 1 mm, followed by manual bonding. The tilt angle was measured to be 20° under resonant conditions, and the resonances were observed to happen at 1.8 and 2.4 kHz for the two axes with the single-crystal silicon actuators. The presented device was integrated in an OCT imaging probe (diameter < 4 mm) to achieve 3D imaging combined with an additional axial scan. The size of the captured volume images was 1 mm × 1 mm × 1.4 mm corresponding to 400 × 200 × 560 pixels, and the 3D OCT imaging successfully captured clear 3D images of tissues with a framerate of 3 frames/s.

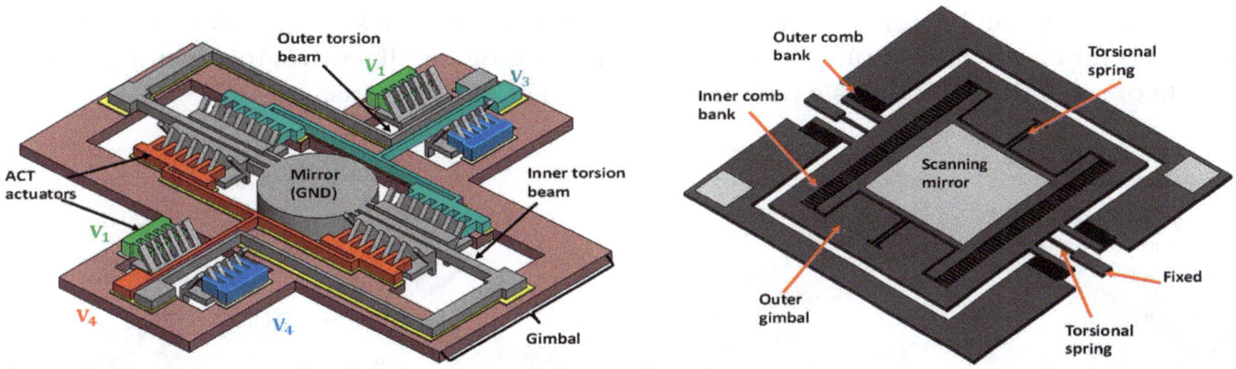

(a) (b)

Figure 2. Schematic drawing of (**a**) the microelectromechanical systems (MEMS) scanner using an angular vertical-comb (AVC) actuator [15] and (**b**) the scanning mirror developed on single-crystal silicon and actuated with two vertical-comb structures [17].

Figure 2b shows another example of a 2D scanning mirror developed on single-crystal silicon for two-photon fluorescence imaging [17]. The mirror with a size of 0.75 mm × 0.75 mm was actuated with two comb banks to achieve a 2D scan, and the resultant scan angle was measured to be about 16°. The fast scanning axis can achieve a scanning frequency of up to 3.5 kHz, and later a similar structure was reported for the construction of a compact dual-axis confocal microscope with a framerate of 8 frames/s. The resonant frequencies were measured to be 500 Hz for the outer axis and 2.9 kHz for the inner axis. The scan angles for these two axes are reported to be ±6.2° and ±3.6°, respectively [9]. Various MEMS scanners have been widely reported in other imaging architectures using this actuation principle, including the OCT [18] and confocal microscopy or endoscop [19–22].

Another scheme is to utilize a fixed electrode to attract the movable micromirror platform to generate the scan motion. In the field of imaging, this type of actuation was firstly adopted to develop a single axis scanner in a confocal microscope where two such scanners were used to achieve a functional 2D scan [23], as described in Figure 1a. Two dimensional scanners can be achieved with quad-electrodes, and these scanners have been reported in miniaturized configurations for confocal microscopy [24] and OCT systems [25]. Figure 3a shows a 2D scanner for OCT imaging application [26], from which it can be seen that the central mirror is connected to the basement through a biaxial gimbal structure, while the quad-electrode pedestals are implemented on the bottom of the mirror with a gap at the static condition. This structure obtained a 2D scan with an achievable angle of ±4° with a 130 V DC power supply, and this device could be operated at its resonant frequency to achieve the same scan angle with 20 V AC plus 60 V DC bias voltage. Compared with the comb-drive actuation, this type of actuation method typically results in a non-linear relationship between the deflection angle and the supplied voltage when DC voltage is used. The resonances of the inner and outer axes were observed to happen at 472 Hz and 399 Hz, respectively. At resonant operation, a linear relationship was obtained between the scan angle and the supplied AC voltage.

It is worth mentioning that such an actuation principle can be extended to develop focus-adjustable MEMS micromirrors by using the attraction force between the mirror and the bottom frame. Such micromirrors have been applied in various OCT imaging systems [27–29], and functional 3D scans can be achieved by integrating this architecture with a quad-electrode based 2D scanner, shown in [30,31]. These architectures are quite similar to the scanner shown in Figure 3a, despite the slightly different mirror geometries and fabrication processes. A quad-electrode pillar was constructed separately and manually inserted to the cavity between the mirror and the underlying frame to achieve a 2D scan, as shown in Figure 3b. Electrostatic attraction is generated between the mirror and its underlying silicon frame to change the focus of the micromirrors. The device [30] was reported to have a scan angle of around ±5° under a 140 V DC voltage supply, while a ±4° scan angle was observed under the resonant frequency at around 216 Hz with 40 V AC voltage. With additional electrostatic actuation, the focus can be adjusted from infinity to 50 mm with less than 100 V. This system was demonstrated for endoscopic applications. In various imaging architectures, this method can provide a framerate of more than 10 frames/s with the resolution of few microns.

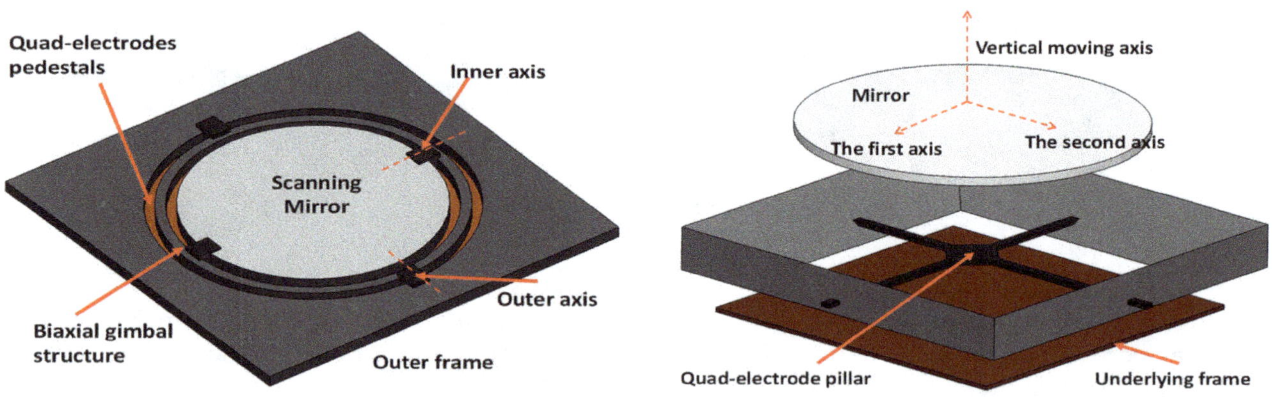

(a) (b)

Figure 3. Mechanical structures of (**a**) the MEMS scanner using quad-electrodes to achieve a 2D scan with a gold-coated mirror [26] and (**b**) the quad-electrode pillar utilized to drive the mirror combined with electrostatic actuation between the mirror and bottom basement for 3D imaging [30].

2.1.2. Electromagnetic Actuation

Electromagnetic actuation is another actuation principle, which utilizes magnetic torque to tilt the microscanner. Two actuation schemes, moving coils and moving magnets, have been applied to develop MEMS scanners. Figure 4a shows an example of moving coils used in a commercial Olympus confocal microscope [32]. External permanent magnets were employed to drive the micromirror on which the driving coils were implemented through electro-plating. The mirror (4.2 mm × 3.0 mm) was constructed on a wafer with 300 μm thickness to maintain the mirror flatness, thus ensuring the imaging quality. The scanner was designed with a resonant frequency of roughly 4 kHz to achieve a fast scan, with its scan angle reaching 8°. It should be noted that the reported scanner was only designed to allow a single-axis scan, and single dual-axis scanners have also been explored for optical coherence tomography, such as the non-resonant scanners shown in [33]. Figure 4b gives the schematic of a single dual-axis scanner using the moving coils scheme, reported in [34], for imaging and display applications. A functional 2D scan was achieved by using mechanical coupling between the mirror (diameter: 1.5 mm) and the outer frame structure. Multi-turn spiral driving coils were implemented within the outer frame through typical bulk MEMS fabrication techniques. An external magnet was set at 45° to the plane of the scanning axis, and thus the outer frame was driven in two orthogonal directions. Such architecture can get full scan angles of 65° and 53°, respectively, and the scan frequency reached up to 20.5 kHz for the fast scan and 60 Hz for the slow scan, respectively. Similar structures can be found in confocal microscopy reported in [35], and Figure 4c shows a two-axis scanning mirror with a thin magnetic layer glued on the backside of the mirror. The depicted mirror is used to construct a MEMS catheter 2.8 mm in diameter for 3D endoscopic OCT and can obtain a scanning range of ±20° in both directions. Additionally, it can be operated at resonant frequencies of 450 Hz and 350 Hz for the depicted inner axis and outer axis, respectively. It is worth mentioning that the required operating voltage is relatively low using this actuation method and thus benefits its applications. Apart from these silicon mirror structures, other types of MEMS scanners have also been explored for imaging applications using this actuation method, such as polydimethylsiloxane-based mirrors [36] and microlenses [37].

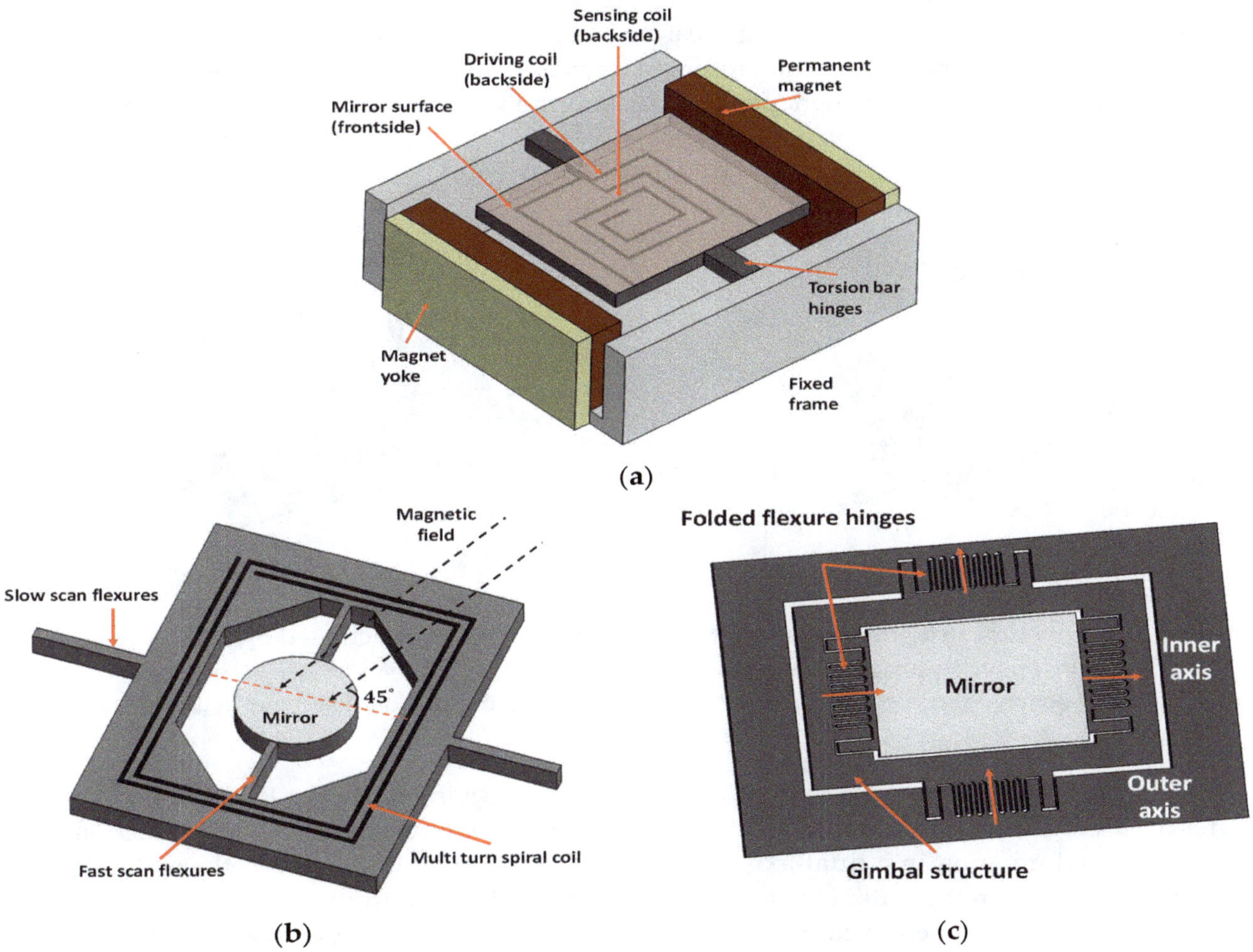

Figure 4. Schematic of the mechanical structures of a (**a**) 1D scanner in Olympus confocal microscope [32]; (**b**) 2D scanner with an external magnet set at 45° to the plane of the scanning axis [34]; (**c**) 2D scanner driven by the glued magnets on the side of the mirror [35].

2.1.3. Piezoelectric Actuation

Piezoelectric actuation provides another solution to develop functional MEMS scanners by incorporating the piezoelectric effect of specific materials, such as lead zirconate titanate (PZT), after PZT was reported to be micromachinable in MEMS devices [38]. This actuation principle typically provides large static deflection and high driving force, and it also allows acceptable resonant frequencies without consuming much power. The original scanner structures were established by incorporating the PZT thin film into a cantilever beam where the mirror was implemented on the topside. Thus, when a voltage was supplied to one side of the PZT, the thin film would expand in a specified direction to generate the driving force, and the whole beam could be titled to obtain a scan angle. In these architectures, there exists a trade-off between actuation angles and the mirror flatness. A fabrication procedure, reported in [39], was designed to independently fabricate the mirror and cantilever beam with defined thickness on a thermal silicon dioxide wafer through a two-step etching and releasing process. Thus, this method could maintain the mirror flatness with a scan angle of ±7° and ±8° at static and resonant conditions, respectively. In this case, the resonant frequency is affected by the length of the beam. More specifically, a shorter beam can result in a higher resonant frequency and reduced scan angle. This PZT cantilever beam structure was employed in a Fourier-domain OCT system to demonstrate its imaging capability. Different from the unit structure, Figure 5a gives another 1D optical scanner where the mirror is connected with two piezoelectric cantilever beams through the folded silicon beams, and thus the scanner is indirectly driven by the PZT beams to ensure the mirror flatness [40]. A so-called 13%-Nb-doped PZT (PNZT) film was employed to actuate such scanners, which shows the potential of achieving large scan angles with piezoelectric actuation by optimizing the properties of applied PZT materials. The presented device, 3.4 mm × 2.5 mm in size, can achieve a scan angle of 152° under a resonant frequency of 394 Hz, and the scanner was successfully demonstrated in a swept-source OCT system.

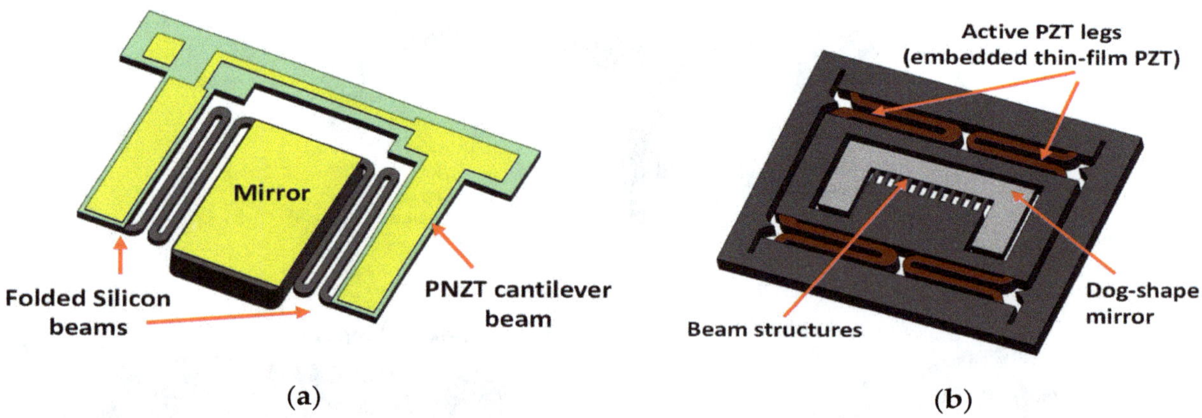

Figure 5. Mechanical structures of (**a**) the MEMS scanners indirectly actuated by a 13%-Nb-doped PZT (PNZT) cantilever beam [40]; (**b**) the MEMS scanners actuated by active lead zirconate titanate (PZT) legs to achieve the vertical translation and rotated by the mechanical couple into the gimbal platform [41].

In addition, a larger scan angle can be achieved by employing a thicker PZT film, and Figure 5b indicates an architecture using a thin PZT film to drive the scanner to rotate and which is suitable for cross-sectional imaging in a dual-axis confocal system [41]. It can be seen that a thin-film PZT was implemented within the outer legs to actuate a gimbal platform in the vertical direction. Specific beam structures were designed to connect the gimbal platform with the mirror, which was designed as dog-bone shape. The inner rotational scanning mirror was actuated through the coupled mechanical motion from the gimbal platform, and the whole device was excited at its resonant frequency. Even though the scanning mirror only resulted in ±5.5° scan angle with 2V AC driving condition,

200 μm displacement could be achieved in the vertical directions owing to the usage of thin-film PZT under 18 V. The resonant frequency of the device was measured at 2.8 kHz and could be increased further by etching holes on the mirror platform. The device consumed power on the order of 30 μW; 2D MEMS scanners using this actuation mechanism can be achieved by modifying the beam structures embedded with the PZT thin film [42,43]. It should be noted that a more complicated fabrication process is required to develop the scanners using piezoelectric actuation, owing to the additional embedded PZT film. In imaging applications, this actuation method can achieve a high framerate with several tens of frames/s, but the resolution may be degraded with high scanning speed in this case.

2.1.4. Electrothermal Actuation

Scanners using electrothermal actuation are generally constructed with thin bimorph structures whose constituent materials have contrasting thermal expansion coefficients. Inspired by the original architecture of thermally actuated micromirrors [44], this type of MEMS scanner was first demonstrated for endoscopic OCT imaging applications with a multilayer Al/silicon oxide mesh structure. The working principles are schematically shown in Figure 6a, where a current was supplied to a polysilicon heater embedded within a beam with mesh structure in this case, and the mesh structure was bent down, and the mesh structure was employed to connect one edge of the mirror and the substrate. Thus, the single-axis scan motion could be realized to get a rotation angle of 17°, and the resonant frequency was observed to be 165 Hz. The reported system consumed 15 mA DC and had an imaging resolution of 20 μm. Later, a dual axis scanner was reported with similar structures for the same application, as shown in Figure 6b [45]. The mirror was connected to the outer frame with electrothermal bimorph beams, while the same beam structure was used to connect the frame to the substrate. Thus, this presented device could be actuated along two orthogonal axes, and the achievable scan angle was up to 40° with the supplied 6.3 mA AC. The resonance of the mirror was measured at 445 Hz and 259 Hz for two separate scanning axes.

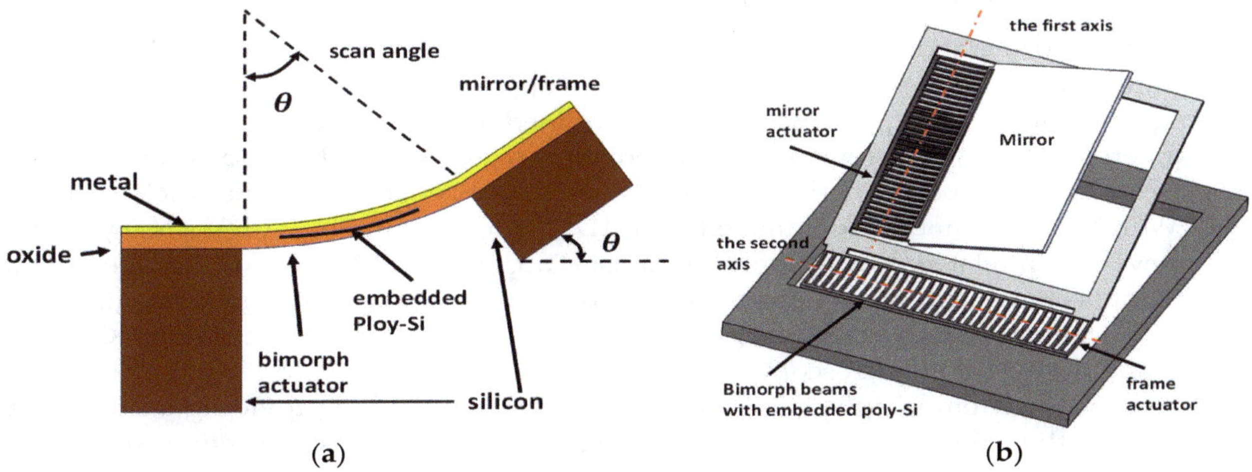

Figure 6. Schematics of (**a**) the working principles of bimorph structures [44]; (**b**) the 2D MEMS scanner using two axial bimorph beams to drive the frame and the mirror [45].

It should be noted that the rotating action along one edge of the mirror may shift the optical path during the scanning process, thus increasing the burden on the optical design for real imaging application. Thus, an alternative architecture was reported to ensure the mirror can rotate along the central axis by modifying the bimorph structures, as shown in Figure 7a [46]. A folded beam with embedded bimorph structure was employed to support and connect the mirror at the central points of its corresponding edge. The micromirror resulted in a ±15° scan angle under a resonant frequency of 400 Hz, and driving condition was set at 5.5V and 15 mA. This micromirror was successfully integrated into a probe (outer diameter: 5.8 mm) for OCT imaging, and the probe size could be further reduced to 2.8 mm using a hidden actuator [47]. Different from fabricating the mirror and actuators as a unit, Figure 7b shows an actuator that utilizes cascaded thermally actuated chevron beams to rotate the central platform with a mounted micro-pyramidal polygon reflector [48]. When current flows through the chevron beams, the beam moves forward owing to the thermal expansion effect, and thus the central platform is driven to rotate. This cascaded structure can achieve a larger rotational angle at 41° compared with the single beam design, and this device was designed to perform circumferential scanning with a 328° scan angle. This device was demonstrated for OCT imaging. Other thermal actuated scanners have also been developed in OCT imaging systems [49] and multiphoton imaging [50] and confocal microscopy [51]. However, the power consumption is still a challenge for this actuation method.

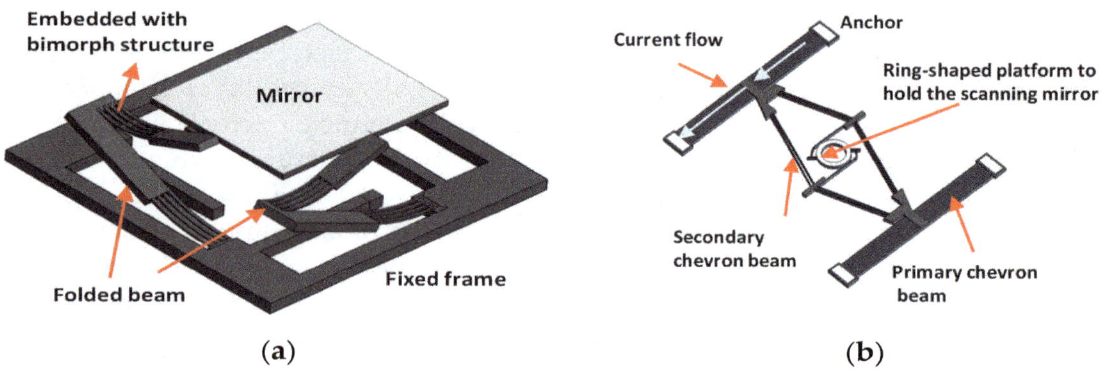

Figure 7. Mechanical structures of (**a**) the 2D scanners with bimorph beam structures to ensure the rotation along the central axes of the mirror [46]; (**b**) the circumferential scanner actuated by cascaded chevron beam to rotate the center ring-shaped platform for the scanning mirror [48].

2.2. Applications of Scanning-Based Single-Pixel Imaging System

The scan-based method typically fits well with the SPI technology, since only one detector is required in these cases to collect the light from the applied MEMS scanners. In these systems, the imaging performance and quality is mainly determined by the applied MEMS scanners. Various MEMS scanners structures were reviewed in the previous sections with the purpose of indicating the performance of such scan-based methods, which are typically dependent on the efficiency of MEMS scanners. With MEMS scanners providing efficient 1D, 2D or 3D scanning, various imaging systems can be achieved with related optical configurations. Thus, the MEMS scanner may be broadened for various applications with proper optical system design. Until now, biological imaging has seen the major application of imaging systems using MEMS scanners, mainly including OCT, confocal microscopy and multiphoton microscopy.

Optical coherence tomography (OCT) is a technology capable of providing a fine resolution with micro-scale; thus, this technology has much significance in disease detection, such as cancer. This system constructs optical scattering image with low-coherence interferometry, and the SPI technology supports the flexibility of the applied light source, which may affect the resolution. By integrating MEMS technology, this system can be miniaturized into a small imaging probe for field applications [52–57]. Figure 8 shows a compact design of an integrated OCT imaging probe constructed with the electrothermal actuators [47]. With hidden actuators, the dimeter of the presented probe is only 2.8 mm, and all required components are integrated to perform OCT scanning. As reviewed, all four predominant actuation methods get their related architectures for OCT imaging, and tunable focal length scanners have also been demonstrated to achieve more functional scanning architectures. More recently, a miniaturized compact OCT catheter was integrated with an array of MEMS scanners based on electrothermal actuation [58]. Adjustable focal length can be implemented with each scanner, which achieves a scan angle at 45°, and thus the reported structure can be adjustable for uneven surfaces, and this catheter was experimentally demonstrated to show its potential in in vivo imaging applications.

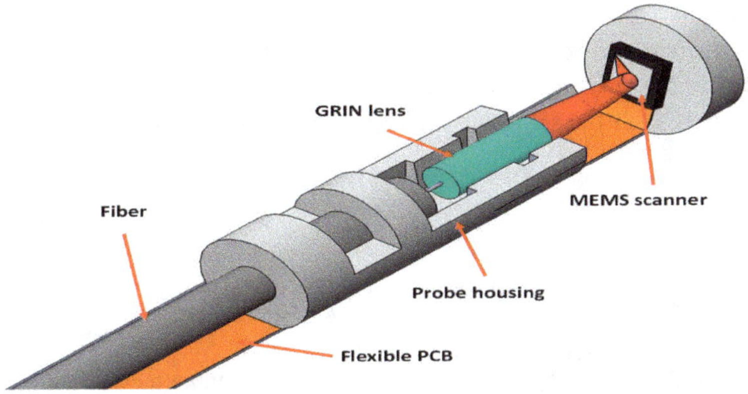

Figure 8. Schematic of a compact optical coherence tomography (OCT) probe (diameter: 2.8mm) with thermoelectric-actuated scanner, hidden actuators, a graded-index (GRIN) lens, a flexible printed circuit board (PCB) and a probe housing made from a fluorinated ethylene [47].

Confocal microscopy is another field where MEMS scanners have been widely explored for several decades, as this technology can provide a subcellular resolution. The exploration of MEMS-based confocal microscopy makes it possible to build portable devices for field testing, considering commercial confocal microscopy is usually limited in lab testing. Figure 9 shows a compact design of confocal microscopy [59], where a single-axis MEMS mirror was adopted to perform scanning. Considering the dynamic range and axial resolution, dual-axis scanning is preferable and also can reduce the complexity of optical systems. In this field, 2D scanners are mainly constructed with electrostatic actuated scanners [60–64], and the scanner, reported in [65], can be switched between the lateral and vertical scanning conditions to support the flexibly of MEMS imaging systems. As we reviewed, the piezoelectric actuation was reported to potentially realize 3D scanning modes [66,67], but the fabrication complexity is still an important consideration to build such PZT-actuated scanners.

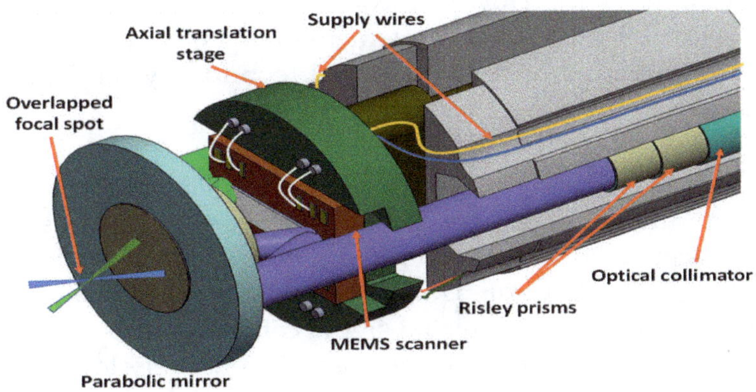

Figure 9. Schematic of a dual-axis confocal microscope with a MEMS scanning mirror and a parabolic mirror to focus two incoming collimated beams [59].

Multiphoton imaging, using non-linear light-tissue interactions to provide in vivo images, also benefits from the MEMS technology. SPI technology shows its advantages in this case, since an efficient detector can be used to detect the applied photons in the near-infrared region. All the mentioned driving mechanisms get their related research work in this application field, and the major architectures are constructed with electrostatic actuators [68] and piezoelectric actuators [69]. In this condition, it is worth mentioning another strategy to build a scanning-based SPI system, which is to utilize a vibrating fiber. One example of the fiber scan system is shown in Figure 10 [70]. Unlike traditional scanning architecture, the presented fiber scan system employs a flexible double cladding fiber to realize the laser excitation and emission. The fiber was driven to be vibrated by the PZT tubular scanner. In addition, a miniaturized objective designed with a focal shift along the longitudinal axis was also employed for two-photon microendoscopy. This mechanism has been widely explored by using different actuation methods for various applications, including OCT [71–75], confocal microscopy [76] and multiphoton imaging [77–79]. However, it should be noted this method cannot provide flexible scanning trajectories.

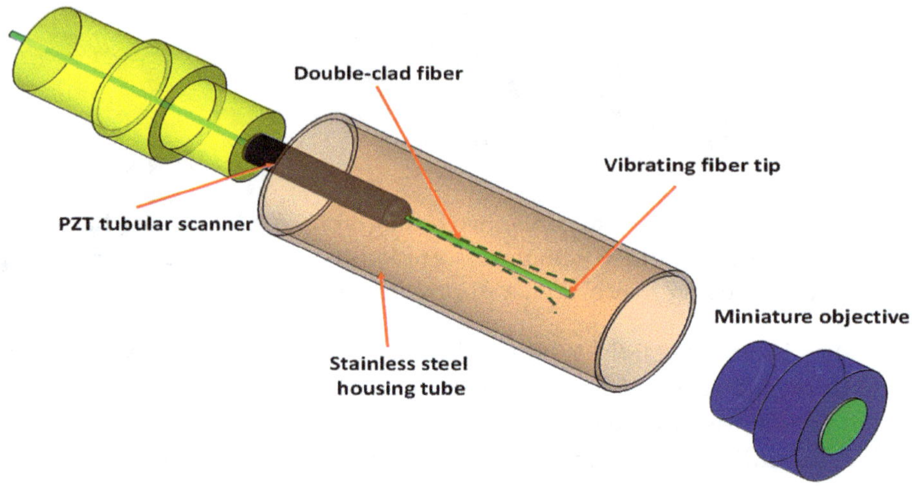

Figure 10. Schematic of the assembly of a fiber scanning system for a two-photon microscope with double-clad fiber actuated by a PZT tubular scanner [70].

It is worth mentioning that MEMS scanners support the flexibility to be employed in various applications through specific optical configurations. Other compact imaging configurations can be found in photoacoustic microendoscopes [80–84], based on the MEMS scanning single-pixel imaging system, to visualize the optical absorption. The scan-based method is also employed in other imaging applications, such as thermal imaging. However, considering the low intensity due to the absorption and scattering, specified algorithms should be implemented in the system to enhance the signal-to-noise ratio [85]. In this case, the potential of computational technology has been shown, which will be discussed in the following section.

3. Encoding-Based Single-Pixel Imaging Systems

Different from the scanning architectures, the encoding-based systems are typically constructed with an SLM to encode the scenery with time-varying patterns. The correlated light intensities are then recorded with a single-pixel photodetector. The light intensities from multiple pixels are collected at each sampling step, and thus the overall detected signal can be increased to make such system viable in these cases where the light intensity from the scenery is relatively low, for example in long-range imaging. In addition, this method is beneficial from the computational technology to allow us to reconstruct an image with a compressive sampling strategy, hence greatly boosting the sampling speed compared with traditional scanning methods. Over the past decades, various compact imaging systems have been demonstrated using this encoding method, due to the availability of commercially miniature devices that can be used to generate time-varying patterns. Despite the advantages, it is noticed that the performance of such imaging systems is limited by the properties of the applied detector, including its dynamic range and associated quantization electronics [3]. Besides, the computational overhead is still an important consideration for anyone planning to construct the encoding based single-pixel imaging system.

3.1. The System Architecture

The fundamental components of an encoding-based imaging system are the SLM to generate time-varying patterns and a photodetector to synchronously collect the encoded light. The performance of such imaging systems is typically decided by the combination of the applied detector and the SLM. Since this paper focuses on these single-pixel imaging systems using MEMS technology, it is noticed that there are two main types of MEMS modulators that have mainly been explored in single-pixel imaging systems, namely digital micromirror devices (DMDs) and liquid crystals on silicon (LCOS), respectively. The LCOS devices utilize the CMOS technology to develop traditional liquid crystals devices (LCD) on a chip, so this paced device can control the amplitude and phase of the incoming light by employing the special light-modulating properties of LCD. The DMD consists of closely packed mirrors, and each mirror can be tilted to two different directions with respect to the direction of the incoming light. One direction can be integrated with the collection system to collect the overall intensity from the mirrors, which are tuned to this direction (on state = 1), while the reflected light from the other direction will not be recorded (off-state = 0). Thus, binary encoding patterns can be conveniently generated on this type of modulator. There are other types of SLMs that can be used to establish a single-pixel imaging system, and one can select the proper modulators in different regions of interest. A summarized table (Table 1) is thus given to compare these modulators, such as DMD [86,87], LCD or LCOS [88,89], mechanical mask [90,91], customized diffuser [92,93], light-emitting diode (LED) arrays [94,95] and optical phase arrays (OPA) [96,97].

Table 1. A summarized table of various modulators applied in single-pixel imaging systems.

Modulators	Compactness and Illumination	Modulation Efficiency	Pixel Resolution and Availability	Operating Wavelengths
Digital micromirror device (DMD)	Miniature device; active/passive illumination.	High speed; simple modulation; programmable.	Flexible pixel resolution; commercially available.	Wide range; micromirrors determined.
(Liquid crystals on sicon(LCOS)/Liquid crystal devices(LCD)	Miniature device; active/passive illumination.	Slow speed; modulate the phase and amplitude of the light; programmable.	Flexible pixel resolution; commercially available.	Wide range; liquid crystals determined.
Customized diffuser	Poor compactness; active/passive illumination.	Slow speed; complicated modulation; not programmable.	Fixed pixel resolution; customized fabrication; costly.	Wide range; materials determined.
Mechanical mask	Can be miniaturized; active/passive illumination.	Slow speed; simple binary modulation patterns; not programmable.	Fixed pixel resolution; customized fabrication; cheap.	Wide range; materials determined.
optical phase arrays (OPA)	On the process of miniaturization; active/passive illumination.	High speed; simple random patterns; controllable.	Flexible pixel resolution; complicated fabrication; costly.	Limited narrow range; light-emitting components determined.
light-emitting diode (LED) arrays	On the process of miniaturization; active illumination.	High speed; simple binary patterns; programmable.	Flexible pixel resolution; commercially available.	Limited narrow range; light-emitting components determined.

From the given table, it can be seen that the LCOS and DMD potentially satisfy the continuously increasing trend of miniature imaging systems due to their compactness. For instance, each side width of the micromirror is almost equal to a tenth of the width of a human hair, and the width of liquid crystals can reach around 6 μm. In an encoding-based SPI system, the resolution of recovered images is typically determined by the spatial resolution of the applied modulators. The LCOS and DMD provide flexible spatial resolution by combining neighboring element [98] as an efficient pixel, compared with some modulators with fixed pixel resolution, such as a diffuser. However, the LCD/LCOS devices usually require longer modulation time to switch different patterns, while DMDs can be operated at a modulation rate in excess of 20 kHz. Besides, recent works indicate that the OPA and LED devices achieve a modulation rate higher than 1 MHz using fast-switching photonics components to meet the requirement of high framerate. It should be noted that a narrow wavelength range usually limits the applications of OPA and LED, and the properties of applied materials determine the operating range of these imaging systems constructed with mechanical masks and a diffuser. Various mechanical masks have also been demonstrated to perform imaging reconstruction, such as coded apertures, but it should be noted that the encoding patterns are fixed and not programmable after the mechanical mask has been fabricated. Even though DMD can only provide simple modulation patterns compared with diffuser and LCOS, DMD is still the most commonly applied element in current imaging systems, due to its availability and relatively wide range. Therefore, this paper reviews the single-pixel imaging systems using DMD.

When reviewing the architectures of the encoding-based SPI systems, it is necessary to consider two similar research communities, namely single-pixel camera and computational ghost imaging [99,100]. Figure 11 gives the general description of these two types of systems using DMDs, from which it can be seen that the single-pixel camera typically sets the SLM (DMDs) at the focal plane of the applied camera lens to modulate the light intensities from the scenery. The encoded light is collected with a single-pixel detector, and this architecture is often referred as focal plane modulation. In the architecture of ghost imaging, on the other hand, SLM (DMDs) is employed to modulate the light from the light source instead, and the photodetector collects the reflected light from the scenery after the scenery is illuminated with special patterns. This is also known as structured light illumination. The two types of systems are essentially the same in terms of optical set-up, but it should be noted that some modulators can only be applied in ghost imaging systems where active illumination is required, such as LED arrays. The inset of Figure 11a schematically shows the structure of DMD, from which it can be seen that binary encoding patterns are generated on the DMD by directing the incoming light to two separate directions.

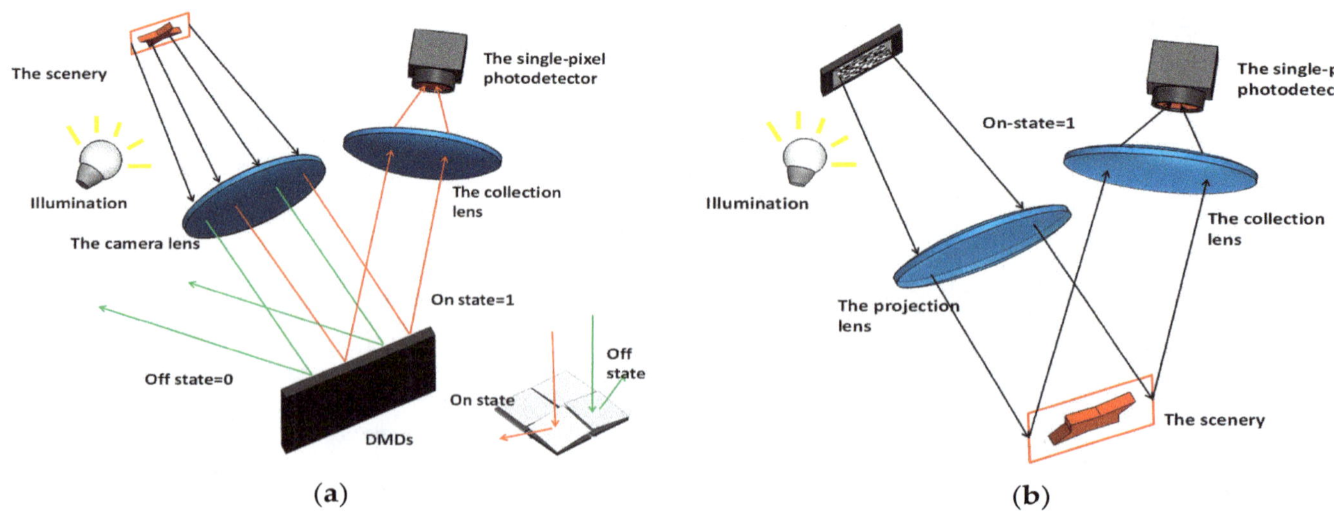

Figure 11. General architectures of two single-pixel imaging systems using digital micromirror devices (DMD): (**a**) the single-pixel camera architecture where the scenery is modulated at the focal plane with inset showing the DMD structure; (**b**) the computational ghost imaging architecture where the scenery is illuminated with the modulated light.

3.2. Single-Pixel Detector Technologies

SPI technology benefits from the development of single-pixel detectors, which have high flexibility in working wavelengths and system configuration. The single-pixel detectors are built with various photoelectric effects to convert the incident light into electrical signals through different materials and structures, and photodiode technology is the most commonly employed detection device in SPI systems [101]. Photodiode technology is capable of a large wavelength spectrum by using a wide range of semiconductor materials, such as Ge, GaP, InAs, InSb, InGaAs and so on, compared with the CMOS and CCD detector array whose operating wavelength range is limited by the applied silicon material. For infrared imaging applications, InGaAs photodiodes provide a reliable method to perform sensing tasks for the range between 0.5 μm and 2.6 μm. The applied materials also affect the resulting gains and response time of different photodiodes, and silicon-based photodiodes usually get high response time and high gains. One can properly select the photodiodes with specific semiconductor materials to meet different applications. It should be noted that the dark current of single-pixel detectors is an important consideration for single-pixel imaging systems, considering that the resulting noise may affect the quality of reconstructed images, especially for the encoding-based approach. Therefore, the operating mode that can result in smaller dark current is desired in this application field, such as photovoltaic mode. Otherwise, proper cooling methods should be applied to reduce the dark current. For example, the photomultiplier tube is an efficient type of single-pixel detector technology, which can achieve low dark current rates with suitable cooling systems, but this technology requires vacuum tube technology despite the provided larger sensitive area [102]. Compared with traditional CCD and CMOS sensor arrays, single-pixel technology also allows the usage of detection a device with high sensitivity to conduct low-level-light detection, such as avalanche photodiode (APD) [103]. In addition, single-pixel detector technologies have also widely been explored to provide single-photon sensitivity, such as the superconducting tunnel junction based detector and the quantum-dot field-effect transistor based detector [104], so the resulted imaging systems are able to realize long-distance imaging tasks that cannot be done in traditional cameras.

Therefore, various detector technologies support the flexibility of SPI systems to work at any wavelengths by using suitable detection devices. In addition, the development of cutting-edge detectors is a popular research direction, so SPI technology also benefits from these newly developed detectors since they are usually demonstrated in the single-pixel form. Furthermore, it is always a challenging task to integrate multiple pixels of a newly constructed detector into an array, especially when non-silicon technology is involved. Therefore, the fabrication of such a detector array will be costly, making this method less attractive in field applications, for example in infrared imaging. It should be noted that traditional cameras are still dominant in the visible range considering cheap detector arrays are available with high pixel resolution up to several megapixels. However, detector arrays are typically expensive or even unavailable for some wavelengths, and thus SPI technology provides a competitive edge over traditional detector array based imagers in terms of detector costs in these cases. For example, an InGaAs IR camera generally costs several thousand dollars, compared with a photodiode, which costs about 100 dollars with satisfactory detection performance.

In addition, the cost of MEMS-based SPI systems also comprises the applied MEMS elements, including the MEMS scanners and modulators. Commercial MEMS scanners using electrostatic actuation cost around 1000 dollars, which still shows the cost advantage over traditional detector arrays. It should be noted that the cost of MEMS scanners may increase with more complicated fabrication processes, for example with piezoelectric actuation based scanners. The scanning-based approach gets its unique applications in biological imaging fields where detector arrays have limited efficiency. For the encoding-based approach, the additional cost comes from the MEMS modulators (DMD), which has been well-established with high pixel resolution and affordable cost. Considering various demonstrations of SPI systems, the average cost of encoding-based systems can be estimated to be around 1000 dollars per megapixel [105], which is generally several times less than that of detector arrays in non-visible ranges. In addition, the cost of such SPI imagers can be maintained over a large wavelength range, compared with the increasing cost of a detector-array camera in the non-visible range. Despite the mentioned advantages of SPI technology, the single-pixel detection element typically requires more sampling time to sequentially record the scanned or encoded light intensities, while traditional cameras capture images in one shot. That is the main reason why MEMS scanners and modulators with higher operating rates are desired in this case to speed up the acquisition. Besides, the encoding-based approach can take advantage of computational technology to reduce sampling time.

3.3. The Mathematical Interpolation and Sampling Strategies

In encoding-based SPI systems, the target image can be considered as a two-dimensional matrix, and each element in the matrix represents the light intensity information at its corresponding location. This matrix can be expanded to a vector $\boldsymbol{X}$ with N unknown light intensities, and the time-varying patterns can be expressed by a matrix Φ with dimension $M \times N$. Each row of the encoding matrix is the patterns $\Phi(j)$ generated by DMD at each sampling step, and thus the detector records the correlated light intensities between the encoding pattern and the target image, which can be mathematically expressed by the inner products of $\Phi(j)$ with $\boldsymbol{X}$. After a complete sampling cycle, M measurements can be obtained to form the measurement vector $\boldsymbol{S}$ as follows:

$$\boldsymbol{S} = \boldsymbol{\Phi X} \tag{1}$$

A complete orthogonal matrix was first employed to construct an encoding-based SPI system, such as Hadamard basis and Fourier basis [106–108]. Despite the fact that this method can reduce the sampling noise [109], this type of system still requires N measurements to reconstruct an N-dimensional image. When the number of measurements is smaller than the signal's dimension ($M < N$), two other types of sampling strategies can be employed to boost the acquisition process, namely compressive sensing and sub-orthogonal sampling, respectively. The sub-orthogonal sampling utilizes a sub-basis Φ ($M < N$) drawn from an orthogonal matrix to compress the signal during the sampling process. The basis is required to be incoherent with the spatial properties of the target images, thus making it possible to reconstruct it through specified algorithms. Compressive sensing (CS) [110] indicates a signal can be accurately recovered with high-probability with much fewer measurements by using its sparsity in some transform bases, after the signal is modulated with pseudo-random patterns.

The efficiency of CS depends on the assumption that the signal $\boldsymbol{X}$ tends to be sparse in a known basis $\boldsymbol{B}$, such as JPEG algorithms. Thus, the sampling process can be modelled as follows after representing the target image with a basis B and sparse vector θ:

$$\boldsymbol{S} = \boldsymbol{\Phi B \theta} \tag{2}$$

where the θ is usually called a K-sparse vector, which means only K elements in the vector are non-zeros. The sparse vector can be efficiently reconstructed through l_1 minimization algorithms with an adequate number of measurements (M), and there are two types of approaches to solve this optimization problem, including the convex optimization algorithms or greedy algorithms. However, it has been proved that pure l_1 minimization algorithms are vulnerable to noise, and thus a more general approach is usually applied to increase its robustness by introducing an additional l_2 minimization term:

$$minimize\ \|\mathbf{X}\|_1 \cdot subject \cdot to \cdot \|\mathbf{S} - \mathbf{\Phi B \theta}\|_2 \leq \delta \tag{3}$$

where δ is the acceptable noise boundary in the real applications. The reconstructed accuracy is ensured by minimizing the l_2 norm function of the measured signals and the signals resulting from the predicted signals, and the l_1 norm guarantees the sparse solution to satisfy the mentioned assumption. Many other types of algorithms can be found in the literature [111–113] to solve such problems, but it can be seen that most algorithms are still based on the l_1 and l_2 minimization problem. It is worth mentioning that an image can be reconstructed by exploring its sparsity in the pixel domain using the minimization of the total variation (TV) or the total curvature (TC) of the images [114,115]. It is worth highlighting that the time required to capture in the encoding systems consists of the sampling time and the data processing time. Even though the usage of CS allows us to speed up the sampling process of a single-pixel imaging system, the described algorithms significantly increase the computational overhead to limit its real-time applications. Typically, this method has been successfully demonstrated in these applications, which allow the post-processing [116,117].

Generally, the single-pixel imaging systems are constructed with three main sampling strategies mentioned above, and a summary of these strategies is given in Table 2. Even though the complete orthogonal sampling could not provide the competitive edges over traditional scanning methods in terms of sampling time, this sampling strategy has wide applications considering its capability of reducing the sources of noise. Additionally, the Hadamard transform sees the major application of DMD to construct a single-pixel imager. Recently a three-step phase-shifting encoding pattern was efficiently generated on DMD to achieve a functional Fourier-transform, despite the fact that the required number of measurements was increased 1.5 times [4]. The efficiency of the sub-orthogonal sampling strategy is dependent on the prior knowledge of the spatial properties of the target scenery, which is required to be incoherent with the chosen sub-basis, and fast reconstruction algorithms can be incorporated with this strategy to significantly boost the reconstruction time. Many imaging architectures have been reported to obtain the prior knowledge in [118–122] before performing the sub-orthogonal sampling. For example, a co-aligned traditional camera was used to get a stream of 2D images continuously [119], and the scenery was sampled with low resolution to get some prediction of the images for later high resolution reconstruction [120]. To optimize the reconstructed results, deep-learning has also been explored to predict the prior information [121]. CS theory has been explored widely in 2D images due to the fact that the natural 2D images tend to be sparse in some domains, especially for visible bandwidths [3,123], but the computational overhead should not be neglected. Additionally, one can select the proper sampling strategy according to the requirements of sampling speed, achievable prior knowledge and reconstruction time.

Table 2. A summarized table of three commonly applied sampling strategies in single-pixel imaging system.

Sampling Strategy	Prior Knowledge	Sampling Speed	Computational Complexity
Orthogonal sampling	No prior knowledge; no signal representation.	Full measurements; slow sampling speed.	Simple computation.
Sub-orthogonal sampling	A specific prior knowledge; no signal representation.	Compressed measurements; high sampling speed.	Not computationally demanding.
Compressive sensing	A general sparse assumption; requires sparse representation.	Compressed measurements; high sampling speed.	Computational overhead.

3.4. Applications of Encoding-Based Single-Pixel Imaging Systems

Compared with the scanning-based SPI systems, the encoding method has wide applications in various fields, and the demonstration for the visible range can be easily found in previously reviewed architectures. However, considering that current cameras efficiently work at the visible range with satisfactory pixel resolution and low computational overhead, in this section we mainly focus on the applications of the MEMS encoding imager in these scenarios where the traditional cameras have limited efficiency, or the detector array based imagers are costly.

3.4.1. One Dimensional Imaging: Spectrometer

Spectral acquisition, commonly conducted with a Fourier-transform spectrometer, plays an important role in various fields, including chemical and biological analysis. However, the FTIR spectrometer is limited to the laboratory testing, owing to its large size and fragile moving optical components. Thus, miniaturized spectrometers have been explored using DMD, owing to the flexibility and advantages of DMD. Figure 12 indicates a typical architecture of the spectrometric system based on DMD, from which it can be seen that a narrow slit is typically employed to select the light into the system, and the incoming light passes through a spectral separation device, such as a prism or grating. The dispersed spectrum is encoded by the encoding patterns generated on the DMD. Finally, a single-pixel detector is used to collect the light from the DMD. The DMD based spectrometer was firstly demonstrated in visible ranges [124], and later this type of spectrometric system began to be reported in non-visible wavelengths. Until now, the DMD has been applied in various fields, including analytical atomic spectrometry [125], chemical sensing [126] and infrared sensing [127]. Besides, CS theory was also utilized to reduce the required number of measurements, thus significantly reducing the sampling time [128,129]. It should be noted that the real resolution of a spectrometric system is also dependent on the optical set-up, so some improvement and analysis have been done by modifying the mask pattern widths to improve the performance of the DMD-based spectrometers in near-infrared sensing applications [130].

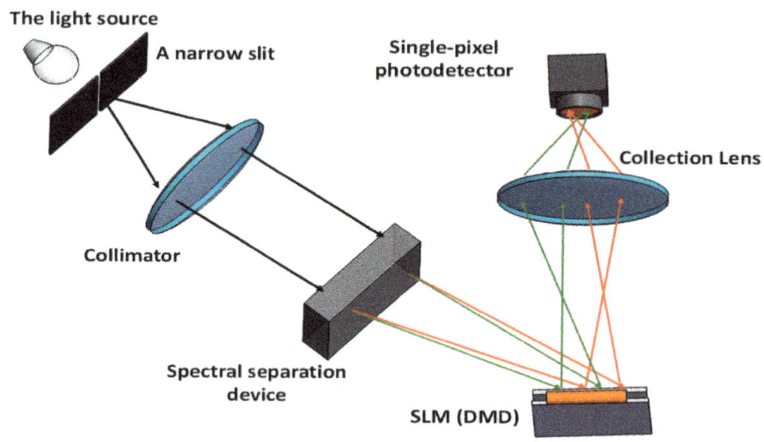

Figure 12. A typical architecture for building a spectrometer using DMD.

More recent explorations have been reported by using the MEMS mechanical mask consisting of sequential encoding rows [131]. Each encoding row contains open pixels and closed pixels, which were fabricated through the typical MEMS fabrication process. The light can pass through the open pixels and be recorded with the applied single-pixel detector, thus representing 1 in the encoding matrix. Thus, binary encoding could be implemented through this structure, and the MEMS mask was driven to scan across a fixed narrow slit, which was just placed in front of the MEMS mask. In this way, time-varying patterns were generated along the slit to encode the dispersed spectrum. This encoding method was firstly demonstrated with the Hadamard transform using an electromagnet actuator. Even though the mask was designed to be operated at its resonant frequency, the travel range was still limited to restrict the number of encoding row to be implemented, thus affecting the achievable pixel resolution. To overcome the limitation, a new mask structure was reported, as shown in Figure 13a [132]. In this design, multiple encoding masks could be cascaded along the slit direction, and each mask was implemented with the Hadamard matrix. This method can potentially increase the dimension of the reconstructed signal by N times with N cascaded MEMS elements, due to the fact that each MEMS mask can achieve a complete orthogonal sampling with a given MEMS travel range. In addition, a compound parabolic concentrator was glued on the single-pixel detectors to collect the encoded light, which can make the system more compact in this case. In addition, another solution has been proposed recently using CS theory for chemical sensing applications; the encoding pattern was designed based on CS theory to reconstruct a higher-dimensional signal with fewer required numbers of measurements [133]. Figure 13b shows the detailed structure of the MEMS mask. It should be noted that an open row was set before all encoding patterns to realize self-triggering, and a gap (shown in the inset) could cause a dip in the measured signal when the gap entered the encoding row, so the mask dynamic positions could be located to determine correct mask patterns. Thus, the reported MEMS device gives the potential to construct a portable and truly miniaturized spectrometer for field applications with satisfactory pixel resolution.

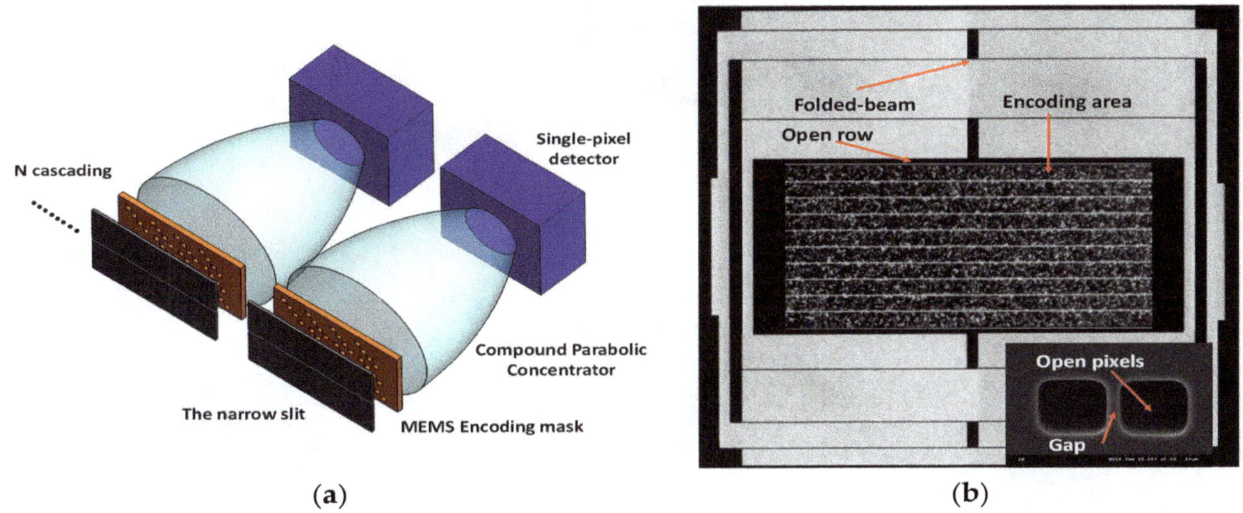

Figure 13. (**a**) The schematic drawing of a MEMS vibrating mask with cascaded structures, with compound parabolic concentrator glued on single-pixel detector [132]; (**b**) The microscopic picture of the compressive sensing (CS) vibrating mask with the inset showing the SEM image of the pixel structures [133].

3.4.2. Non-Visible Imaging

Non-visible imaging systems have much significance in different sensing applications, as some unique properties can be obtained at a certain wavelength range. An infrared imager was reported to detect the leakage of methane gas using DMD [134] illuminated by a 1.651 um infrared laser diode. Sequential Hadamard encoding patterns were generated by the DMD with a pixel resolution of 16×16. This architecture was successfully used to capture methane gas leakage of 0.2 L/minute from a distance of 1 m. The framerate was reported to be 25 frame/s owing to the high switch speed of the DMD. Figure 14 depicts a single-pixel imager that was designed to capture the visible images and the short-wave infrared images at the same time [87]. Similar with the standard architecture shown in Figure 9, the scenery was focused onto the DMD where Hadamard encoding patterns were implemented. The encoded light passed through a hot-mirror to separate the short-wave infrared image from the encoded light beam. The infrared image was captured with InGaAs photodiode, while the visible images were recorded with visible red, blue and green channels after the images were separated with a dichroic prism. By utilizing the programmable ability of DMD, a fast optimization method was constructed to result in a framerate of 10 Hz in this case. CS theory was also incorporated with DMD-based infrared imager [135], and 64×64 pixels near-infrared images (830 nm) were captured from half of the required measurements. In addition, non-visible image capture has also been explored in multispectral imaging systems [136–139]. For example, the near-infrared images of colorful target objects were obtained in a polarimetric spectral imaging system [128]. In addition, DMD was also employed in other imaging fields to overcome the limitations of traditional imagers, such as photoacoustic microscopy systems [140]. A DMD-based photoacoustic motionless system was thus demonstrated to result in better performance than traditional systems, and its achievable axis range could achieve 1.8 m without sacrificing the resolution. It is noticed that a single-pixel imager obtains the potential to be operated for any wavelengths by conveniently changing the applied photodetector, but the properties of the applied SLM become a limiting factor for the achievable operating range of a specified imager. With special SLM, terahertz imaging can be achieved using the single-pixel imaging technology [92,141].

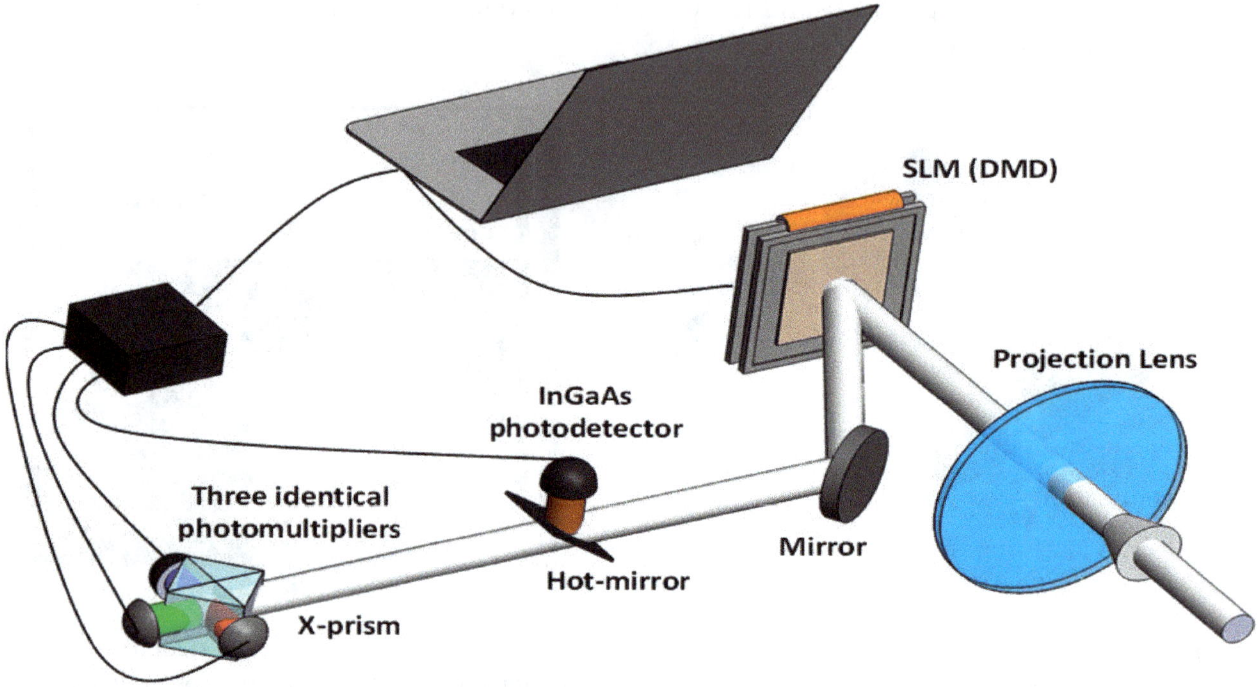

Figure 14. The schematic drawing of a DMD-based single-pixel imaging system to capture the visible images and infrared images at the same time [87].

3.4.3. Hyperspectral Imaging

Hyperspectral imaging is a method to capture continuous 2D images over a wide spectral range, and thus specific properties of a 2D scenery can be extracted at a certain wavelength. The traditional way to construct a hyperspectral imager is to utilize mechanical slit scanning across the target or the object to capture its 3D information. This methodology requires a moving slit to realize the scanning motion, and limited amount of light that comes through the slit may affect the SNR. Thus, snapshot hyperspectral imagers were developed to capture 3D information in a single image. After the coded aperture was reported in a hyperspectral imager [142,143], computational technology became preferable in this field. Meanwhile, the DMD provides a more flexible choice in this field to replace the coded aperture in modulating spatial information. Single-pixel hyperspectral imaging systems can be found in [144–148]. Compressive sensing has also been explored to reduce the required number of measurements to speed up the acquisition time. However, it is noticed that the majority of hyperspectral imaging systems still utilizes sensor arrays to record the encoded signal. Thus, more recent research has been done by using the two separate encoding mechanisms to perform hyperspectral sampling, as shown in Figure 15 [149]. The incoming light was first modulated with an encoding mask before being dispersed to provide the spectral information. The encoded light containing spectral and spatial information was collected with a single-pixel detector, and a special Hadamard transform was conducted to perform the reconstruction. The applied resonant scanner can ensure a high operating speed, and the whole system could be constructed within a small package size

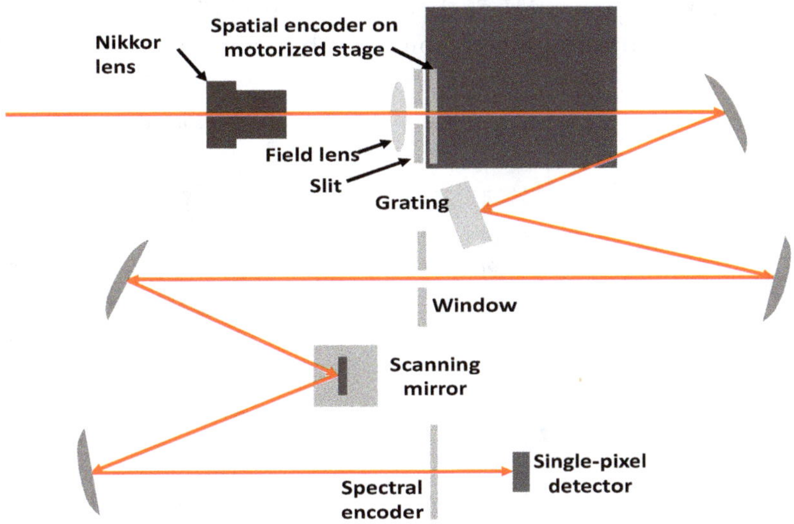

Figure 15. Schematic of a single-pixel hyperspectral imager in [149].

3.4.4. Three-Dimensional Imaging and Lensless Imaging

Another advantage associated with the encoding-based single-pixel imaging system is that the single-pixel detector can be fabricated with a very high timing resolution. With the advancement in technology, the time-of-flight approach has been developed to benefit the robotics, security and medical fields. Figure 16a shows a typical 3D imaging system using the time-of-flight approach, and such an imager can be found in [150], which gives a 10 Hz framerate using the Hadamard basis. When a short-pulsed light is supplied as the illumination light source, the signals captured by the detector are not only determined by the overlapping intensity between the encoding patterns and the scenery, but also the distance information. Since single-pixel detectors with picosecond response time are available, the distance information of each pixel can be distinguished using such detectors. From the given example, the reflected light from the red star and yellow ball is separately recorded by the detector. Thus, a 3D image can be constructed with the image of the scene and additional 2D depth information. It is worth mentioning that only one signal can be obtained with its corresponding encoding patterns in traditional 2D single-pixel imaging. In this case, one encoding pattern can generate a variety of measured signals by shifting the depth, thus befitting the development of a 3D data cube. Various research works have been devoted to this field [151–153]. Another method is to utilize more than one camera structure to capture the image of the scenery at different views or use different illumination patterns at one viewpoint. The performance of this 3D imager is typically determined by its viewpoints and the stereo vision geometry. Based on this concept, many single-pixel imaging systems have been reported for 3D imaging applications [154–156] with various mathematical models. It should also be noted that this system gets a stable depth resolution through an absolute measurement process, thus giving rise to the potential for long-distance measurements.

Similar to 3D imaging systems, single-pixel technology also befits the development of a potential imaging approach called lensless imaging. Figure 16b shows the typical architecture of lensless imaging systems, and no imaging and collection components are required in this case [157]. From the mentioned applications above, it should be noted that the imaging quality is highly affected by the properties of the applied optical components, especially when the system works in the non-visible range. For example, the aberrations of the lens may distort the resultant images. Using the power of computational technology, specific mathematical models can be established to describe the optical field after the scenery is modulated with special patterns, and a single-pixel detector is placed within its light field to collect a signal. Based on the measured signals and computational optics, the system can reconstruct a target image. Recently, a lensless imaging system was successfully demonstrated with an LCD device, which shows the potential of this technology [158]. With the development of sensor fabrication technology and computational technology, it has the potential to be a miniaturized imager.

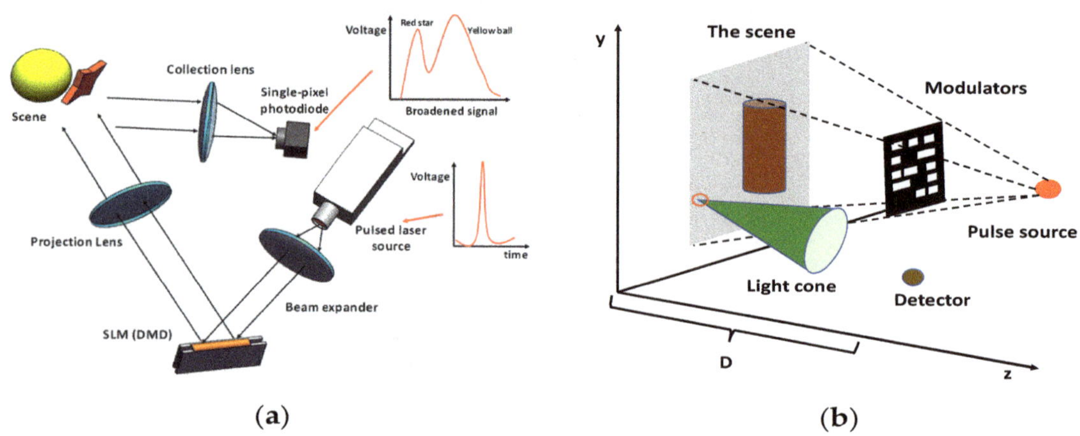

Figure 16. General architecture of (**a**) the time-of-flight approach to construct a 3D imaging with a pulsed laser source and high timing resolution detector [150] and (**b**) the lensless imaging system [157].

4. Summary

In this paper, we review two main research directions for single-pixel imaging systems utilizing MEMS technology. The first methodology employs MEMS scanners to capture images, while the second method reconstructs the images through specified algorithms with the encoded signals. In terms of system configurations, the performance of the scanning systems is typically determined by the applied scanners. Four predominant actuation principles were reviewed, and each one has its potential and limitations. In general, higher scan angles and higher axial translation can increase the field-of-view of the imager, while higher frequency can increase its frame rate. Its power consumption is also an important factor for consideration. Electrostatic actuation has low power consumption despite the high voltage required, but the high voltage limits its applications. The comb-drive actuator is more commonly used compared to the parallel plate actuator as it has larger scan angles. Electromagnetic actuation can reach large scan angles with additional magnets, but this increases the package size and thus makes it less suitable for integration into imaging probes. PZT actuators can provide good scan frequency and scan angles, but its fabrication is more complex as the PZT film needs to be embedded within the beam actuators. Electrothermal actuation can obtain large scan angles and is more compact, but it consumes more power.Besides, the scan-based method can realize 3D imaging with the appropriate actuator design, such as in a focus-adjustable MEMS micromirror, while for the encoding-based approach, 3D images are usually obtained with the power of an applied detector and computational technology.

Considering the miniaturization, scan-based MEMS imagers can be constructed in a more compact size, but the field-of-view is limited compared with encoding-based MEMS imagers. Encoding-based MEMS imagers can also collect more light in each sampling process, thus the detected signal may be boosted, making it more desirable in long range imaging. In terms of cost, the SPI technology also provides the competitive edge over the detector array based camera in non-visible imaging applications, considering that the detector-array is expensive or unavailable in these wavelength ranges. It should be noted that although the detected signal is increased, the encoded information is affected by the detector noise, which varies about a mean value. Thus, to ensure the recovered image quality, the detector and light source have to be stable during the acquisition process. Regarding the applications of these two methodologies, scanning-based single-pixel imaging systems see major use in the biological imaging field. In this field, MEMS technology provides an efficient way to construct a miniaturized imager for different applications. While it may be quite difficult to further integrate a DMD-based imager, it benefits from both single-pixel imaging technology and computational technology, thus providing competitive edges over the traditional scanning method in terms of sampling time, but the post processing required may be longer than the scan-based method due to the computational overhead.

Overall, the scan-based MEMS system is widely expected to be a highly useful tool in biomedical imaging applications in the future, owing to its ability for miniaturization, while encoding-based MEMS systems have the potential for long range imaging, 3D imaging and lensless imaging due to the rapid advancement of single-pixel detector technology and computational technology.

Author Contributions: Conceptualization, G.Z. (Guangcan Zhou) and G.Z. (Guangya Zhou); investigation, G.Z. (Guangcan Zhou); resources, G.Z. (Guangcan Zhou), Z.H.L and Y.Q.; writing-original draft preparation, G.Z. (Guangcan Zhou), Z.H.L and Y.Q.; writing—review and editing, G.Z. (Guangcan Zhou), Z.H.L., Y.Q. and G.Z. (Guangya Zhou); supervision, G.Z. (Guangya Zhou); funding acquisition, G.Z. (Guangya Zhou). All authors have read and agreed to the published version of the manuscript.

References

1. Baird, J.L. Apparatus for Transmitting Views or Images to a Distance. U.S. Patent 1,699,270, 15 January 1929.
2. Goldberg, E. Nipkow Disk for Television (1934). U.S. Patent 1,973,203, 11 September 1934.
3. Duarte, M.F.; Davenport, M.A.; Takhar, D.; Laska, J.N.; Sun, T.; Kelly, K.F. Single-pixel imaging via compressive sampling. *IEEE Signal Process. Mag.* **2008**, *25*, 83–91. [CrossRef]
4. Zhang, Z.; Wang, X.; Zheng, G.; Zhong, J. Fast fourier single-pixel imaging via binary illumination. *Sci. Rep.* **2017**, *7*, 12029. [CrossRef] [PubMed]
5. Studer, V.; Jérome, B.; Chahid, M.; Mousavi, H.S.; Candes, E.; Dahan, M. Compressive fluorescence microscopy for biological and hyperspectral imaging. *Proc. Natl. Acad. Sci. USA* **2012**, *109*, E1679–E1687. [CrossRef] [PubMed]
6. Petersen, K. Silicon Torsional Scanning Mirror. *IBM J. Res. Dev.* **1980**, *24*, 631–637. [CrossRef]
7. Conant, R.; Hagelin, P.; Krishnamoorthy, U.; Hart, M.; Lau, K.; Muller, R. A Raster-scanning full-motion video display using polysilicon micromachined mirrors. *Sens. Actuators A Phys.* **2000**, *83*, 291–296. [CrossRef]
8. Do, D.; Yoo, H.; Gweon, D.G. Fiber-optic raster scanning two-photon endomicroscope using a tubular piezoelectric actuator. *J. Biomed. Opt.* **2014**, *19*, 066010. [CrossRef]
9. Hyejun, R.; Piyawattanametha, W.; Taguchi, Y.; Lee, S.; Mandella, M.J.; Solgaard, O. Two-dimensional mems scanner for dual-axis confocal microscopy. *J. Microelectromech. Syst.* **2007**, *16*, 969–976.
10. Hwang, K.; Seo, Y.H.; Jeong, K.H. Microscanners for optical endomicroscopic applications. *Micro Nano Syst. Lett.* **2017**, *5*, 1. [CrossRef]
11. Myaing, M.T.; MacDonald, D.J.; Li, X.D. Fiber-optic scanning two-photon fluorescence endoscope. *Opt. Lett.* **2006**, *31*, 1076–1078. [CrossRef]
12. Engelbrecht, C.J.; Johnston, R.S.; Seibel, E.J.; Helmchen, F. Ultra-compact fiber-optic two-photon microscope for functional fluorescence imaging *in vivo*. *Opt. Express* **2008**, *16*, 5556–5564. [CrossRef]
13. Liang, W.; Murari, K.; Zhang, Y.; Chen, Y.; Li, M.J.; Li, X.; Liang, W.X. Increased illumination uniformity and reduced photodamage offered by the Lissajous scanning in fiber-optic two-photon endomicroscopy. *J. Biomed. Opt.* **2012**, *17*, 021108. [CrossRef] [PubMed]
14. Hwang, K.; Seo, Y.; Ahn, J.; Kim, P.; Jeong, K. Frequency selection rule for high definition and high frame rate Lissajous scanning. *Sci. Rep.* **2017**, *7*, 14075. [CrossRef] [PubMed]
15. Aguirre, A.D.; Hertz, P.R.; Chen, Y.; Fujimoto, J.G.; Piyawattanametha, W.; Fan, L.; Wu, M.C. Two-axis mems scanning catheter for ultrahigh resolution three-dimensional and en face imaging. *Opt. Express* **2007**, *15*, 2445–2453. [CrossRef] [PubMed]
16. Jung, W.; McCormick, D.T.; Zhang, J.; Wang, L.; Tien, N.C.; Chen, Z. Three-dimensional endoscopic optical coherence tomography by use of a two-axis microelectronmechanical scanning mirror. *Appl. Phys. Lett.* **2006**, *88*, 163901. [CrossRef]
17. Piyawattanametha, W.; Barretto, R.P.J.; Ko, T.H.; Flusberg, B.A.; Cocker, E.D.; Ra, H.; Lee, D.; Solgaard, O.; Schnitzer, M.J. Fast-scanning two-photon fluorescence imaging based on a microelectromechanical systems two-dimensional scanning mirror. *Opt. Lett.* **2006**, *31*, 2018–2020. [CrossRef]

18. Karthik, K.; Jonathan, C.C.; Austin, M.; Nate, J.K.; Kazunori, H.; Thomas, E.M.; Xiaojing, Z. Fast 3d in vivo swept-source optical coherence tomography using a two-axis mems scanning micromirror. *J. Opt. A Pure Appl. Opt.* **2008**, *10*, 044013.
19. Piyawattanametha, W.; Hyejun, R.; Mandella, M.J.; Loewke, K.; Wang, T.D.; Kino, G.S.; Solgaard, O.; Contag, C.H. 3D near-infrared fluorescence imaging using an In miniature dual-axis confocal microscope. *IEEE J. Sel. Top. Quantum Electron.* **2009**, *15*, 1344–1350. [CrossRef]
20. Maitland, K.C.; Shin, H.J.; Ra, H.; Lee, D.; Solgaard, O.; Richards-Kortum, R. Single fiber confocal microscope with a two-axis gimbaled mems scanner for cellular imaging. *Opt. Express* **2006**, *14*, 8604–8612. [CrossRef]
21. Liu, J.T.C.; Mandella, M.J.; Ra, H.; Wong, L.K.; Solgaard, O.; Kino, G.S.; Piyawattanametha, W.; Contag, C.H.; Wang, T.D. Miniature near-infrared dual-axis confocal microscope utilizing a two-dimensional microelectromechanical systems scanner. *Opt. Lett.* **2007**, *32*, 256–258. [CrossRef]
22. Piyawattanametha, W.; Wang, T.D. Mems-based dual-axis confocal microendoscopy. *IEEE J. Sel. Top. Quantum Electron.* **2010**, *16*, 804–814. [CrossRef] [PubMed]
23. Dickensheets, D.L.; Kino, G.S. Silicon-micromachined scanning confocal optical microscope. *J. Microelectromech. Syst.* **1998**, *7*, 38–47. [CrossRef]
24. Arrasmith, C.L.; Dickensheets, D.L.; Mahadevan-Jansen, A. Mems-based handheld confocal microscope for in vivo skin imaging. *Opt. Express* **2010**, *18*, 3805–3819. [CrossRef] [PubMed]
25. Yeow, J.T.W.; Yang, V.X.D.; Chahwan, A.; Gordon, M.L.; Qi, B.; Vitkin, I.A.; Wilson, B.C.; Goldenberg, A.A. Micromachined 2D scanner for 3D optical coherence tomography. *Sens. Actuators A Phys.* **2005**, *117*, 331–340. [CrossRef]
26. Strathman, M.; Liu, Y.; Keeler, E.G.; Song, M.; Baran, U.; Xi, J.; Sun, M.-T.; Wang, R.; Li, X.; Lin, L.Y. Mems scanning micromirror for optical coherence tomography. *Biomed. Opt. Express* **2015**, *6*, 211–224. [CrossRef]
27. Qi, B.; Himmer, P.A.; Gordon, M.L.; Yang, V.X.D.; Dickensheets, D.L.; Vitkin, I.A. Dynamic focus control in high-speed optical coherence tomography based on a microelectromechanical mirror. *Opt. Commun.* **2004**, *232*, 123–128. [CrossRef]
28. Yang, V.X.D.; Mao, Y.; Standish, B.A.; Munce, N.R.; Chiu, S.; Burnes, D.; Wilson, B.C.; Vitkin, I.A.; Himmer, P.A.; Dickensheets, D.L. Doppler optical coherence tomography with a micro-electro-mechanical membrane mirror for high-speed dynamic focus tracking. *Opt. Lett.* **2006**, *31*, 1262–1264. [CrossRef]
29. Dickensheets, D.L. Requirements of mems membrane mirrors for focus adjustment and aberration correction in endoscopic confocal and optical coherence tomography imaging instruments. *J. Micro Nanolithogr. MEMS MOEMS* **2008**, *7*, 021008. [CrossRef]
30. Strathman, M.; Liu, Y.; Li, X.; Lin, L.Y. Dynamic focus-tracking mems scanning micromirror with low actuation voltages for endoscopic imaging. *Opt. Express* **2013**, *21*, 23934–23941. [CrossRef]
31. Shao, Y.; Dickensheets, D.L. Moems 3D scan mirror for single-point control of beam deflection and focus. *MOEMS* **2005**, *4*, 041502. [CrossRef]
32. Miyajima, H.; Asaoka, N.; Isokawa, T.; Ogata, M.; Aoki, Y.; Imai, M.; Fujimori, O.; Katashiro, M.; Matsumoto, K. A mems electromagnetic optical scanner for a commercial confocal laser scanning microscope. *J. Microelectromech. Syst.* **2003**, *12*, 243–251. [CrossRef]
33. Mitsui, T.; Takahashi, Y.; Watanabe, Y. A 2-axis optical scanner driven non-resonantly by electromagnetic force for OCT imaging. *J. Micromech. Microeng.* **2016**, *16*, 2482. [CrossRef]
34. Yalcinkaya, A.D.; Urey, H.; Brown, D.; Montague, T.; Sprague, R. Two-axis electromagnetic microscanner for high resolution displays. *J. Microelectromech. Syst.* **2006**, *15*, 786–794. [CrossRef]
35. Kim, K.H.; Park, B.H.; Maguluri, G.N.; Lee, T.W.; Rogomentich, F.J.; Bancu, M.G.; Bouma, B.E.; de Boer, J.F.; Bernstein, J.J. Two-axis magnetically-driven mems scanning catheter for endoscopic high-speed optical coherence tomography. *Opt. Express* **2007**, *15*, 18130–18140. [CrossRef] [PubMed]
36. Kim, S.; Lee, C.; Kim, J.Y.; Kim, J.; Lim, G.; Kim, C. Two-axis polydimethylsiloxane-based electromagnetic microelectromechanical system scanning mirror for optical coherence tomography. *J. Biomed. Opt.* **2016**, *21*, 106001. [CrossRef] [PubMed]
37. Siu, C.P.B.; Zeng, H.; Chiao, M. Magnetically actuated MEMS microlens scanner for in vivo medical imaging. *Opt. Express* **2007**, *15*, 11154–11166. [CrossRef]
38. Beeby, S.P.; Blackburn, A.; White, N.M. Processing of PZT piezoelectric thick films on silicon for microelectromechanical systems. *J. Micromech. Microeng.* **1999**, *9*, 218–229. [CrossRef]

39. Gilchrist, K.H.; McNabb, R.P.; Izatt, J.A.; Grego, S. Piezoelectric scanning mirrors for endoscopic optical coherence tomography. *J. Micromech. Microeng.* **2009**, *19*, 095012. [CrossRef]
40. Naono, T.; Fujii, T.; Esashi, M.; Tanaka, S. A large-scan-angle piezoelectric MEMS optical scanner actuated by a Nb-doped PZT thin film. *J. Micromech. Microeng.* **2014**, *24*, 015010. [CrossRef]
41. Qiu, Z.; Rhee, C.-H.; Choi, J.; Wang, T.D.; Oldham, K.R. Large stroke verticle pzt microactuator with high-speed rotational scanning. *J. Microelectromech. Syst.* **2014**, *23*, 256–258. [CrossRef]
42. Koh, K.H.; Kobayashi, T.; Lee, C. A 2-D MEMS scanning mirror based on dynamic mixed mode excitation of a piezoelectric PZT thin film S-shaped actuator. *Opt. Express* **2011**, *19*, 13812–13824. [CrossRef]
43. Naono, T.; Fujii, T.; Esashi, M.; Tanaka, S. Non-resonant 2-D piezoelectric MEMS optical scanner actuated by Nb doped PZT thin film. *Sens. Actuator A Phys.* **2015**, *233*, 147–157. [CrossRef]
44. Xie, H.; Pan, Y.; Fedder, G.K. Endoscopic optical coherence tomographic imaging with a cmos-mems micromirror. *Sens. Actuators A* **2003**, *103*, 237–241. [CrossRef]
45. Jain, A.; Kopa, A.; Pan, Y.; Fedder, G.K.; Xie, H. A two-axis electrothermal micromirror for endoscopic optical coherence tomography. *IEEE J. Sel. Top. Quantum Electron.* **2004**, *10*, 636–642. [CrossRef]
46. Sun, J.; Guo, S.; Wu, L.; Liu, L.; Choe, S.-W.; Sorg, B.S.; Xie, H. 3D in vivo optical coherence tomography based on a low-voltage, large-scan-range 2D mems mirror. *Opt. Express* **2010**, *18*, 12065–12075. [CrossRef]
47. Samuelson, S.R.; Wu, L.; Sun, J.; Choe, S.-W.; Sorg, B.S.; Xie, H. A 2.8-mm imaging probe based on a high-fill-factor mems mirror and wire-bonding-free packaging for endoscopic optical coherence tomography. *J. Microelectromech. Syst.* **2012**, *21*, 1291–1302. [CrossRef]
48. Mu, X.; Zhou, G.; Yu, H.; Du, Y.; Feng, H.; Tsai, J.M.; Chau, F.S. Compact MEMS-driven pyramidal polygon reflector for circumferential scanned endoscopic imaging probe. *Opt. Express.* **2012**, *20*, 6325–6339. [CrossRef]
49. Pan, Y.; Xie, H.; Fedder, G.K. Endoscopic optical coherence tomography based on a microelectromechanical mirror. *Opt. Lett.* **2001**, *26*, 1966–1968. [CrossRef]
50. Chen, S.C.; Choi, H.; So, P.T.; Culpepper, M.L. Thermomechanical actuator-based three-axis optical scanner for high-speed two-photon endomicroscope imaging. *J. Microelectromech. Syst.* **2014**, *23*, 570–578. [CrossRef]
51. Liu, L.; Wang, E.; Zhang, X.; Liang, W.; Li, X.; Xie, H. MEMS-based 3D confocal scanning microendoscope using MEMS scanners for both lateral and axial scan. *Sens. Actuators A Phys.* **2014**, *215*, 89–95. [CrossRef]
52. Sun, J.; Xie, H. MEMS-based endoscopic optical coherence tomography. *Int. J. Opt.* **2011**. [CrossRef]
53. Yuan, W.; Brown, R.; Mitzner, W.; Yarmus, L.; Li, X. Super-achromatic monolithic microprobe for ultrahigh-resolution endoscopic optical coherence tomography at 800 nm. *Nat. Commun.* **2017**, *8*, 1531. [CrossRef] [PubMed]
54. Zara, J.M.; Yazdanfar, S.; Rao, K.D.; Izatt, J.A.; Smith, S.W. Electrostatic micromachine scanning mirror for optical coherence tomography. *Opt. Lett.* **2003**, *28*, 628–630. [CrossRef] [PubMed]
55. Gora, M.J.; Suter, M.J.; Tearney, G.J.; Li, X. Endoscopic optical coherence tomography: Technologies and clinical applications [Invited]. *Biomed. Opt. Express* **2017**, *8*, 2405–2444. [CrossRef] [PubMed]
56. Wang, D.; Fu, L.; Wang, X.; Gong, Z.; Samuelson, S.R.; Duan, C.; Jia, H.; Ma, J.S.; Xie, H. Endoscopic swept-source optical coherence tomography based on a two-axis microelectromechanical system mirror. *J. Biomed. Opt.* **2013**, *18*, 086005. [CrossRef] [PubMed]
57. Tran, P.H.; Mukai, D.S.; Brenner, M.; Chen, Z. In vivo endoscopic optical coherence tomography by use of a rotational microelectromechanical system probe. *Opt. Lett.* **2004**, *29*, 1236–1238. [CrossRef]
58. Luo, S.; Wang, D.; Tang, J.; Zhou, L.; Duan, C.; Wang, D.; Liu, H.; Zhu, Y.; Li, G.; Zhao, H.; et al. Circumferential-scanning endoscopic optical coherence tomography probe based on a circular array of six 2-axis MEMS mirrors. Biomed. *Opt. Express* **2018**, *9*, 2104–2114. [CrossRef]
59. Piyawattanametha, W.; Ra, H.; Qiu, Z.; Friedland, S.; Liu, J.T.C.; Loewke, K.; Kino, G.S.; Solgaard, O.; Wang, T.D.; Mandella, M.J.; et al. In vivo near-infrared dual-axis confocal microendoscopy in the human lower gastrointestinal tract. *J. Biomed. Opt.* **2012**, *17*, 0211021–0211024. [CrossRef]
60. Shin, H.J.; Pierce, M.C.; Lee, D.; Ra, H.; Solgaard, O.; Richards-Kortum, R. Fiber-optic confocal microscope using a MEMS scanner and miniature objective lens. *Opt. Express* **2007**, *15*, 9113–9122. [CrossRef]
61. Li, H.; Duan, X.; Qiu, Z.; Zhou, Q.; Kurabayashi, K.; Oldham, K.R.; Wang, T.D. Integrated monolithic 3D MEMS scanner for switchable real time vertical/horizontal cross-sectional imaging. *Opt. Express* **2016**, *24*, 2145–2155. [CrossRef]

62. Qiu, Z.; Liu, Z.; Duan, X.; Khondee, S.; Joshi, B.; Mandella, M.J.; Oldham, K.; Kurabayashi, K.; Wang, T.D. Targeted vertical cross-sectional imaging with handheld near-infrared dual axes confocal fluorescence endomicroscope. *Biomed. Opt. Express* **2013**, *4*, 322–330. [CrossRef]
63. Qiu, Z.; Khondee, S.; Duan, X.; Li, H.; Mandella, M.J.; Joshi, B.P.; Zhou, Q.; Owens, S.R.; Kurabayashi, K.; Oldham, K.R.; et al. Vertical cross-sectional imaging of colonic dysplasia in vivo with multi-spectral dual axes confocal endomicroscopy. *Gastroenterology* **2014**, *146*, 615–617. [CrossRef] [PubMed]
64. Li, H.; Qiu, Z.; Duan, X.; Oldham, K.R.; Kurabayashi, K.; Wang, T.D. 2D resonant microscanner for dual axes confocal fluorescence endomicroscope. In Proceedings of the 2014 IEEE 27th International Conference on Micro Electro Mechanical Systems (MEMS), San Francisco, CA, USA, 26–30 January 2014; pp. 805–808.
65. Yao, J.; Wang, L.; Yang, J.M.; Maslov, K.I.; Wong, T.T.; Li, L.; Huang, C.H.; Zou, J.; Wang, L.V. High-speed label-free functional photoacoustic microscopy of mouse brain in action. *Nat. Methods* **2015**, *12*, 407. [CrossRef] [PubMed]
66. Liu, L.; Xie, H. 3-D confocal lasers canning microscopy based on a full-MEMS scanning system. *IEEE. Photonics Technol. Lett.* **2013**, *25*, 1478–1480. [CrossRef]
67. Choi, J.; Qiu, Z.; Rhee, C.H.; Wang, T.; Oldham, K. A three-degree-of-freedom thin-film PZT-actuated microactuator with large out-of-plane displacement. *J. Micromech. Microeng.* **2014**, *24*, 075017. [CrossRef] [PubMed]
68. Piyawattanametha, W.; Cocker, E.D.; Burns, L.D.; Barretto, R.P.; Jung, J.C.; Ra, H.; Solgaard, O.; Schnitzer, M.J. In vivo brain imaging using a porTable 2.9 g two-photon microscope based on a microelectromechanical systems scanning mirror. *Opt. Lett.* **2009**, *34*, 2309–2311. [CrossRef] [PubMed]
69. Rivera, D.R.; Brown, C.M.; Ouzounov, D.G.; Pavlova, I.; Kobat, D.; Webb, W.W.; Xu, C. Compact and flexible raster scanning multiphoton endoscope capable of imaging unstained tissue. *Proc. Natl. Acad. Sci. USA* **2011**, *108*, 17598–17603. [CrossRef] [PubMed]
70. Liang, W.; Hall, G.; Messerschmidt, B.; Li, M.J.; Li, X. Nonlinear optical endomicroscopy for label-free functional histology in vivo. *Light Sci. Appl.* **2017**, *6*, e17082. [CrossRef]
71. Liu, X.; Cobb, M.J.; Chen, Y.; Kimmey, M.B.; Li, X. Rapid-scanning forward-imaging miniature endoscope for real-time optical coherence tomography. *Opt. Lett.* **2004**, *29*, 1763–1765. [CrossRef]
72. Zhang, N.; Tsai, T.H.; Ahsen, O.O.; Liang, K.; Lee, H.C.; Xue, P.; Li, X.; Fujimoto, J.G. Compact piezoelectric transducer fiber scanning probe for optical coherence tomography. *Opt. Lett.* **2014**, *39*, 186–188. [CrossRef]
73. Park, H.C.; Song, C.; Kang, M.; Jeong, Y.; Jeong, K.H. Forward imaging OCT endoscopic catheter based on MEMS lens scanning. *Opt. Lett.* **2012**, *37*, 2673–2675. [CrossRef]
74. Park, H.C.; Seo, Y.H.; Hwang, K.; Lim, J.K.; Yoon, S.Z.; Jeong, K.H. Micromachined tethered silicon oscillator for an endomicroscopic Lissajous fiber scanner. *Opt. Lett.* **2014**, *39*, 6675–6678. [CrossRef] [PubMed]
75. Chen, T.; Zhang, N.; Huo, T.; Wang, C.; Zheng, J.G.; Zhou, T.; Xue, P. Tiny endoscopic optical coherence tomography probe driven by a miniaturized hollow ultrasonic motor. *J. Biomed. Opt.* **2013**, *18*, 086011. [CrossRef] [PubMed]
76. Seo, Y.H.; Hwang, K.; Jeong, K.H. 1.65 mm diameter forward-viewing confocal endomicroscopic catheter using a flip-chip bonded electrothermal MEMS fiber scanner. *Opt. Express* **2018**, *26*, 4780–4785. [CrossRef] [PubMed]
77. Zhao, Y.; Sheng, M.; Huang, L.; Tang, S. Design of a fiber-optic multiphoton microscopy handheld probe. *Biomed. Opt. Express* **2016**, *7*, 3425–3437. [CrossRef]
78. Huang, L.; Mills, A.K.; Zhao, Y.; Jones, D.J.; Tang, S. Miniature fiber-optic multiphoton microscopy system using frequency-doubled femtosecond Er-doped fiber laser. *Biomed. Opt. Express* **2016**, *7*, 1948–1956. [CrossRef] [PubMed]
79. Savastano, L.E.; Zhou, Q.; Smith, A.; Vega, K.; Murga-Zamalloa, C.; Gordon, D.; McHugh, J.; Zhao, L.; Wang, M.M.; Pandey, A.; et al. Multimodal laser-based angioscopy for structural, chemical and biological imaging of atherosclerosis. *Nat. Biomed. Eng.* **2017**, *1*, 0023. [CrossRef]
80. Guo, H.; Song, C.; Xie, H.; Xi, L. Photoacoustic endomicroscopy based on a MEMS scanning mirror. *Opt. Lett.* **2017**, *42*, 4615–4618. [CrossRef]
81. Park, K.; Kim, J.Y.; Lee, C.; Jeon, S.; Lim, G.; Kim, C. Handheld Photoacoustic Microscopy Probe. *Sci. Rep.* **2017**, *7*, 13359. [CrossRef]
82. Dong, B.; Chen, S.; Zhang, Z.; Sun, C.; Zhang, H.F. Photoacoustic probe using a microring resonator ultrasonic sensor for endoscopic applications. *Opt. Lett.* **2014**, *39*, 4372–4375. [CrossRef]

83. Hsieh, B.Y.; Chen, S.L.; Ling, T.; Guo, L.J.; Li, P.C. All-optical scanhead for ultrasound and photoacoustic dual-modality imaging. *Opt. Express* **2012**, *20*, 1588–1596. [CrossRef]
84. Zaman, R.T.; Yousefi, S.; Long, S.R.; Saito, T.; Mandella, M.; Qiu, Z.; Chen, R.; Contag, C.H.; Gambhir, S.S.; Chin, F.T.; et al. A Dual-Modality Hybrid Imaging System Harnesses Radioluminescence and Sound to Reveal Molecular Pathology of Atherosclerotic Plaques. *Sci. Rep.* **2018**, *8*, 1–13. [CrossRef] [PubMed]
85. Li, L.; Stankovic, V.; Stankovic, L.; Li, L.; Cheng, S.; Uttamchandani, D. Single pixel optical imaging using a scanning MEMS mirror. *J. Micromech. Microeng.* **2011**, *21*, 025022. [CrossRef]
86. Gibson, G.M.; Edgar, M.P.; Bowman, R.; Padgett, M.J. Single-pixel infrared and visible microscope. *Optica* **2014**, *1*, 285–289.
87. Edgar, M.P.; Gibson, G.M.; Bowman, R.W.; Sun, B.; Radwell, N.; Mitchell, K.J. Simultaneous real-time visible and infrared video with single-pixel detectors. *Sci. Rep.* **2015**, *5*, 10669. [CrossRef] [PubMed]
88. Zhang, Z.; You, Z.; Chu, D. Fundamentals of phase-only liquid crystal on silicon (LCOS) devices. *Light Sci. Appl.* **2014**, *3*, e213. [CrossRef]
89. Nagahara, H.; Zhou, C.; Watanabe, T.; Ishiguro, H.; Nayar, S.K. Programmable Aperture Camera Using LCoS. In *European Conference on Computer Vision*; Springer: Berlin/Heidelberg, Germany, 2010; pp. 337–350.
90. Thibault, P.; Dierolf, M.; Menzel, A.; Bunk, O.; David, C.; Pfeiffer, F. High-resolution scanning x-ray diffraction microscopy. *Science* **2008**, *321*, 379–382. [CrossRef] [PubMed]
91. Marcia, R.F.; Willett, R.M. COMPRESSIVE CODED APERTURE SUPERRESOLUTION IMAGE RECONSTRUCTION. In Proceedings of the IEEE International Conference on Acoustics, Speech and Signal Processing, Las Vegas, NV, USA, 31 March–4 April 2008.
92. Gong, W.; Zhao, C.; Yu, H.; Chen, M.; Xu, W.; Han, S. Three-dimensional ghost imaging lidar via sparsity constraint. *Sci. Rep.* **2016**, *6*, 26133. [CrossRef]
93. Zhao, C.; Gong, W.; Chen, M.; Li, E.; Wang, H.; Xu, W. Ghost imaging LIDAR via sparsity constraints. *Appl. Phys. Lett.* **2012**, *101*, 141123. [CrossRef]
94. Xu, Z.H.; Chen, W.; Penuelas, J.; Padgett, M.; Sun, M.J. 1000 fps computational ghost imaging using led-based structured illumination. *Opt. Express* **2018**, *26*, 2427–2434. [CrossRef]
95. Salvador-Balaguer, E.; Latorre-Carmona, P.; Chabert, C.; Pla, F.; Lancis, J.; Enrique Tajahuerce, E. Low-cost single-pixel 3D imaging by using an LED array. *Opt. Express* **2018**, *26*, 15623–15631. [CrossRef]
96. Komatsu, K.; Ozeki, Y.; Nakano, Y.; Tanemura, T. Ghost imaging using integrated optical phased array. In Proceedings of the Optical Fiber Communication Conference 2017, Los Angeles, CA, USA, 19–23 March 2017.
97. Li, L.J.; Chen, W.; Zhao, X.Y.; Sun, M.J. Fast Optical Phased Array Calibration Technique for Random Phase Modulation LiDAR. *IEEE Photonics J.* **2018**, *11*, 6900410. [CrossRef]
98. Philiips, D.B.; Sun, M.J.; Taylor, J.M.; Edgar, M.P.; Barnett, S.M.; Gibson, G.M.; Padgett, M.J. Adaptive foveated single-pixel imaging with dynamic super-sampling. *Sci. Adv.* **2017**, *3*, e1601782. [CrossRef] [PubMed]
99. Pittman, T.B.; Shih, Y.H.; Strekalov, D.V.; Sergienko, A.V. Optical imaging by means of two-photon quantum entanglement. *Phys. Rev. A* **1995**, *52*, R3429. [CrossRef] [PubMed]
100. Shapiro, J.H. Computational ghost imaging. *Phys. Rev. A* **2008**, *78*, 061802. [CrossRef]
101. Sang, L.; Liao, M.; Sumiya, M. A Comprehensive Review of Semiconductor Ultraviolet Photodetectors: From Thin Film to One-Dimensional Nanostructures. *Sensors* **2013**, *13*, 10482–10518. [CrossRef]
102. Martinenghi, E.; Di Sieno, L.; Contini, D.; Sanzaro, M.; Pifferi, A.; Dalla Mora, A. Time-resolved single-photon detection module based on silicon photomultiplier: A novel building block for time-correlated measurement systems. *Rev. Sci. Instrum.* **2016**, *87*, 073101. [CrossRef]
103. Singh, A.; Srivastav, V.; Pal, R. HgCdTe avalanche photodiodes: A review. *Opt. Laser Technol.* **2011**, *43*, 1358–1370. [CrossRef]
104. Eisaman, M.D.; Fan, J.; Migdall, A.; Polyakov, S.V. Invited Review Article: Single-photon sources and detectors. *Rev. Sci. Instrum.* **2011**, *87*, 071101. [CrossRef]
105. Edgar, M.P.; Gibson, G.M.; Padgett, M.J. Principles and prospects for single-pixel imaging. *Nat. Photonics* **2019**, *13*, 13–20. [CrossRef]
106. Pratt, W.K.; Kane, J.; Andrews, H.C. Hadamard transform image coding. *Proc. IEEE* **1969**, *57*, 58–68. [CrossRef]
107. Sloane, N.J.A.; Harwit, M. Masks for Hadamard transform optics, and weighing designs. *Appl. Opt.* **1976**, *15*, 107–114. [CrossRef] [PubMed]

108. Zhang, Z.; Ma, X.; Zhong, J. Single-pixel imaging by means of fourier spectrum acquisition. *Nat. Commun.* **2015**, *6*, 6225. [CrossRef]
109. Dabov, K.; Foi, A.; Katkovnik, V.; Egiazarian, K. Image denoising by sparse 3D transform-domain collaborative filtering. *IEEE Trans. Image Process.* **2007**, *16*, 2080–2095. [CrossRef] [PubMed]
110. Donoho, D.L. Compressed sensing. *IEEE Inf. Theory* **2006**, *52*, 1289–1306. [CrossRef]
111. Noor, I.; Jacobs, E.L. Adaptive compressive sensing algorithm for video acquisition using a single-pixel camera. *J. Electron. Imaging* **2013**, *22*, 021013. [CrossRef]
112. Candes, E.J.; Tao, T. Near-optimal signal recovery from random projections: Universal encoding strategies? *IEEE. Trans. Inf. Theory* **2006**, *52*, 5406–5425. [CrossRef]
113. Zheng, J.; Jacobs, E.L. Video compressive sensing using spatial domain sparsity. *Opt. Eng.* **2009**, *48*, 087006. [CrossRef]
114. Rudin, L.I.; Osher, S.; Fatemi, E. Nonlinear total variation based noise removal algorithms. *Phys. D Nonlinear Phenom.* **1992**, *60*, 259–268. [CrossRef]
115. Goldluecke, B.; Cremers, D. Introducing total curvature for image processing. In Proceedings of the 2011 International Conference on Computer Vision, Barcelona, Spain, 6–13 November 2011; pp. 1267–1274.
116. Sankaranarayanan, A.C.; Studer, C.; Baraniuk, R.G. CS-MUVI: Video compressive sensing for spatial-multiplexing cameras. In Proceedings of the IEEE International Conference on Computational Photography, Sesttle, WA, USA, 28–29 April 2012.
117. Xu, L.; Sankaranarayanan, A.; Studer, C.; Li, Y.; Baraniuk, R.; Kelly, K.F. *Multi-Scale Compressive Video Acquisition*; Optical Society of America: Washington, DC, USA, 2013.
118. Soldevila, F.; Salvador-Balaguer, E.; Clemente, P.; Tajahuerce, E.; Lancis, J. High-resolution adaptive imaging with a single photodiode. *Sci. Rep.* **2015**, *5*, 14300. [CrossRef]
119. Edgar, M.P.; Sun, M.J.; Gibson, G.M.; Spalding, G.C.; Phillips, D.B.; Padgett, M.J. Real-time 3D video utilizing a compressed sensing time-of-flight single-pixel camera. In *Optical Trapping and Optical Micromanipulation XIII*; International Society for Optics and Photonics: San Diego, CA, USA, 2016.
120. Czajkowski, K.M.; Pastuszczak, A.; Kotynski, R. Real-time single-pixel video imaging with fourier domain regularization. *Opt. Express* **2018**, *26*, 20009–20022. [CrossRef]
121. Higham, C.F.; Murray-Smith, R.; Padgett, M.J.; Edgar, M.P. Deep learning for real-time single-pixel video. *Sci. Rep.* **2018**, *8*, 2369. [CrossRef] [PubMed]
122. Rousset, F.; Ducros, N.; Farina, A.; Valentini, G.; Andrea, C.D.; Peyrin, F. Adaptive basis scan by wavelet prediction for single-pixel imaging. *IEEE Trans. Comput.* **2017**, *3*, 36–46. [CrossRef]
123. Sen, P.; Chen, B.; Garg, G.; Marschner, S.R.; Horowitz, M.; Levoy, M.; Lensch, H.P.A. Dual photography. *ACM Trans. Graph.* **2005**, *24*, 745–755. [CrossRef]
124. Wagner, E.P.; Smith, B.W.; Madden, S.; Winefordner, J.D.; Mignatdi, M. Construction and Evaluation of a Visible Spectrometer Using Digital Micromirror Spatial Light Modulation. *Appl. Spectrosc. Rev.* **1995**, *49*, 1715–1719. [CrossRef]
125. Batchelor, J.D.; Jones, B.T. Development of a Digital Micromirror Spectrometer for Analytical Atomic Spectrometry. *Anal. Chem.* **1998**, *23*, 4907–4914. [CrossRef]
126. Xiang, D.; Arnold, M.A. Solid-State Digital Micro-Mirror Array Spectrometer for Hadamard Transform Measurements of Glucose and Lactate in Aqueous Solutions. *Appl. Spectrosc.* **2011**, *10*, 1170–1180. [CrossRef] [PubMed]
127. Dudley, D.; Duncan, W.M.; Slaughter, J. Emerging digital micromirror device (DMD) applications. In *MOEMS Display and Imaging Systems*; International Society for Optics and Photonics: San Jose, CA, USA, 2003.
128. Oldevila, F.; Irles, E.; Durán, V.; Clemente, P.; Mercedes, F.; Enrique, T.; Jesús, L. Single-pixel polarimetric imaging spectrometer by compressive sensing. *Chin. Phys. B* **2013**, *113*, 551–558.
129. Starling, D.; Storer, I.; Howland, G. Compressive sensing spectroscopy with a single pixel camera. *Appl. Opt.* **2016**, *55*, 5198–5202. [CrossRef]
130. Xu, J.L.; Liu, J.; Lin, C.B.; Sun, Q. SNR analysis and Hadamard mask modification of DMD Hadamard Transform Near-Infrared spectrometer. *Opt. Commun.* **2017**, *383*, 250–254. [CrossRef]
131. Du, Y.; Zhou, G.Y. A MEMS-driven Hadamard transform spectrometer. In *MOEMS and Miniaturized Systems XVII*; International Society for Optics and Photonics: San Francisco, CA, USA, 2018.
132. Li, L.; Qi, Y.; Lim, Z.H.; Zhou, G.; Chau, F.S.; Zhou, G. MEMS-based self-referencing cascaded line-scan camera using single-pixel detectors. *Opt. Express* **2019**, *27*, 25457–25469. [CrossRef]

133. Zhou, G.; Qi, Y.; Lim, Z.H.; Zhou, G. Single-pixel MEMS Spectrometer based on Compressive Sensing. *IEEE Photon. Technol. Lett.* **2020**, *32*, 287–290. [CrossRef]
134. Gibson, G.M.; Sun, B.; Edgar, M.P.; Philips, D.B.; Hempler, H.; Maker, G.T.; Malcolm, G.P.; Padgett, M.J. Real-time imaging of methane gas leaks using a single-pixel camera. *Opt. Express* **2017**, *24*, 2998–3005. [CrossRef] [PubMed]
135. Miao, J.; Song, B.; Cai, L.; Zhang, S.; Dong, L.; Wang, C. Single Pixel Black Phosphorus Photodetector for Near-Infrared Imaging. *Small* **2018**, *2*, 1702082. [CrossRef]
136. Welsh, S.S.; Edgar, M.P.; Bowman, R.; Jonathan, P.; Sun, B.; Padgett, M.J. Fast full-color computational imaging with single-pixel detectors. *Opt. Express* **2013**, *21*, 23068–23074. [CrossRef]
137. Bian, L.; Suo, J.; Situ, G.; Li, Z.; Fan, J.; Chen, F.; Dai, Q. Multispectral imaging using a single bucket detector. *Sci. Rep.* **2016**, *6*, 24752. [CrossRef]
138. Rousset, F.; Ducros, N.; Peyrin, F.; Valentini, G.; D'Andrea, C.; Farina, A. Time-resolved multispectral imaging based on an adaptive single-pixel camera. *Opt. Express* **2018**, *26*, 10550–10558. [CrossRef]
139. Zhang, Z.B.; Liu, S.J.; Peng, J.Z.; Yao, M.H.; Zheng, G.; Zhong, H.G. Simultaneous spatial, spectral, and 3d compressive imaging via efficient fourier single-pixel measurements. *Optica* **2018**, *5*, 315–319. [CrossRef]
140. Yang, J.M.; Gong, L.; Xu, X.; Hai, P.F.; Shen, Y.C.; Suzuki, Y.; Wang, L.H.V. Motionless volumetric photoacoustic microscopy with spatially invariant resolution. *Nat. Commun.* **2017**, *8*, 780. [CrossRef]
141. Yu, W.K.; Liu, X.F.; Yao, X.R.; Wang, C.; Zhai, Y.; Zhai, G.J. Complementary compressive imaging for the telescopic system. *Sci. Rep.* **2014**, *4*, 5834. [CrossRef]
142. Arguello, H.; Rueda, H.; Wu, Y.; Prather, D.W.; Arce, G.R. Higher-order computational model for coded aperture spectral imaging. *Appl. Opt.* **2013**, *52*, D12–D21. [CrossRef]
143. Martín, G.; Bioucas-Dias, J.M.; Plaza, A. Hyperspectral coded aperture (HYCA): A new technique for hyperspectral compressive sensing. In Proceedings of the 21st European Signal Processing Conference EUSIPCO, Marrakech, Morocco, 9–13 September 2013.
144. Wu, Y.; Mirza, I.O.; Arce, G.R.; Prather, D.W. Development of a digital-micromirror-device-based multishot snapshot spectral imaging system. *Opt. Lett.* **2011**, *14*, 2692–2694. [CrossRef] [PubMed]
145. Lin, X.; Wetzstein, G.; Lin, Y.; Dai, Q. Dual-coded compressive hyperspectral imaging. *Opt. Lett.* **2014**, *7*, 2044–2047. [CrossRef] [PubMed]
146. Pian, Q.; Yao, R.; Zhao, L.; Intes, X. Hyperspectral time-resolved wide-field fluorescence molecular tomography based on structured light and single-pixel detection. *Opt. Lett.* **2015**, *40*, 431–434. [CrossRef]
147. Sun, T.; Kelly, K. Compressive Sensing Hyperspectral Imager. In *Computational Optical Sensing and Imaging*; Optical Society of America: Washington, DC, USA, 2009.
148. Jin, S.; Hui, W.; Wang, Y.; Huang, K.; Shi, Q.; Ying, C.; Liu, D.; Ye, Q.; Zhou, W.; Tian, J. Hyperspectral imaging using the single-pixel Fourier transform technique. *Sci. Rep.* **2017**, *7*, 45209. [CrossRef] [PubMed]
149. Qi, Y.; Li, L.; Zhou, G.; Lim, Z.H.; Chau, F.S.; Zhou, G. A single-pixel Hyperspectral imager using two-stage Hadamard Encoding. **2019**. under review.
150. Sun, M.J.; Edgar, M.P.; Gibson, G.M.; Sun, B.; Radwell, N.; Lamb, R. Single-pixel three-dimensional imaging with time-based depth resolution. *Nat. Commun.* **2016**, *7*, 12010. [CrossRef] [PubMed]
151. Howland, G.A.; Dixon, P.B.; Howell, J.C. Photon-counting compressive sensing laser radar for 3D imaging. *Appl. Opt.* **2011**, *50*, 5917–5920. [CrossRef]
152. Howland, G.A.; Lum, D.J.; Ware, M.R.; Howell, J.C. Photon counting compressive depth mapping. *Opt. Express* **2013**, *21*, 23822. [CrossRef]
153. Yu, H.; Li, E.; Gong, W.; Han, S. Structured image reconstruction for three-dimensional ghost imaging lidar. *Opt. Express* **2015**, *23*, 14541. [CrossRef]
154. Zhang, Y.; Edgar, M.P.; Sun, B.; Radwell, N.; Gibson, G.M.; Padgett, M.J. 3D single-pixel video. *J. Opt.* **2016**, *18*, 035203. [CrossRef]
155. Woodham, R.J. Photometric method for determining surface orientation from multiple images. *Opt. Eng.* **1980**, *19*, 139–144. [CrossRef]
156. Sun, B.; Edgar, M.P.; Bowman, R.; Vittert, L.E.; Welsh, S.; Bowman, A. 3D computational imaging with single-pixel detectors. *Science* **2013**, *340*, 844–847. [CrossRef] [PubMed]

157. Satat, G.; Tancik, M.; Raskar, R. Lensless Imaging With Compressive Ultrafast Sensing. *IEEE. Trans. Comput. Imaging* **2017**, *3*, 398–407. [CrossRef]
158. Jiang, H.; Huang, G.; Wilford, P. Multi-view in lensless compressive imaging. *APSIPA Trans. Signal Inf. Process.* **2014**, *3*, E15. [CrossRef]

4

Ultrahigh Frequency Ultrasonic Transducers Design with Low Noise Amplifier Integrated Circuit

Di Li [1,2,*,†], Chunlong Fei [1,*,†], Qidong Zhang [1], Yani Li [1], Yintang Yang [1] and Qifa Zhou [2]

1 School of Microelectronics, Xidian University, Xi'an 710071, China; qdzhang@xidian.edu.cn (Q.Z.); yanili@mail.xidian.edu.cn (Y.L.); ytyang@xidian.edu.cn (Y.Y.)

2 Department of Ophthalmology and Biomedical Engineering, University of Southern California, Los Angeles, CA 90089-1111, USA; qifazhou@usc.edu

* Correspondence: lidi2004@126.com (D.L.); clfei@xidian.edu.cn (C.F.)

† The authors contributed equally to this work.

Abstract: This paper describes the design of an ultrahigh frequency ultrasound system combined with tightly focused 500 MHz ultrasonic transducers and high frequency wideband low noise amplifier (LNA) integrated circuit (IC) model design. The ultrasonic transducers are designed using Aluminum nitride (AlN) piezoelectric thin film as the piezoelectric element and using silicon lens for focusing. The fabrication and characterization of silicon lens was presented in detail. Finite element simulation was used for transducer design and evaluation. A custom designed LNA circuit is presented for amplifying the ultrasound echo signal with low noise. A Common-source and Common-gate (CS-CG) combination structure with active feedback is adopted for the LNA design so that high gain and wideband performances can be achieved simultaneously. Noise and distortion cancelation mechanisms are also employed in this work to improve the noise figure (*NF*) and linearity. Designed by using a 0.35 μm complementary metal oxide semiconductor (CMOS) technology, the simulated power gain of the echo signal wideband amplifier is 22.5 dB at 500 MHz with a capacitance load of 1.0 pF. The simulated *NF* at 500 MHz is 3.62 dB.

Keywords: ultrahigh frequency ultrasonic transducer; Si lens; tight focus; finite element simulation; low noise amplifier (LNA); noise figure

1. Introduction

Ultrahigh frequency ultrasound has recently been investigated as a tool in the field of microbiology. Applications include acoustic microscopy for the non-invasive investigation of biological tissue and living cells [1–4] and non-contact manipulation of microparticles or cells that are based on radiation force principle [5–7]. State of the art in acoustic microscopy is to work with single element focusing transducers. In most cases, the transducers in the ultrahigh frequency range are based on ZnO thin films on sapphire with a grind spherical cavity as a focusing element on the opposite side of the ZnO layer.

The attenuation of generated signal in water is proportional to the covered distance and the square of the frequency. With the increasing operation frequency, the focus distance of the transducer should decrease, thus demand smaller radius and higher sphericity of the lens. When comparing with a sapphire lens for ultrahigh frequency ultrasonic transducer design, a silicon lens might be more appropriate for the following reasons: (1) the silicon wafer is cheaper than the sapphire crystal; (2) good uniformity can be utilized using microelectromechanical systems (MEMS) lithography and etching techniques for the silicon lens rather than the grinding method for the sapphire lens;

and, (3) it is possible to make multi lens on a silicon lens body for advanced transducer configurations. In addition, the signal amplitude of the ZnO based transducer is rather low for a good performance in acoustic microscopy due to the weak piezoelectric behavior. Another important non-ferroelectric piezoelectric material, Aluminum nitride (AlN), possess better chemical and thermal stabilization, better compatibility with the complementary metal oxide semiconductor (CMOS) technology than ZnO [8–10]. Furthermore, the much higher longitudinal wave velocity benefits AlN for ultrahigh frequency application.

Figure 1 shows a schematic diagram of an ultrahigh frequency ultrasonic transducer that is based on the silicon acoustic lens. The ultrasound is generated by an AlN thin piezoelectric layer with electrode on both sides. The AlN layer is sputtered on the silicon lens body according to special designed pattern to reduce the rim echo around the lens cavity. Two lead wires are electrical connected with the bottom and top electrodes. The whole device was encased in a brass tube to provide RF shielding. The gap between the brass tube and the device was filled by insulating epoxy.

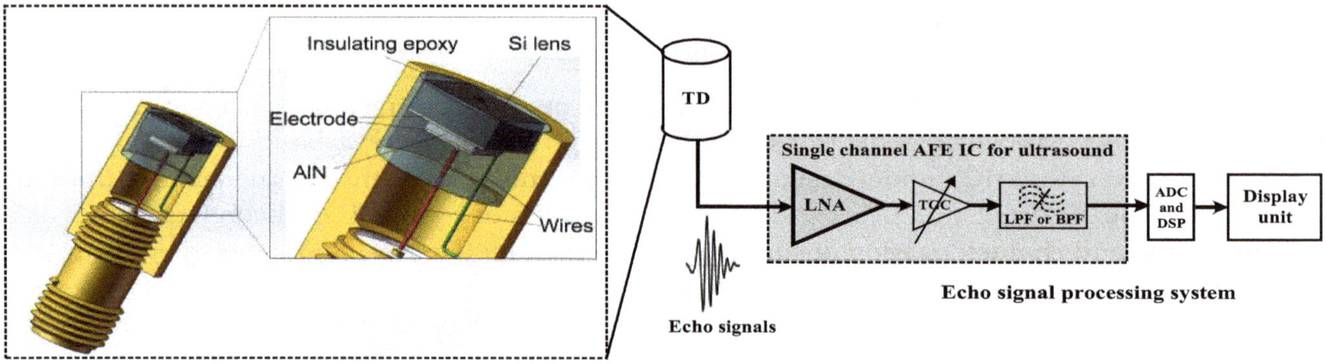

Figure 1. Schematic diagram of the AlN ultrahigh frequency ultrasonic transducer and the echo signal processing system.

Miniaturization and performance improvement of the ultrasound system have been developed in the past several years. One of the driving forces is the improvement of the transducer technology, and the other one is the advanced semiconductor technology based on which the integrated circuits (IC) for ultrasound application could further enhance the system sensitivity and reduce the cost. The transducer front-end, especially the analog receiving portion, plays a significant role in the overall performance of the system. Low noise, large bandwidth, high frequency, and linearity are the important aspects that should be considered carefully. The typical ultrasound receiving analog front-end (AFE) IC, as shown in Figure 1 consists of a low noise amplifier (LNA), a time-gain-compensation (TGC) amplifier and a low-pass or band-pass filter, and generally these blocks are arranged in a cascade scheme to make up the AFE receiver chain [11]. The amplified and filtered echo signals will be finally converted to be digital signals by an analog-to-digital converter (ADC) and processed by the digital signal processing (DSP) block. In fact, performances of the first block LNA including bandwidth, noise figure, gain and linearity have a decisive impact on the performances of the overall AFE receiver chain. The noise figure (*NF*) of an n-cascaded structure receive chain can be expressed as

$$NF = NF_1 + \frac{NF_2 - 1}{G_1} + \frac{NF_3 - 1}{G_2} + \cdots + \frac{NF_n - 1}{G_{n-1}} \tag{1}$$

where NF_i and G_i stands, respectively, for the noise figure and gain of the ith circuit block in the chain. It is obvious that high gain (G_1) of the LNA could reduce the noise contribution of the following stages, and low noise figure (NF_1) of the LNA could result in a low *NF* of the whole receiver chain. Meanwhile, high gain of the LNA could also relax the circuit complexity of the other gain blocks in the AFE. Since the real medical ultrasound echo signal is not a signal with only one single frequency, large bandwidth of the first block LNA is desirable to guarantee the integrity of the information carried in the ultrasonic echoes. The linearity of the LNA should also be considered and simulated carefully since the distortions and nonlinearities introduced by the LNA are unlikely to be removed by the following stages in the AFE [12–14]. Although some well-known chip design companies, such as the ADI (Analog Devices Inc., Norwood, MA. USA), MAXIM (MAXIM integrated Inc., Sunnyvale, CA, USA), and TI (Texas Instruments Inc., Dallas, TX, USA) had designed a series of low noise LNA chips which can be used for the ultrahigh frequency ultrasonic applications, a good trade-off, especially between the noise and gain, were not achieved. Most of the chips were featured with good noise performance while poor gain performance.

In this work, we presented the design of 500 MHz ultrasonic transducers using AlN piezoelectric thin film as the piezoelectric element and using silicon lens for focusing. The fabrication and characterization of silicon lens was presented in detail. As the most important circuit block in the AFE for echo signal processing, a wideband and high gain LNA with an inductor-less CS-CG combination structure was also designed in this work. The LNA that was proposed in this work featured low noise figure, high gain, and good linearity characteristics.

2. Fabrication and Characterization of Silicon Lens

The isotropic XeF_2 dry etch process was chosen for etching silicon cavity over the conventional isotropic wet etch. Previously we used $HF:HNO_3:CH_3COOH$ = 1:2:3 (HNA) solution wet etching [3]. The dry etch process has several advantages over it: (1) photoresist can be directly used as etching mask while an additional hard mask (SiN) that is grown by low pressure chemical vapor deposition LPCVD is necessary in the wet etch process. Therefore, fabrication time is reduced. (2) XeF_2 etching can be realized at a slower etching rate than wet etching, leading to better half sphere shape and better surface smoothness. (3) XeF_2 etching process is more controllable. We can control the etching depth easily by just changing the number of etching cycles. Contrarily, wet etching is very sensitive to the HNA solution's composition (the ratio of hydrofluoric acid, nitric acid, and acetic acid), which cannot be controlled accurately. (4) All reactions happen inside closed chamber which enables people to avoid handling toxic or corrosive chemical.

The reactant, XeF_2, is in a solid crystalline form at room temperature. When exposed to low pressure, the XeF_2 crystal sublimates to gas phase. It has high selectivity on silicon over other materials, such as most photoresist, oxides, nitrides, and many metals. The chemical reaction involved is:

$$2XeF_2 + Si \rightarrow 2Xe\ (g) + SiF_4\ (g) \tag{2}$$

Photolithography was used to transfer patterns onto photoresist for the fabrication of the cavity. The mask pattern designed is 4 mm × 4 mm arrays of circles with diameter ranging from 50 μm to 300 μm (25 μm step from row to row) in order to obtain silicon lens of different size. The photolithography process is: Firstly, the silicon wafer was spin coated photoresist (AZ MIR701, 3000 rpm, 40 s, postbake: 90 °C, 1 min; MicroChemicals GmbH, Ulm, Germany). Then mask aligner was used to expose the coated wafers for 20 s at power of 3.75 mW/cm^2 (postbake 110 °C, 1 min). Next, the exposed wafer was developed by an AZ 300 developer for one minute, and the pattern was successfully transferred onto the photoresist. The wafer was put into XeF_2 etcher chamber and went through 125 etch cycles (about 4 h). At last, residual coating on samples was removed by acetone with ultrasound agitation.

The final diameter of silicon lens ranges from 200 μm to 540 μm, depending on the original mask pattern size. Figure 2 shows a cross section of the silicon lenses and a zoom-in image of a corner of the lens, by which we can inspect the shape and surface smoothness. As can be seen, the hemispherical shape is clear and the surface smoothness is at hundred nanometer level.

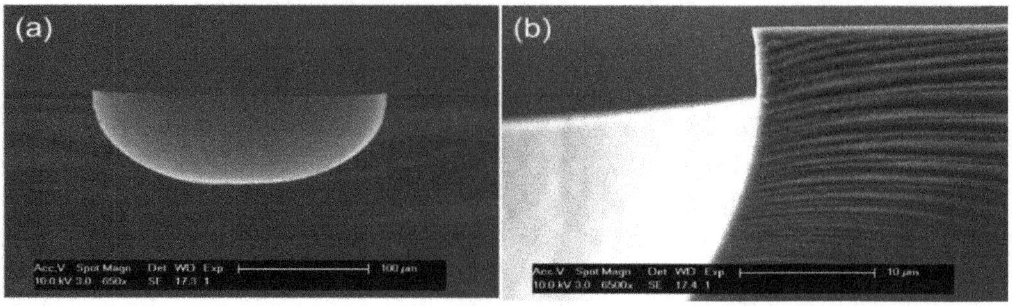

Figure 2. (**a**) Scanning electron microscope (SEM) image of a cross section of a dry etched Si cavity; (**b**) SEM image of a corner of a dry etched Si cavity.

3. Transducer Design and Finite Element Simulation

Aluminum nitride was selected for piezoelectric layer of the ultrahigh frequency transducer duo to it excellent properties, such as a high longitudinal velocity (~11,000 m/s), high thermal stability (melting point ~2100 °C and piezoelectric effect application up to 1150 °C), relatively high electromechanical coupling coefficient ((k_t ~0.28), and low dielectric constant ($\varepsilon^s/\varepsilon$ ~8). Furthermore, AlN is compatible with the complementary metal oxide semiconductor (CMOS) technology. Specific design parameters and performance of the transducer were simulated through a finite element model-based simulation software PZFlex (PZFlex2016, Weidlinger Associates, Inc., Mountain View, CA, USA). The main materials that were used for the simulation are listed at Table 1.

Table 1. Materials used for the transducer simulation consideration.

Material	Function	c (m/s)	ρ(kg/m^3)	Z(MRayl)
AlN	Piezoelectric element	11,000	3260	35.86
Si	Lens	8430	2340	19.8
Water	Front load	1540	1000	1.54
EPO-TEK 301	Backing	2650	1150	3.05

Figure 3a gives the designed specification of the AlN stack together with the lens and backing material. The thickness of AlN film was 9 μm in order to achieve center frequency of 500 MHz. AlN film was connected series to a 50 Ω resistor during the simulation process, and the transducer was driven by a sinusoidal signal with excitation frequency of 500 MHz and peak-to-peak voltage of 1 V. Box size was chosen to be 1/20 wavelength at both the axial and lateral direction. Simulation time was set to be 0.22 μs for signal sending and receiving. Figure 3b shows the pulse-echo waveform and frequency spectrum that were achieved from the finite element simulation. The center frequency (f_c) and −6 dB bandwidth (BW) were determined by the following equations:

$$f_c = \frac{f_l + f_u}{2} \tag{3}$$

$$BW = \left(\frac{f_u - f_l}{f_c}\right) \times 100\% \tag{4}$$

where f_l and f_u are defined as lower and upper −6 dB frequencies, respectively, at which the magnitude of the amplitude in the spectrum is 50% (−6 dB) of the maximum. The center frequency and −6 dB bandwidth were calculated to be 559 MHz and 40%. In the simulation, the focal depth was determined from the acoustic pressure pattern (Figure 3c). The focal depth of the AlN transducer was calculated as 143.6 μm, assuming a value of 1490 m/s for the speed of sound in water. The on focus lateral beam profile (Figure 3d) demonstrated the −6 dB beam width simulated to be 2.7 μm. The finite element simulation results demonstrate that, based on this AlN transducer with silicon lens, it is possible to design and fabricate ultrasonic transducer with high center frequency and narrow −6 dB beam width.

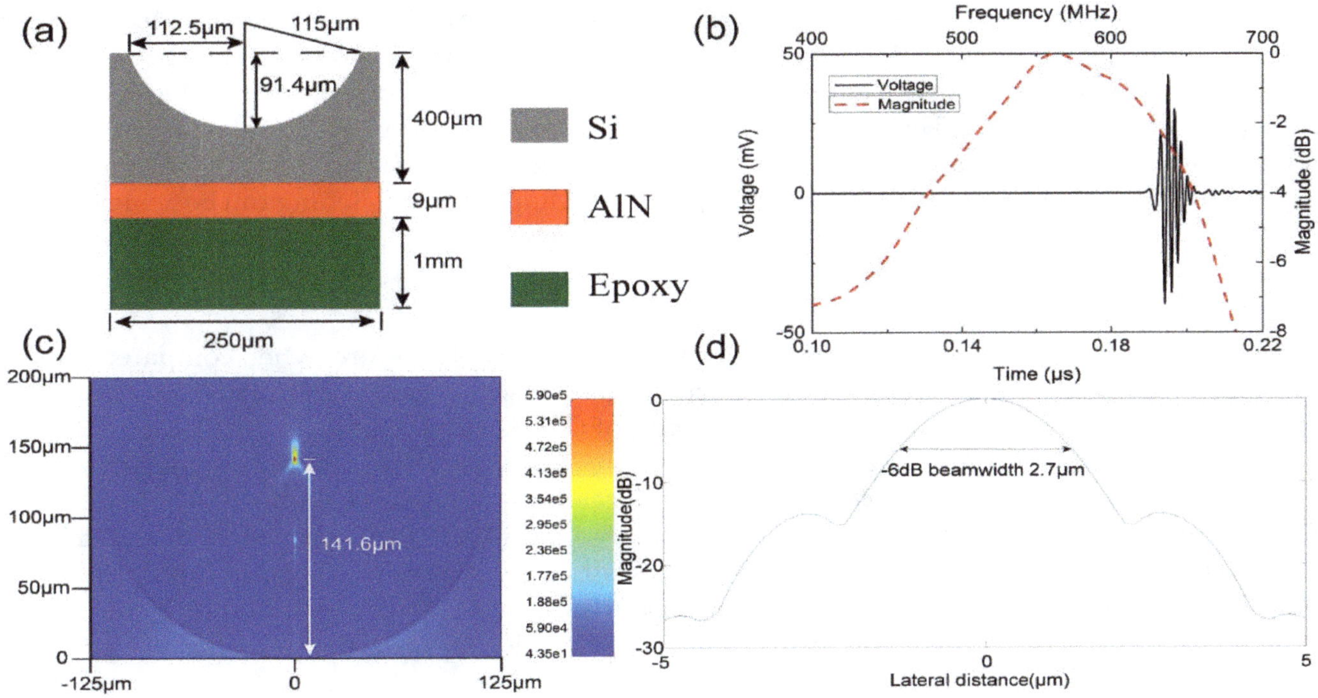

Figure 3. (**a**) Design specifications of the Aluminum Nitride (AlN) stack with lens and backing material; (**b**) the simulated pulse-echo waveform and frequency spectrum of the silicon lens transducer; (**c**) the acoustic pressure pattern generated by the transducer; and, (**d**) The on focus lateral beam profile of the silicon lens transducer.

4. The Echo Signal LNA Integrated Circuit Design

The LNA used for the ultrasound echo signals processing should be featured with low noise figure, wideband, high gain, and good linearity characteristics, as mentioned in the first section. These performance requirements can be well met by the traditional inductor-based LNAs. However, the on-chip bulky inductors occupy very large area which counters the purpose of high integration required in the ultrasound systems and many other applications. In addition, accurate inductor models are very difficult to build, which may lead to many times of tape-out and thus greatly increasing of the cost [15–18]. Therefore, inductor-less LNA has become more attractive in these years and several topologies had been proposed in the published literatures [19–25]. These topologies can be in fact divided into three categories, including common-source (CS) structure with resistor-terminated [15,26], shunt-feedback (SFB) amplifier [27], and common-gate (CG) structure with capacitive cross-coupling or gain boosting techniques [28–31]. The resistor-terminated CS scheme as shown in Figure 4a provides the input impedance by using a 50-Ω shunt resistor. However, large transconductance (g_m) of input transistor (M1) is needed to achieve low noise performance. For both the SFB (Figure 4b) and CG (Figure 4c) schemes, low noise figure can be achieved with small g_m of the input transistor, but the power consumption is generally high to achieve the input matching. The g_m-boosting technique is popular in these years and its basic idea is using an auxiliary voltage gain to simultaneously apply signal on both gate and source of the input transistors (Figure 4d). The g_m of the CG transistor (M1) can be boosted, since it forms a negative feedback loop with the amplifier. This technique offers a low noise figure of the LNA and meanwhile a favorable power consumption-input matching tradeoff.

Inductor-less scheme and CS-CG combination structure are employed in this work for the LNA integrated circuit design to meet the small chip area and high performance requirements. The generations of CMOS technologies exhibit excellent performances, such as low noise figure, high characteristic frequency, and so on, and could also provide larger margin for the design of high performance integrated circuits with low cost. The medical input ultrasound signal frequency in this work is centered at 500 MHz, and since most current CMOS processes can handle this easily, a 0.35 μm

CMOS process is adopted for the LNA design with better integration and power reduction being achieved. The single-end schematic of the proposed LNA in this work is shown in Figure 5a. The input resistor R_{in} is the source impedance and it equals typically 50 Ω. The first stage is in fact a CG amplifier using g_m-boosting technique. The active feedback amplifier is realized by a common-source amplifier consisted by transistor M4 and load resistor R_{L1}, and the gain of the amplifier can be expressed as $-g_{m4}R_{L1}$. If A_v is expressed as the local open loop gain, the impedance matching can be achieved when

$$R_{in} = \frac{1}{g_{m1}(1 + A_v)} \tag{5}$$

where g_{m1} is the transconductance of the feedback transistor M1. Therefore, when compared with the traditional common-mode or common-gate structure, the transconductance of the LNA needed for the input impedance matching can be reduced by a factor of (1 + A_v) [32]. Since a fully differential scheme will be adopted in this design, the circuit could also provide a negative gain for the negative output V_{out-} to form a positive feedback when the whole differential circuits are realized. The input signal is firstly amplified by the CS transistor M4 and then injected into the CG amplifier consisted by M2, M3, and diode transistor load M6. The folded-cascode structure is also employed in this design where transistor M5 is stacked on the top of M1 and M3 on the top of M2 to provide high reverse isolation and therefore the power gain. For the positive gain path from V_{in} to V_{out+}, the gain can be expressed as

$$A_{v,out+} = g_{m1}(1 + g_{m4}R_{L1})\left(g_{m5}r_{O5}r_{O1}\left|\right|\frac{1}{g_{m7}}\right) \tag{6}$$

and for the negative gain path from V_{in} to V_{out-}

$$A_{v,out-} = -g_{m4}R_{L1}g_{m2}\left(g_{m3}r_{O3}r_{O2}\left|\right|\frac{1}{g_{m6}}\right) \tag{7}$$

where r_{Oi} are drain-to-source resistance of transistor Mi.

In the proposed LNA, noise contributions from transistors M1 and M2, as shown in Figure 5b can be canceled. Taking noise contribution from M2 as the example and similar analysis can also be applied for the one from M1. The noise that is generated by transistors M2 can be modeled as a current source $i_{n,2}$, which will both generate a noise voltage $v_{n,2}$ at point X and the negative output $v_{n,out-}$, which can be given by

$$v_{n,out-} = -\frac{i_{n,2}}{g_{m6}} \tag{8}$$

The $v_{n,2}$ will be also amplified by the CS amplifier consisted by M1, M5, and M7, and the noise voltage at the V_{out+} end can be given by

$$v_{n,out+} = -i_{n,2}R_{L1}g_{m1}\left(g_{m5}r_{O5}r_{O1}\left|\right|\frac{1}{g_{m7}}\right) \tag{9}$$

The noise contribution from M2 can be cancelled when $v_{n,out+} = v_{n,out-}$, since it becomes a purely common-mode signal and it will finally undergo subtraction at the output ends V_{out+} and V_{out-}. Therefore, parameters of the related devices in the circuits should be designed to satisfy

$$R_{L1}g_{m1}g_{m6}\left(g_{m5}r_{O5}r_{O1}\left|\right|\frac{1}{g_{m7}}\right) = 1 \tag{10}$$

Noise cancelation mechanism greatly improves the noise performance of the whole circuits [32,33]. The thermal noise of resistor R_{L1} and channel thermal noise of transistor M4 then take up the primary part of the whole LNA noise.

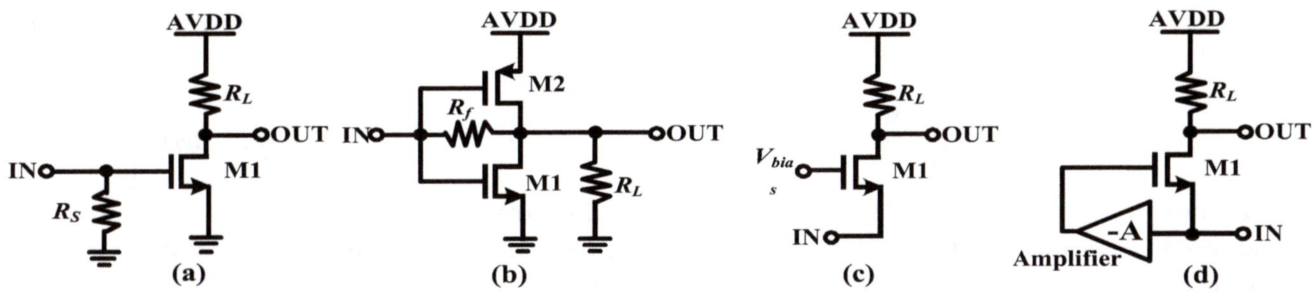

Figure 4. Inductor-less wideband low noise amplifier (LNA) (**a**) common-source (CS) amplifier (**b**) shunt-feedback (SFB) amplifier (**c**) common-gate (CG) amplifier and (**d**) CG amplifier with gm-boosting technique.

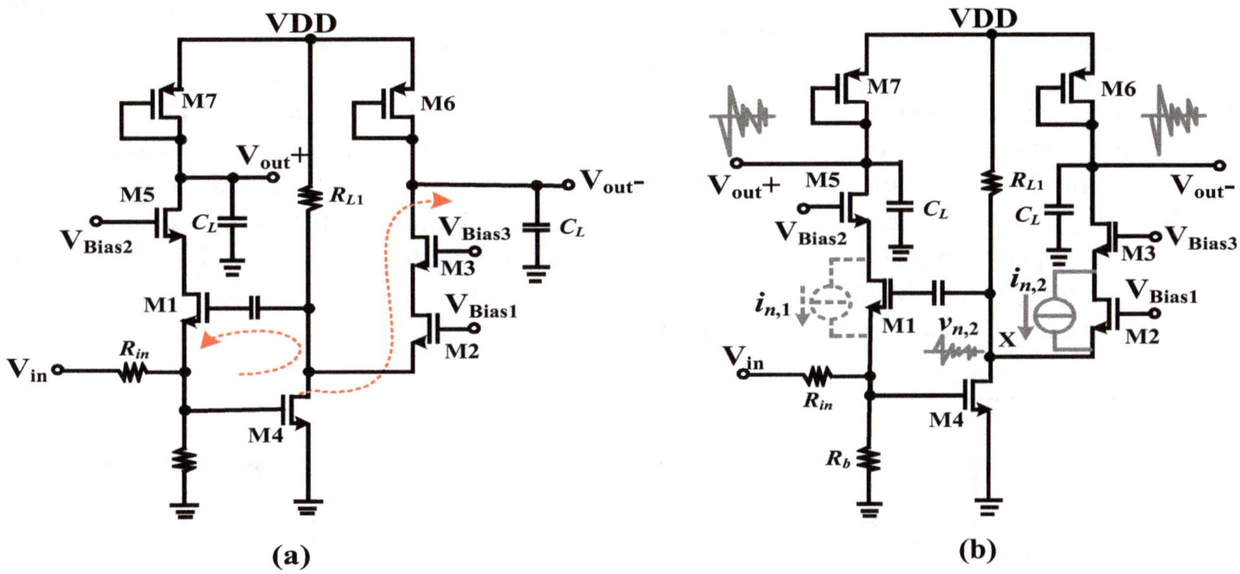

Figure 5. The proposed LNA (**a**) single-end schematic and signal propagation paths and (**b**) noise model of the key devices and analysis of noise cancelation mechanism.

High order harmonic distortions have a much smaller contribution to the nonlinearities of the LNA due to their low power while the low order ones, especially the 2nd and 3rd harmonics are the prominent components that should be considered. Fully differential structure has the advantage of ideally canceling the even order harmonics, which can be considered as common-mode components that appeared at the balanced differential output ends. The 3rd harmonics distortion components can be partly cancelled in this work. The distortion currents of the transistors can be modeled as current sources paralleled with the transistors and the distortions from M1 and M2 can be eliminated by the similar mechanism of noise canceling. Attention should be paid that the distortion and noise cancelation might lose effect at a very high frequency due to the phase shift.

The schematic of the whole differential LNA that was used in this work is shown in Figure 6. Fully differential and symmetrical scheme will not only double the gain, but also achieve a better common mode noise rejection and overcome the performance deterioration of the analog front-end circuits resulted by noise coupling through the substrate from the digital circuits. Bias voltages V_{Bias1}~V_{Bias5} are provided through bias resistors R_1 and R_2 to make sure that the transistors in the circuits could operate in saturate states. The coupling capacitances C_1 and C_2 are designed to be much greater than the parasitical capacitances of the input transistors. The cross-coupled scheme at the output ends could further enhance the voltage gain of the differential LNA, and the gain of the differential circuits can be expressed as

$$A_{v,diff} = g_{m1}(1 + g_{m4}R_{L1})\left[\frac{1}{g_{m7}}||r_{O5}||(g_{m10}r_{O10}r_{O9})\right] + g_{m4}R_{L1} + g_{m2}\left[\frac{1}{g_{m6}}||r_{O12}||(g_{m3}r_{O3}r_{O2})\right] \quad (11)$$

Common-mode feedback (CMFB) circuits consisted by transistors M13–M23 is also employed to stabilise the dc operating voltages of the LNA core. It provides a common mode feedback voltage for the gates of M2 and M9 after detecting the common mode voltages of V_{DP} and V_{DN}. The voltage test points are located at the drains of M5 and M8 rather than the output ends (V_{out+} and V_{out-}) for not introducing noise in the outputs. Simple low-pass filters consisted by R_f and C_f are used to remove the high frequency noise. CTRL1 and CTRL2 are two control signals with complementary phases, and transistors M16 to M19 are acted as switches under these two control signals. When CTRL1 is high and CTRL2 is low, the two inputs of the CMFB block are in fact both the sum of the DC voltages of V_{DP} and V_{DN} (the AC components are filtered by the RC filters). If the common-mode voltage, for example, is higher than the expected one, the V_{CMFB} and the currents flowing through M2 and M9 will be decreased. Then, the currents flowing through M5 and M12 will be increased and the common-mode voltage of V_{DP} and V_{DN} decreased. Since a current mirror is constructed by transistors M14 and M15, Currents I_1 and I_2 on the two branches in the CMFB are equal and the difference between input DC voltages that are applied onto the gates of M20–M23 can then be detected. Therefore, when CTRL1 is low and CTRL2 is high, the CMFB will detect the difference between the DC voltages of V_{DP} and V_{DN}. With the feedback loop, the DC offset will then be corrected.

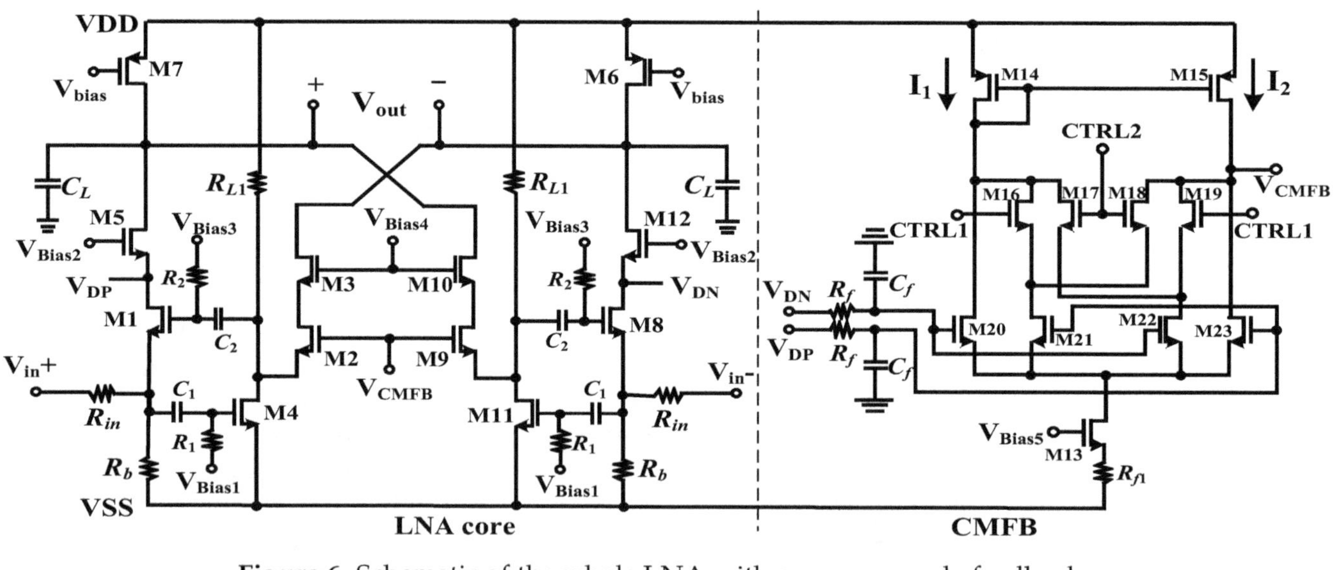

Figure 6. Schematic of the whole LNA with common-mode feedback.

The proposed differential LNA was designed by using a 0.35 μm CMOS technology and it consumes a current of 2.5 mA from a 3.3 V power supply. Generally, the capacitance load of the LNA (C_L in Figure 6) which is also the input capacitance of the next stage in the AFE chain may vary over a certain range, and therefore simulations of the gain and bandwidth with different capacitances load should be considered. Figure 7 shows the simulated AC response of the LNA with the capacitances load tuning from 0.1 pF to 1.0 pF. The bandwidth decreases with the increase of the C_L. The maximum gain of the LNA is about 23.2 dB, and at 500.023 MHz the gain is about 22.5 dB. The gain variation retains a flatness of smaller than 0.7 dB over the frequency range from 400 MHz to 700 MHz with a capacitance load of 1.0 pF.

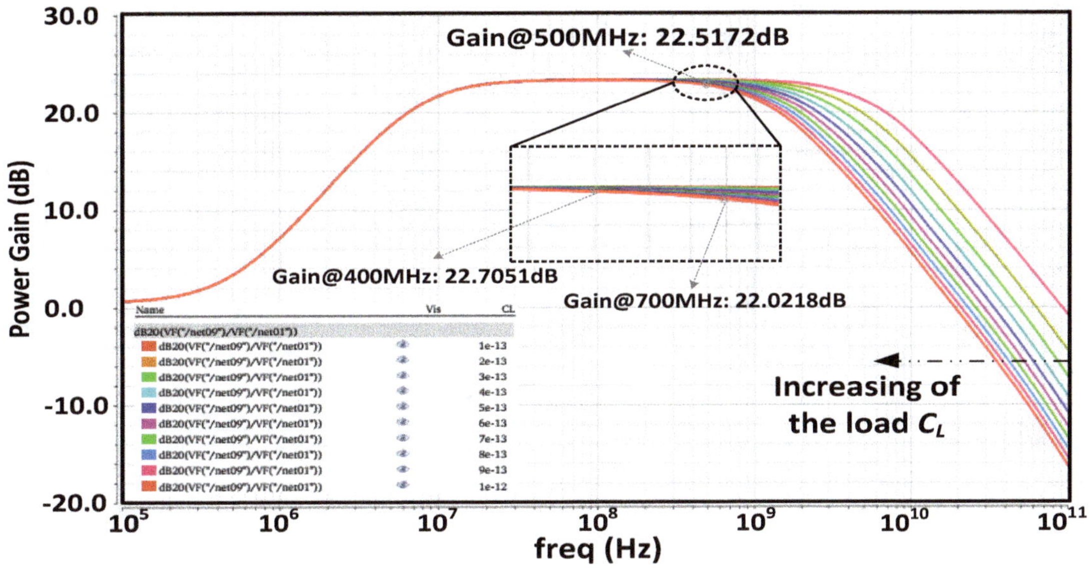

Figure 7. The simulated AC response of the LNA with different C_L.

Figure 8 presents the transient simulation result of the LNA. The peak-to-peak amplitude of the input signal is about 90 mV and the fundamental frequency 500 MHz. After being amplified by the LNA, the magnitude is from −0.58 to 0.61 V and the power gain is about 22.43 dB, which is consistent with the AC simulation results that are shown in Figure 7. Figure 9a presents the simulated noise figure (*NF*) and input reflection coefficient (S11) of the LNA versus the input frequency. The *NF* is about 3.62 dB at 500 MHz and the minimum is about 3.5 dB from 0.1 to 1 GHz. The increase of *NF* at low frequencies is due to the flicker noise ($1/f$ noise), and due to the drop in gain, it increases at high frequencies. The S11 is lower than −10 dB over the bandwidth, which implies that good matching performance of the LNA input is achieved. Two-tone test is done for measuring the input 1 dB compression point (P_{1dB}) and third-order intermodulation (IM3) distortion of the LNA, which are shown in Figure 9b. The P_{1dB} and the input third-order intercept point (IIP3) at 500 MHz are respectively −20 dBm and −11 dBm, which imply that the LNA could accommodate input echo signals with large amplitudes and linearity performance.

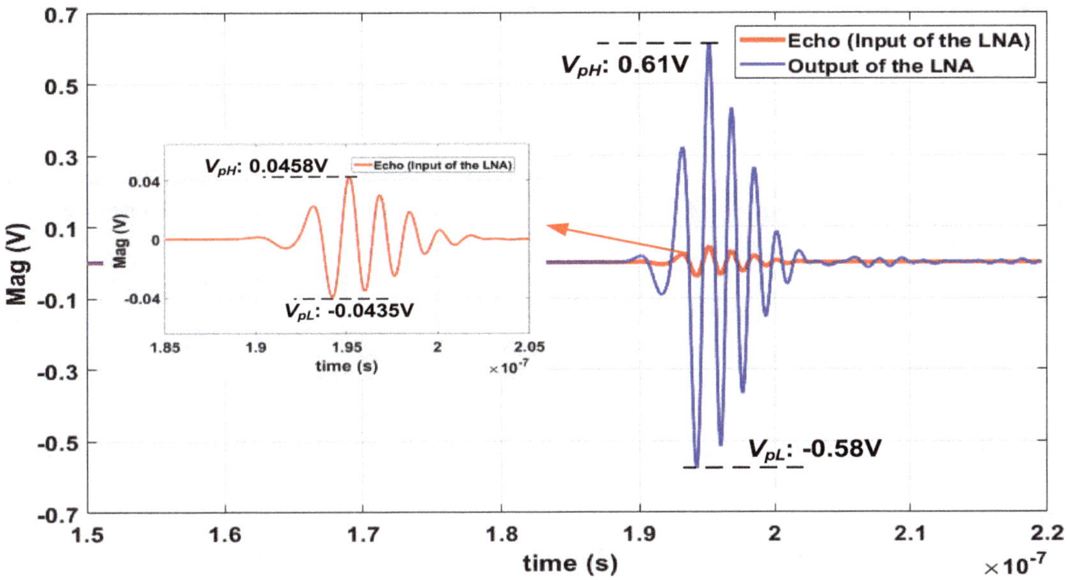

Figure 8. Transient simulation waveform of the LNA output.

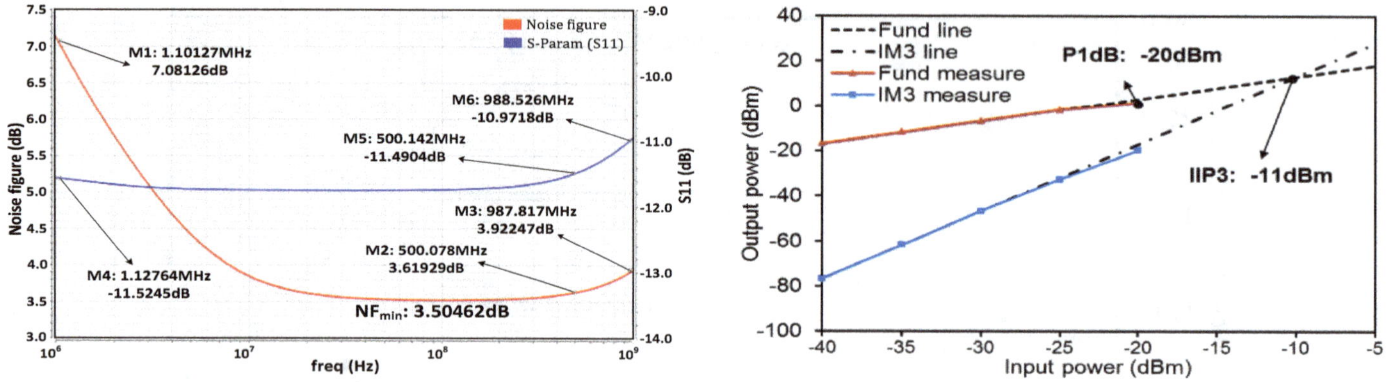

(a) (b)

Figure 9. Simulated results of (**a**) *NF* and S11 versus input frequency (**b**) distortion performance in terms of the input-referred P_{1dB} and IIP3.

5. Conclusions

In this work, ultrahigh frequency ultrasonic transducers are designed using AlN piezoelectric thin film as the piezoelectric element and using silicon lens for focusing. The fabrication and characterization of silicon lens was presented in detail. Finite element simulation was used for transducer design and evaluation. The results demonstrate that, based on this AlN transducer with silicon lens, it is possible to design and fabricate ultrasonic transducer with high center frequency and narrow −6 dB beam width. A wideband inductor-less LNA with CS-CG combination structure for the ultrasonic medical echo signal processing was also proposed in this work. Active feedback structure and noise cancelation mechanism were employed and the LNA featured wideband coverage while maintaining low noise figure, high gain, and good linearity. Designed by using a 0.35 μm CMOS technology, the simulation results show that the LNA achieves a power gain of 22.5 dB at 500 MHz and remains a gain flatness of smaller than 0.7 dB over a frequency range from 400 MHz to 700 MHz. The simulated noise figure is 3.62 dB at 500 MHz, and the P_{1dB}, IIP3 at 500 MHz are, respectively, −20 dBm, −11 dBm.

Author Contributions: Methodology, D.L., C.F. and Q.Z. (Qifa Zhou); Formal analysis, Q.Z. (Qidong Zhang) and Y.Y.; Software, Y.L.; Writing—original draft, D.L. and C.F.; Writing—review & editing, D.L., Y.Y. and Q.Z. (Qifa Zhou). All authors reviewed the manuscript.

References

1. Jakob, A.; Weiss, E.C.; Knoll, T.; Bauerfeld, F.; Hermann, J.; Lemor, R. P2E-5 Silicon Based GHz Acoustic Lenses For Time Resolved Acoustic Microscopy. In Proceedings of the 2007 IEEE Ultrasonics Symposium Proceedings, New York, NY, USA, 28–31 October 2007; IEEE: Piscataway, NJ, USA, 2007. [CrossRef]
2. Jakob, A.; Bender, M.; Knoll, T.; Lemor, R.; Zhou, Q.F.; Zhu, B.P.; Han, J.X.; Shung, K.K.; Lehnert, T.; Koch, M.; et al. Comparison of different piezoelectric materials for GHz acoustic microscopy transducers. In Proceedings of the 2009 IEEE International Ultrasonics Symposium, Rome, Italy, 20–23 September 2009; IEEE: Piscataway, NJ, USA, 2009. [CrossRef]
3. Fei, C.L.; Hsu, H.S.; Vafanejad, A.; Li, Y.; Lin, P.F.; Li, D.; Yang, Y.T.; Kim, E.S.; Shung, K.K.; Zhou, Q.F. Ultrahigh frequency ZnO silicon lens ultrasonic transducer for cell-size microparticle manipulation. *J. Alloys Compd.* **2017**, *729*, 556–562. [CrossRef]
4. Rohrbach, D.; Jakob, A.; Lloyd, H.O.; Tretbar, S.H.; Silverman, R.H.; Mamou, J. A Novel Quantitative 500-MHz Acoustic Microscopy System for Ophthalmologic Tissues. *IEEE Trans. Biomed. Eng.* **2017**, *64*, 715–724. [CrossRef] [PubMed]

5. Fei, C.L.; Chiu, C.T.; Ma, J.G.; Zhu, B.P.; Xiong, R.; Shi, J.; Shung, K.K.; Zhou, Q.F. Ultrahigh frequency (100 MHz–300 MHz) ultrasonic transducers for optical resolution medical imaging. *Sci. Rep.* **2016**, *6*, 28360. [CrossRef] [PubMed]
6. Fei, C.L.; Li, Y.; Zhu, B.P.; Chiu, C.T.; Chen, Z.Y.; Li, D.; Yang, Y.T.; Shung, K.K.; Zhou, Q.F. Contactless microparticle control via ultrahigh frequency needle type single beam acoustic tweezers. *Appl. Phys. Lett.* **2016**, *109*, 288–290. [CrossRef] [PubMed]
7. Zhu, B.P.; Fei, C.L.; Wang, C.; Zhu, Y.H.; Yang, X.F.; Zheng, H.R.; Zhou, Q.F.; Shung, K.K. Self-focused AlScN film ultrasound transducer for individual cell manipulation. *ACS Sens.* **2017**, *2*, 172–177. [CrossRef] [PubMed]
8. Fei, C.L.; Liu, X.L.; Zhu, B.P.; Li, D.; Yang, Y.T.; Zhou, Q.F. AlN Piezoelectric Thin Films for Energy Harvesting and Acoustic Devices. *Nano Energy* **2018**, *51*, 146–162. [CrossRef]
9. Chen, B.Z.; Chu, F.T.; Liu, X.Z.; Li, Y.R.; Rong, J.; Jiang, H.B. AlN-based piezoelectric micromachined ultrasonic transducer for photoacoustic imaging. *Appl. Phys. Lett.* **2013**, *103*, 031118. [CrossRef]
10. Lu, Y.P.; Heidari, A.; Horsley, D.A. A high fill factor annular array of high frequency piezoelectric micromachined ultrasonic transducers. *J. Microelectromech. Syst.* **2015**, *24*, 904–913. [CrossRef]
11. Elkim, R.; Kim, B.; Mohan, C. A 16-channel 38.6 mW/ch Fully Integrated Analog Front-end for Handheld Ultrasound Imaging. In Proceedings of the 2014 IEEE Biomedical Circuits and Systems Conference (BioCAS) Proceedings, Lausanne, Switzerland, 22–24 October 2014; IEEE: Piscataway, NJ, USA, 2014.
12. Stephan, C.B.; Eric, A.M.K.; Domine, M.W.L.; Bram, N. Wideband Balun-LNA With Simultaneous Output Balancing, Noise-Canceling and Distortion-Canceling. *IEEE J. Solid-State Circuits* **2008**, *43*, 1341–1350. [CrossRef]
13. Xu, X.C.; Harish, V.; Sandeep, O.; Eduardo, B.; Karthik, V. Challenges and Considerations of Analog Front-ends Design for Portable Ultrasound Systems. In Proceedings of the 2010 IEEE International Ultrasonics Symposium, San Diego, CA, USA, 11–14 October 2010; IEEE: Piscataway, NJ, USA, 2010. [CrossRef]
14. Tommaso, D.I.; Martin, C.H.; Pere, L.M.; Ivan, H.H.J.; Jorgen, A.J. System-Level Design of an Integrated Receiver Front End for a Wireless Ultrasound Probe. *IEEE Trans. Ultrason. Ferroelectr. Freq. Control* **2016**, *63*, 1935–1946. [CrossRef]
15. Lee, K.; Nam, I.; Kwon, I.; Gil, J.; Han, K.; Park, S.; Seo, B.-I. The impact of semiconductor technology scaling on CMOS RF and digital circuits for wireless application. *IEEE Trans. Electron. Devices* **2005**, *52*, 1415–1422. [CrossRef]
16. Mahdi, P.; Karim, A.; Mourad, N.E.-G. Short Channel Output Conductance Enhancement Through Forward Body Biasing to Realize a 0.5 V 250 µW 0.6–4.2 GHz Current-Reuse CMOS LNA. *IEEE J. Solid-State Circuits* **2016**, *51*, 574–586. [CrossRef]
17. Zhang, H.; Fan, X.H.; Edgar, S.S. A Low-Power, Linearized, Ultra-Wideband LNA Design Technique. *IEEE J. Solid-State Circuits* **2009**, *44*, 320–330. [CrossRef]
18. Wang, H.R.; Zhang, L.; Yu, Z.P. A Wideband Inductorless LNA With Local Feedback and Noise Cancelling for Low-Power Low-Voltage Applications. *IEEE Trans. Circuits Syst. I* **2010**, *57*, 1993–2005. [CrossRef]
19. Mohamed, E.-N.; Ahmed, A.H.; Edgar, S.-S.; Kamran, E. An Inductor-Less Noise-Cancelling Broadband Low Noise Amplifier with Composite Transistor Pair in 90 nm CMOS Technology. *IEEE J. Solid-State Circuits* **2011**, *46*, 1111–1122. [CrossRef]
20. Zhan, J.-H.C.; Taylor, S.S. An inductor-less broadband LNA with gain step. In Proceedings of the 2006 Proceedings of the 32nd European Solid-State Circuits Conference, Montreux, Switzerland, 19–21 September 2006; IEEE: Piscataway, NJ, USA, 2006. [CrossRef]
21. Vidojkovic, M.; Sanduleanu, M.; Tang, J.V.D.; Baltus, P.; Roermund, A.V. A 1.2 V, inductorless, broadband LNA in 90 nm CMOS LP. In Proceedings of the 2007 IEEE Radio Frequency Integrated Circuits (RFIC) Symposium, Honolulu, HI, USA, 3–5 June 2007; IEEE: Piscataway, NJ, USA, 2007. [CrossRef]
22. Ramzan, R.; Andersson, S.; Dabrowski, J. A 1.4 V 25 mW inductorless wideband LNA in 0.13 CMOS. In Proceedings of the 2007 IEEE International Solid-State Circuits Conference. Digest of Technical Papers, San Francisco, CA, USA, 11–15 February 2007; IEEE: Piscataway, NJ, USA, 2007. [CrossRef]
23. Baakmeer, S.C.; Klumperink, E.A.M.; Nauta, B.; Leenaerts, D.M.W. An inductorless wideband balun-LNA in 65 nm CMOS with balanced output. In Proceedings of the ESSCIRC 2007—33rd European Solid-State Circuits Conference, Munich, Germany, 11–13 September 2007; IEEE: Piscataway, NJ, USA, 2007. [CrossRef]

24. Hampel, S.K.; Schmitz, O.; Tiebout, M.; Rolfes, I. Inductorless 1–10.5 GHz wideband LNA for multistandard applications. In Proceedings of the 2009 IEEE Asian Solid-State Circuits Conference, Taipei, Taiwan, 16–18 November 2009; IEEE: Piscataway, NJ, USA, 2009. [CrossRef]
25. Zhan, J.-H.C.; Taylor, S.S. A 5 GHz resistive-feedback CMOS LNA for low-cost multi-standard applications. In Proceedings of the 2006 IEEE International Solid State Circuits Conference—Digest of Technical Papers, San Francisco, CA, USA, 6–9 February 2006; IEEE: Piscataway, NJ, USA, 2006. [CrossRef]
26. Linten, D.; Thijs, S.; Natarajan, M.I.; Wambacq, P.; Jeamsaksiri, W.; Ramos, J.; Mercha, A.; Jenei, S.; Donnay, S.; Decoutere, S. An ESD-protected DC-to-6 GHz 9.7 mW LNA in 90 nm digital CMOs. *IEEE J. Solid-State Circuits* **2005**, *40*, 1434–1442. [CrossRef]
27. Wang, S.B.T.; Niknejad, A.M.; Brodersen, R.W. Design of a Sub-mW 960-MHz UWB CMOS LNA. *IEEE J. Solid-State Circuits* **2006**, *41*, 2449–2456. [CrossRef]
28. Zhuo, W.; Embabi, S.; Gyvez, J.P.D.; Sinencio, E.S. Using capacitive cross-coupling technique in RF low noise amplifiers and down-conversion mixer design. In Proceedings of the Proceedings of the 26th European Solid-State Circuits Conference, Stockholm, Sweden, 19–21 September 2000; IEEE: Piscataway, NJ, USA, 2000.
29. Zhuo, W.; Li, X.; Shekhar, S.; Embabi, S.H.K.; Gyvez, J.P.D.; Allstot, D.J.; Sinencio, E.S. A capacitor cross-coupled common-gate low-noise amplifier. *IEEE Trans. Circuits Syst. II* **2005**, *52*, 875–879. [CrossRef]
30. Li, X.Y.; Shekhar, S.; Allstot, D.J. Gm-boosted common-gate LNA and differential colpitts VCO/QVCO in 0.18-m CMOS. *IEEE J. Solid-State Circuits* **2005**, *40*, 2609–2619. [CrossRef]
31. Woo, S.; Kim, W.; Lee, C.-H.; Lim, K.; Laskar, J. A 3.6 mW differential common-gate CMOS LNA with positive-negative feedback. In Proceedings of the 2009 IEEE International Solid-State Circuits Conference—Digest of Technical Papers, San Francisco, CA, USA, 8–12 February 2009; IEEE: Piscataway, NJ, USA, 2009. [CrossRef]
32. Chehrazi, S.; Mirzaei, A.; Bagheri, R.; Abidi, A.A. A 6.5 GHz wideband CMOS low noise amplifier for multi-band use. In Proceedings of the IEEE 2005 Custom Integrated Circuits Conference, San Jose, CA, USA, 21–21 September 2005; IEEE: Piscataway, NJ, USA, 2005. [CrossRef]
33. Bruccoleri, F.; Klumperink, E.A.M.; Nauta, B. Wide-band CMOS low-noise amplifier exploiting thermal noise cancelling. *IEEE J. Solid-State Circuits* **2004**, *39*, 275–282. [CrossRef]

5

High Frequency Needle Ultrasonic Transducers Based on Lead-Free Co Doped $Na_{0.5}Bi_{4.5}Ti_4O_{15}$ Piezo-Ceramics

Chunlong Fei [1,†], Tianlong Zhao [1,†], Danfeng Wang [1,2], Yi Quan [3], Pengfei Lin [1], Di Li [1], Yintang Yang [1], Jianzheng Cheng [2], Chunlei Wang [4], Chunming Wang [4,*] and Qifa Zhou [5,*]

1. School of Microelectronics, Xidian University, Xi'an 740071, China; clfei@xidian.edu.cn (C.F.); zhaotl@xidian.edu.cn (T.Z.); jikedandan@163.com (D.W.); pflinxidian@163.com (P.L.); lidi2004@126.com (D.L.); yangyt@xidian.edu.cn (Y.Y.)
2. School of Electronic and Electrical Engineering, Wuhan Textile University, Wuhan 430200, China; jzcheng@wtu.edu.cn
3. Electronic Materials Research Laboratory, Key Laboratory of the Ministry of Education & International Center for Dielectric Research, Xi'an Jiaotong University, Xi'an 740049, China; quanyi@stu.xjtu.edu.cn
4. School of Physics, State Key Laboratory of Crystal Materials, Shandong University, Jinan 250100, China; wangcl@sdu.edu.cn
5. Department of Ophthalmology and Biomedical Engineeing, University of Southern California, Los Angeles, CA 90089-1111, USA

* Correspondence: wangcm@sdu.edu.cn (C.W.); qifazhou@usc.edu (Q.Z.)

† The authors contributed equally to this work.

Abstract: This paper describes the design, fabrication, and characterization of tightly focused (f-number close to 1) high frequency needle-type transducers based on lead-free $Na_{0.5}Bi_{4.5}Ti_{3.975}Co_{0.025}O_{15}$ (NBT-Co) piezo-ceramics. The NBT-Co ceramics, are fabricated through solid-state reactions, have a piezoelectric coefficient d_{33} of 32 pC/N, and an electromechanical coupling factor k_t of 35.3%. The high Curie temperature (670 °C) indicates a wide working temperature range. Characterization results show a center frequency of 70.4 MHz and a −6 dB bandwidth of 52.7%. Lateral resolution of 29.8 μm was achieved by scanning a 10 μm tungsten wire target, and axial resolution of 20.8 μm was calculated from the full width at half maximum (FWHM) of the pulse length of the echo. This lead-free ultrasonic transducer has potential applications in high resolution biological imaging.

Keywords: lead-free piezoelectric materials; high frequency ultrasonic transducer; needle-type; high spatial resolution

---

1. Introduction

Tightly focused high frequency ultrasonic transducers have many clinical applications, ranging from imaging the skin and eye to small animal imaging, because of their improved image resolution [1–4]. The improvement of axial resolution is due to a reduction in wavelength, and thus pulse duration, for a fixed number of cycles per pulse. The improvement of on-focus lateral resolution is due to the small f-number, defined as the ratio of the focal distance to the spatial dimension of the transducer, of the tightly focused transducer and the wavelength. As the key component of ultrasonic transducers, piezoelectric materials such as zinc oxide (ZnO) and aluminum nitride (AlN) piezoelectric films [5,6], lead oxide based ferroelectrics, especially the lead zirconate titanate (PZT) system, lead niobiumzine zirconate titanate (PMN-PT) crystal [7–9], lithium niobate ($LiNbO_3$) single crystal [4], and lead-free piezoelectric ceramics [10–12] have been investigated extensively. Among them, due to their environmental friendliness, simple preparation methods, and relatively low cost, lead-free piezoelectric ceramics have attracted significant interest.

Lead-free $Na_{0.5}Bi_{4.5}Ti_4O_{15}$ (abbreviated as NBT) based materials have been studied recently for their interesting properties, such as high Curie temperature, low dielectric loss, and reasonable piezoelectric behaviors [13–15]. However, the piezoelectric performance of pure NBT ceramics is quite weak; the value of piezoelectric coefficient d_{33} is 16 pC/N [16]. Researchers have made many attempts, such as A- or B-site modification and grain orientation techniques, to overcome these shortcomings and improve the piezoelectric and ferroelectric properties of NBT ceramics [13,17,18]. In these studies, the B-site acceptor modification improved the piezoelectricity of NBT ceramics significantly [15]. For example, the value of d_{33} of Co-doped NBT (NBT-Co) piezoelectric ceramics is over 30 pC/N, which is almost twice of the value of pure NBT ceramics.

To the best of the authors' knowledge, transducers based on NBT-based ceramics for high frequency ultrasound applications have rarely been reported. In this paper, NBT-Co ceramics were prepared and systematically investigated. A tightly focused needle-type ultrasonic transducer with center frequency of 70 MHz was designed and fabricated based on the performance of the NBT-Co ceramics. The electrical and acoustic properties of the transducer were investigated in detail, which demonstrated the great potential of this lead-free transducer for application in high resolution biological and medical imaging.

2. Fabrication and Characterization of Co-Doped $Na_{0.5}Bi_{4.5}Ti_4O_{15}$ Ceramics

2.1. Fabrication

A conventional mixed-oxide technique was used to prepare sodium-potassium bismuth titanate (NBT-Co) piezoelectric ceramics. Analytical grade Na_2CO_3 (99.9%), Bi_2O_3 (99.9%), TiO_2 (99.9%), and Co_2O_3 (99.9%) were selected as starting materials. The composition investigated in the present work is $Na_{0.5}Bi_{4.5}Ti_{3.975}Co_{0.025}O_{15}$ (abbreviated as NBT-Co). The mixture was wet milled in polyethylene bottles with ZrO_2 balls for 12 h in ethanol and calcined at 800 °C for 2 h. Then the mixture was milled again in the same conditions. The milled powders were dried, ground, and granulated with polyvinyl alcohol (PVA) binder, then pressed into disks at a pressure of 150 MPa. The green compacts were put into a sealed crucible fully surrounded with powder having the same composition and sintered at 1080–1100 °C for 3 h. After cooling to room temperature freely, the size of the final samples was 13 mm in diameter and 0.5 mm in thickness.

Phase structure was determined by X-ray diffraction technology with $CuK\alpha_1$ (λ = 1.540596 Å) radiation (D8 Advance; Bruker AXS GMBH, Karlsruhe, Germany). Surface micromorphology of the sintered ceramics was detected by scanning electron microscopy (SEM, S-4800, Hitachi, Tokyo, Japan). The piezoelectric coefficient d_{33} was measured by a quasi-static d_{33} meter (ZJ-2, Institute of Acoustics, Academia Sinica, Taipei, Taiwan). Dielectric measurements were performed with a 4294A impedance analyzer (Agilent Technologies, Santa Clara, CA, USA). The electromechanical coupling factors (k_p, k_t), and frequency constants (N_p, N_t) were calculated according to IEEE standards [19].

2.2. Characterization

Figure 1 shows the X-ray diffraction pattern of the NBT-Co piezoelectric ceramic powder. The diffraction pattern is in agreement with the diffraction data for NBT ceramics, indicating that the Co doping does not change the crystal structure of NBT ceramics. The surface of the NBT-Co piezoelectric ceramics is shown in the inset scanning electron microscopy (SEM) image. As shown, the sample has a dense structure and plate-like morphology, corresponding with the high anisotropy of NBT-Co ceramics.

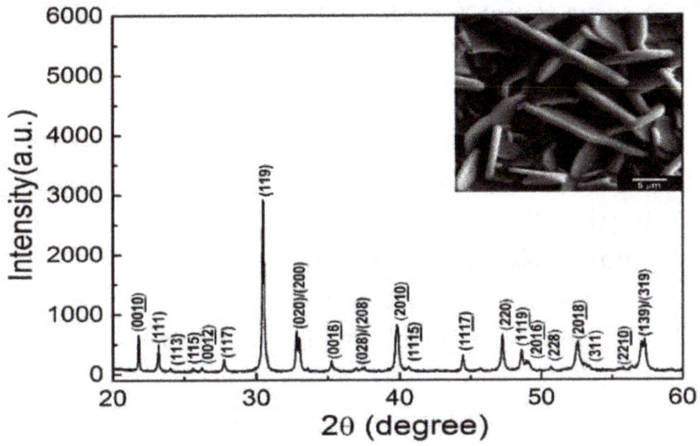

Figure 1. The X-ray diffraction pattern and scanning electron microscopy (SEM) image (embedded) of the Co-doped $Na_{0.5}Bi_{4.5}Ti_4O_{15}$ (NBT-Co) sample.

Detailed room temperature electrical properties of the NBT-Co polycrystalline piezoelectric ceramics are in Table 1. The piezoelectric coefficient d_{33} of NBT-Co ceramics was found to be 32 pC/N, with a large enhancement of double that of pure NBT ceramics. In addition, the relative permittivity ε and dielectric loss tan δ at 1 MHz are 148 and 0.26%, respectively. Furthermore, the planar electromechanical coupling factor (k_p) and thickness electromechanical coupling factor (k_t) were calculated according to the resonance method and found to be 5.2% and 35.3%, respectively. In addition, the planar frequency constant (N_p) and thickness frequency constant (N_t) makes little difference and were found to be 2320 and 2280, respectively.

Table 1. Electrical properties of Co-doped $Na_{0.5}Bi_{4.5}Ti_4O_{15}$ (NBT-Co) ceramics.

T_c (°C)	$\varepsilon_{33}{}^T$	Tan δ (%)	d_{33} (pC/N)	k_p (%)	k_t (%)	N_p (Hz·m)	N_t (Hz·m)
670	148	0.26	32	5.2	35.3	2320	2280

Figure 2 shows the relative permittivity ε and dielectric loss tan δ measured at 1 kHz, 10 kHz, 100 kHz, and 1 MHz as a function of temperature for the cobalt-modified NBT piezoelectric ceramics. The Curie temperature was found to be 670 °C and remains unchanged at all measured frequencies, indicating typical diffuse phase transition characteristics. It can be seen that the dielectric loss tan δ is lower than 1% even when the temperature reached 400 °C; this is important for high temperature piezoelectric applications.

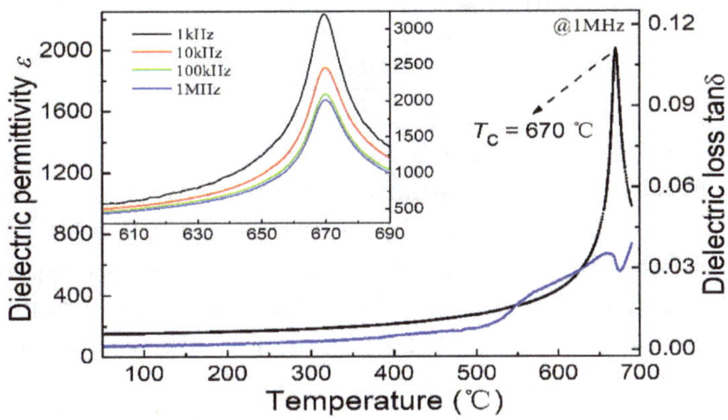

Figure 2. The relative permittivity (black curve) and dielectric loss (blue curve) of the Co-doped $Na_{0.5}Bi_{4.5}Ti_4O_{15}$ (NBT-Co) ceramic measured at 1 MHz and other frequencies (embedded) as a function of temperature.

3. Design, Fabrication, and Characterization of Tightly Focused Needle Ultrasonic Transducer

3.1. Transducer Design and Fabrication

Krimholtz, Leadom, and Mettaei (KLM) model-based simulation software PiezoCAD (Sonic Concepts, Woodinville, WA, USA) was used for transducer design. Finite element modeling software Field II was utilized to give the theoretical analysis of imaging performance by simulating the intensity profile in the X-Z plane. Key parameters of NBT-Co ceramics used for simulation are in Table 2. During the simulation, E-solder 3022 and Parylene C were selected as backing and matching materials, respectively, which is consistent with the experiment. The pulse-echo simulation results (shown in Figure 3a) show transducer design with center frequency of 76.2 MHz and −6 dB bandwidth of 31.8%; the Field II simulation results (shown in Figure 3b) show the on-focus −6 dB beam width to be less than 30 μm for NBT-Co transducer with *f*-number = 1. All these results suggest that NBT-Co ceramics can be used for high frequency and high resolution transducer applications.

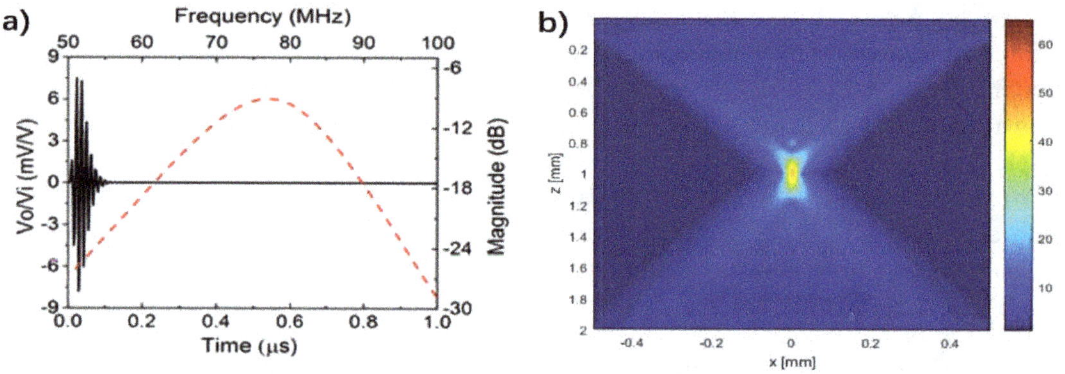

Figure 3. (**a**) Modelling results of Co-doped $Na_{0.5}Bi_{4.5}Ti_4O_{15}$ (NBT-Co) single element transducer from Krimholtz, Leadom, and Mettaei (KLM) model-based simulation software PiezoCAD. (**b**) Simulated intensity profile in X-Z plane of NBT-Co transducer with *f*-number of 1.

Table 2. Parameters of Co-doped $Na_{0.5}Bi_{4.5}Ti_4O_{15}$ (NBT-Co) ceramics used for PiezoCAD modeling.

Property	NBT-Co
Longitudinal velocity v	4600 m/s
Density ρ	6500 kg/m^3
Acoustic impedance Z	29.9 MRayl
Clamped relative dielectric constant ε_r	20
Dielectric loss tan δ	0.0026
Thickness electromechanical coupling k_t	0.353
Piezoelectric coefficient d_{33}	32 pC/N

Based on the prepared NBT-Co piezoelectric ceramics, a high frequency press-focused needle-type transducer was design and fabricated. The schematic diagram and photograph of the designed NBT-Co high frequency ultrasonic transducer are shown in Figure 4. Firstly, the NBT-Co ceramic was manually lapped to around 30 μm, per the design. Au (100 nm) electrodes were sputtered on one side of the NBT-Co ceramic; E-solder 3022 was then cast on this side as the backing material, which was lapped to 2 mm. The sample was diced to 0.7 × 0.7 mm^2 posts using a dicing saw (DAD 323, Disco, Tokyo, Japan) and housed inside a polyimide tube, which provided electrical isolation for the element. The entire assembly was sealed in a steel needle. A lead wire was connected to the backing layer at one side and a SubMiniature version A (SMA) connector at the other side. Then a 100 nm Au layer was sputtered across the front surface to form the ground plane connection. The transducer was press-focused at 90 °C by a highly polished chrome/steel ball bearings with diameter of 2 mm using a set of customer designed fixtures. Finally, a PDS 2010 Labcoator (Specialty Coating Systems, Indianapolis, IN, USA) was used to vapor-deposit a ~8 μm layer of Parylene C on the front face of the transducer to serve as an acoustic matching layer.

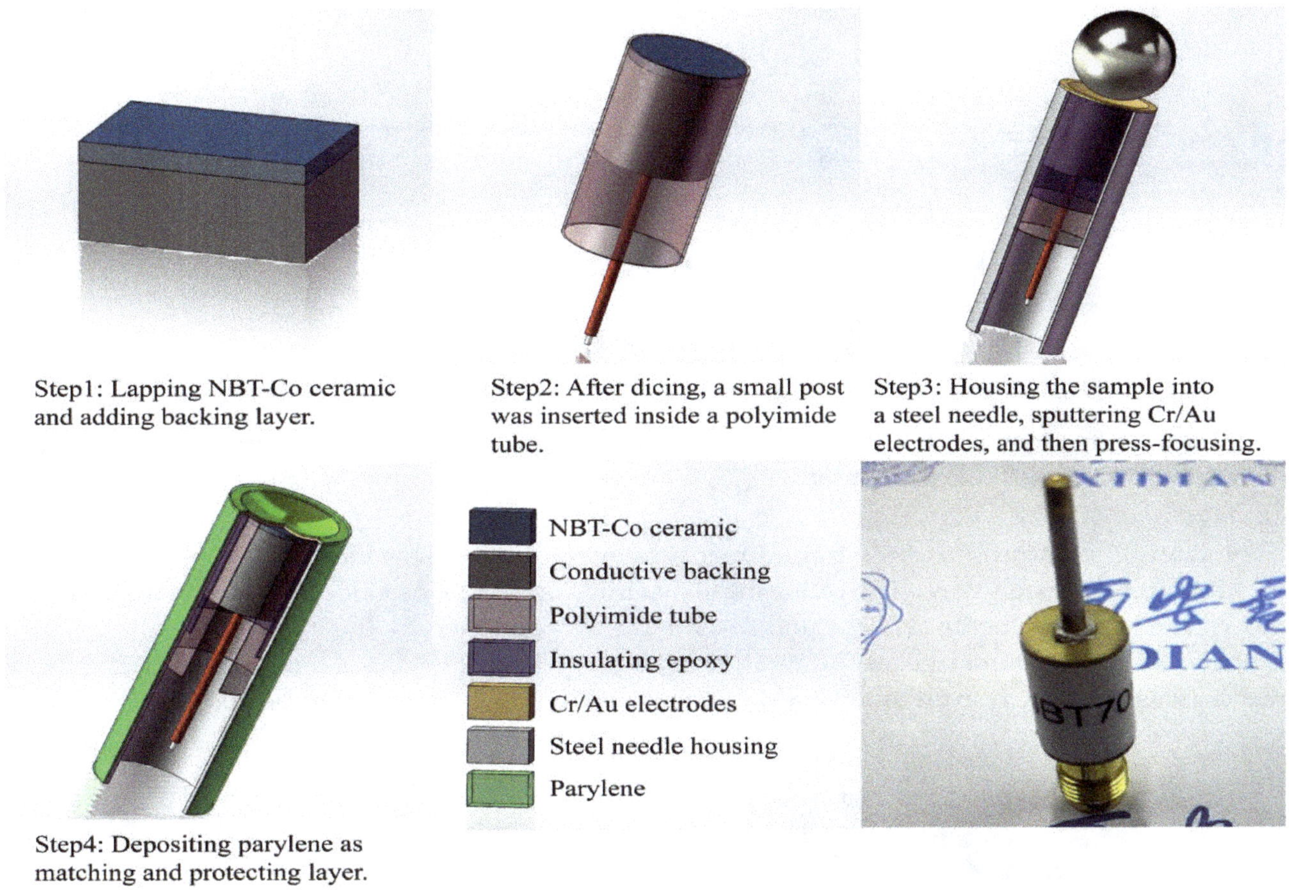

Figure 4. The schematic diagram and photograph of the Co-doped $Na_{0.5}Bi_{4.5}Ti_4O_{15}$ (NBT-Co) needle transducer.

3.2. Transducer Characterization

The pulse-echo response of the NBT-Co needle transducer was measured in distilled water through conventional means [4]. The pulse-echo response and frequency spectrum of the NBT-Co press-focused transducer are shown in Figure 5. The measured transducer performance is in Table 3. As can be seen, the NBT-Co transducer exhibits center frequency of 70.4 MHz and a −6 dB bandwidth of 52.7%. The f-number was calculated to be 1.03. The small f-number, which leads to narrow beam width, is expected to yield high lateral resolution.

Table 3. Measured Co-doped $Na_{0.5}Bi_{4.5}Ti_4O_{15}$ (NBT-Co) transducer performance.

Property	NBT-Co Transducer
Center frequency (MHz)	70.4
Peak to peak Voltage (mV) @ 0 dB gain	123
−6dB Bandwidth	52.7%
Focus depth (mm)	1.02
f-number	1.03

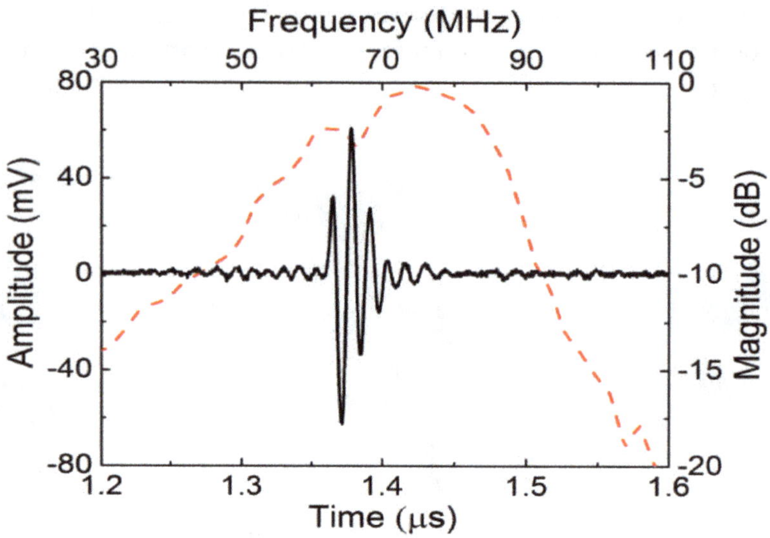

Figure 5. Time-domain pulse/echo response and normalized frequency spectrum of Co-doped $Na_{0.5}Bi_{4.5}Ti_4O_{15}$ (NBT-Co) transducers.

The lateral beam profile of the transducer was evaluated by scanning a wire phantom made of 10 μm diameter tungsten wire. The pulse intensity integral (PII) was calculated from the wire target. As shown in Figure 6, a beam width equal to 29.8 μm was obtained by the NBT-Co needle transducer in detecting a spatial point target at full width at half maximum (FWHM, −6 dB). In addition, the axial resolution was calculated from the FWHM of the pulse length of the echo to be 20.8 μm.

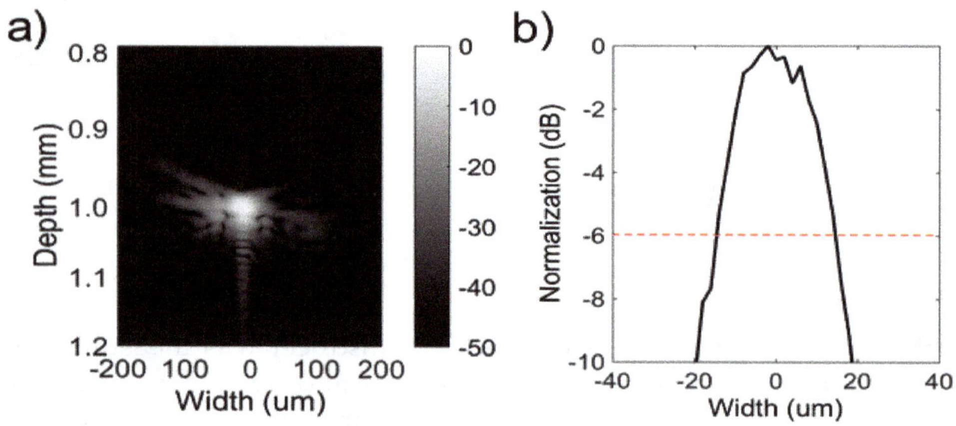

Figure 6. (**a**) Image of 10 μm tungsten wire target; (b) Lateral beam profile of the Co-doped $Na_{0.5}Bi_{4.5}Ti_4O_{15}$ (NBT-Co) transducers.

4. Conclusions

Lead-free NBT-Co ceramics were fabricated and investigated systematically. Based on the prepared NBT-Co ceramics, a high frequency and small *f*-number transducer was designed and fabricated. The fabricated transducer has center frequency of 70.4 MHz, −6 dB bandwidth of 52.7%, and *f*-number close to 1. Axial resolution of 20.8 μm was calculated from the FWHM of the pulse length of the echo, and lateral resolution of 29.8 μm was achieved using tungsten wire imaging. These results illustrate that lead-free NBT-Co ceramics have great potential for high frequency ultrasonic applications.

Author Contributions: C.F., T.Z., C.M.W. and Q.Z. conceived and designed the experiments; D.W., Y.Q. and P.L. performed the experiments; C.F., T.Z and J.C. analyzed the data; D.L., Y.Y. and C.L.W. contributed reagents/materials/analysis tools; C.F. and T.Z. wrote the paper. All authors reviewed the manuscript.

Acknowledgments: Financial support from the National Natural Science Foundations of China (11604251, 11174230), the National Key Project of Intergovernmental Cooperation in International Scientific and Technological Innovation (2016YFE0107900), the Natural Science Foundations of Shannxi Province (2017JQ1006), and Xidian University (XJS16034, XJS17026, JBG161101, JBX171106) , the Fundamental Research Funds of Shandong University (2016JC036, 2017JC032), and a foundation under the Grant No. 2015JMRH0103 are greatly appreciated.

References

1. Pavlin, C.J.; Harasiewicz, K.; Sherar, M.D.; Foster, F.S. Clinical use of ultrasound biomicroscopy. *Ophthalmology* **1991**, *98*, 287–295. [CrossRef]
2. Foster, F.S.; Lockwood, G.R.; Ryan, L.K.; Harasiewicz, K.A.; Berube, L.; Rauth, A.M. Principles and applications of ultrasound backscatter microscopy. *IEEE Trans. Ultrason. Ferroelectr. Freq. Control* **1993**, *40*, 608–617. [CrossRef] [PubMed]
3. Khairy, H.A.; Atta, H.R.; Green, F.D.; Van der Hoek, J.; Azuara-Blanco, A. Ultrasound biomicroscopy in deep sclerectomy. *Eye* **2005**, *19*, 555. [CrossRef] [PubMed]
4. Fei, C.L.; Chiu, C.T.; Chen, X.Y.; Chen, Z.Y.; Ma, J.G.; Zhu, B.P.; Shung, K.K. and Zhou, Q.F. Ultrahigh frequency (100–300MHz) ultrasonic transducers for optical resolution medical imagining. *Sci. Rep.* **2016**, *6*, 20360. [CrossRef] [PubMed]
5. Zhu, B.; Fei, C.; Wang, C.; Zhu, Y.; Yang, X.; Zheng, H.; Zhou, Q.; Shung, K.K. Self-Focused AlScN Film Ultrasound Transducer for Individual Cell Manipulation. *ACS Sens.* **2017**, *2*, 172–177. [CrossRef] [PubMed]
6. Fei, C.; Hsu, H.S.; Vafanejad, A.; Li, Y.; Lin, P.; Li, D.; Yang, Y.; Kim, E.; Shung, K.K.; Zhou, Q. Ultrahigh frequency ZnO silicon lens ultrasonic transducer for cell-size microparticle manipulation. *J. Alloys Compd.* **2017**, *729*, 556–562. [CrossRef]
7. Zhou, Q.F.; Lau, S.; Wu, D.W.; Shung, K.K. Piezoelectric films for high frequency ultrasonic transducers in biomedical applications. *Prog. Mat.Sci.* **2011**, *56*, 139–174. [CrossRef] [PubMed]
8. Zhu, F.; Qiu, J.; Ji, H.; Zhu, K.; Wen, K. Comparative investigations on dielectric, piezoelectric properties and humidity resistance of PZT-SKN and PZT-SNN ceramics. *J. Mater. Sci. Mater. Electron.* **2015**, *26*, 2897–2904. [CrossRef]
9. Zhou, Q.; Lam, K.H.; Zheng, H.; Qiu, W.; Shung, K.K. Piezoelectric single crystal ultrasonic transducers for biomedical applications. *Prog. Mater. Sci.* **2014**, *66*, 87–111. [CrossRef] [PubMed]
10. Saito, Y.; Takao, H.; Tani, T.; Nonoyama, T.; Takatori, K.; Homma, T.; Nagaya, T.; Nakamura, M. Lead-free piezoceramics. *Nature* **2004**, *432*, 84. [CrossRef] [PubMed]
11. Ringgaard, E.; Wurlitzer, T. Lead-free piezoceramics based on alkali niobates. *J. Eur. Ceram. Soc.* **2005**, *25*, 2701–2706. [CrossRef]
12. Maeder, M.D.; Damjanovic, D.; Setter, N. Lead free piezoelectric materials. *J. Electroceram.* **2004**, *13*, 385–392. [CrossRef]
13. Gao, D.; Kwok, K.W.; Lin, D. Microstructure, piezoelectric and ferroelectric properties of Mn-added $Na_{0.5}Bi_{4.5}Ti_4O_{15}$ ceramics. *Curr. Appl. Phys.* **2011**, *11*, S124–S127. [CrossRef]
14. Peng, Z.; Chen, Q.; Wu, J.; Liu, D.; Xiao, D.; Zhu, J. Dielectric properties and impedance analysis in Aurivillius-type ($Na_{0.25}K_{0.25}Bi_{0.5}$) 1 − x (LiCe) x/2 [] x/2$Bi_4Ti_4O_{15}$ ceramics. *J. Alloys Compd.* **2012**, *541*, 310–316.
15. Zhao, T.L.; Guo, Z.L.; Wang, C.M. The Effects of Na/K Ratio on the Electrical Properties of Sodium-Potassium Bismuth Titanate $Na_{0.5}Bi_{4.5}Ti_4O_{15}$-$K_{0.5}Bi_{4.5}Ti_4O_{15}$. *J. Am. Ceram. Soc.* **2012**, *95*, 1062–1067. [CrossRef]
16. Zhao, L.; Xu, J.X.; Yin, N.; Wang, H.C.; Zhang, C.J.; Wang, J.F. Microstructure, dielectric, and piezoelectric properties of Ce-modified $Na_{0.5}Bi_{4.5}Ti_4O_{15}$ high temperature piezoceramics. *Phys. Status Solidi (RRL)-Rapid Res. Lett.* **2008**, *2*, 111–113. [CrossRef]
17. Wang, C.M.; Wang, J.F.; Zhang, S.; Shrout, T.R. Electromechanical properties of a-site (LiCe)-modified sodium bismuth titanate ($Na_{0.5}Bi_{4.5}Ti_4O_{15}$) piezoelectric ceramics at elevated temperature. *J. Appl. Phys.* **2009**, *105*, 094110. [CrossRef]

18. Chen, H.; Shen, B.; Xu, J.; Zhai, J. Textured $Ca_{0.85}(Li, Ce)_{0.15}Bi_4Ti_4O_{15}$ ceramics for high temperature piezoelectric applications. *Mater. Res. Bull.* **2012**, *47*, 2530–2534. [CrossRef]
19. IEEE Standard on Piezoelectricity (ANSI/IEEE Standard No. 176, 1987).

6

Scanning MEMS Mirror for High Definition and High Frame Rate Lissajous Patterns

Yeong-Hyeon Seo [1,2], Kyungmin Hwang [1,2], Hyunwoo Kim [1,2] and Ki-Hun Jeong [1,2,*]

1 Department of Bio and Brain Engineering, KAIST, Daejeon 34141, Korea; yseo@kaist.ac.kr (Y.-H.S.); k.hwang@kaist.ac.kr (K.H.); hkim151@kaist.ac.kr (H.K.)

2 KAIST Institute for Health Science and Technology, Daejeon 34141, Korea

* Correspondence: kjeong@kaist.ac.kr

Abstract: Scanning MEMS (micro-electro-mechanical system) mirrors are attractive given their potential use in a diverse array of laser scanning display and imaging applications. Here we report on an electrostatic MEMS mirror for high definition and high frame rate (HDHF) Lissajous scanning. The MEMS mirror comprised a low Q-factor inner mirror and frame mirror, which provided two-dimensional scanning at two similar resonant scanning frequencies with high mechanical stability. The low Q inner mirror enabled a broad frequency selection range. The high definition and high frame rate (HDHF) Lissajous scanning of the MEMS mirror was achieved by selecting a set of scanning frequencies near its resonance with a high greatest common divisor (GCD) and a high total lobe number. The MEMS mirror had resonant scanning frequencies at 5402 Hz and 6702 Hz in x and y directions, respectively. The selected pseudo-resonant frequencies of 5450 Hz and 6700 Hz for HDHF scanning provided 50 frames per second with 94% fill factor in 256 × 256 pixels. This Lissajous MEMS mirror could be utilized for assorted HDHF laser scanning imaging and display applications.

Keywords: MEMS mirror; Lissajous scanning; pseudo-resonant; sensing; imaging; display

---

1. Introduction

Microscanners play a vital role in various low-power and compact scanning applications, including in display [1–4], sensing [5–8], and biomedical imaging [9–16]. In particular, resonant MEMS (micro-electro-mechanical system) mirrors provide a focus beam with a small size and high energy efficiency at any distance [17–20] and the monolithic fabrication facilitates low-cost commercialization [21,22]. Unlike raster scanning MEMS mirrors, Lissajous MEMS mirrors operate at high scanning frequencies in both axes and also offer simple fabrication [3,23], high mechanical stability [17,24], and uniform scanning quality [21,25]. However, in MEMS mirrors, there is still a trade-off between the frame rate (FR) and the fill factor (FF) for high quality laser scanning.

This trade-off relationship restricts the implementation of high definition and high frame rate (HDHF) Lissajous scanning. The FF increases as the ratio of two scanning frequencies becomes more complex, whereas the pattern repeat rate is lessened. Full-repeated Lissajous scanning often has a low frame rate, which is determined by the pattern repeat rate. In contrast, non-repeated Lissajous scanning provides a higher frame rate than the pattern repeat rate [26]. However, non-repeated scanning exacerbates the trade-off relationship between the FF and the FR. Besides, the frame rate can be determined by the ratio of two scanning frequencies [2,3], but the frame rate is usually a non-integer. The resonant frequency of Lissajous MEMS mirrors is highly dependent on the physical dimension and, thus, an integer frame rate is barely obtained due to the microfabrication tolerance. Furthermore, some technical artifacts, such as flickering phenomenon, occur [2]. Recently, the frequency selection rule for HDHF Lissajous scanning has been reported to overcome the trade-off relationship [27]. The FR increases the greatest common divisor (GCD), while the FF increases with the total lobe number, i.e., divided by the sum of two scanning frequencies as the GCD of the two scanning frequencies. The frequency selection should satisfy a high GCD and high total lobe number results in HDHF Lissajous scanning. HDHF Lissajous scanning with 10 frames per seconds and 92% fill factor was demonstrated with a 1 kHz scanning frequency. HDHF Lissajous scanning has been successfully implemented in PZT (piezo-tube) fiber scanners; however, it has not yet been achieved with MEMS mirrors. PZT fiber scanners have been widely used for endomicroscopic applications [16,28,29]; however, they still have some technical limitations including a high cost and the need for further miniaturization. The conventional Lissajous mirror has a high Q-factor, which substantially changes the scanning amplitude depending on the scanning frequency. For this reason, the conv-entional Lissajous mirror still has technical limitations for HDHF Lissajous scanning applications.

Here we report an electrostatic MEMS mirror capable of high definition and high frame rate (HDHF) Lissajous scanning. Figure 1 indicates a schematic illustration of the high definition and high frame rate (HDHF) Lissajous MEMS scanner. The HDHF Lissajous MEMS mirror features an inner mirror with a low Q-factor, which allowed a broad selection range of scanning frequencies. A low Q-factor of the inner mirror was realized by using a thin and short torsion bar. The selection of scanning frequencies at pseudo-resonance with a high GCD and high total lobe number (N, $(f_x + f_y)/\text{GCD}$), which is larger than the minimum total lobe number (N_{min}) for the targeted FF, allowed HDHF Lissajous scanning. Note that f_x and f_y infer the resonant frequencies of the inner mirror and frame mirror, respectively, whilst f_x' and f_y' infer the selected scanning frequencies of the inner mirror and frame mirror, respectively, as determined by the frequency selection rule.

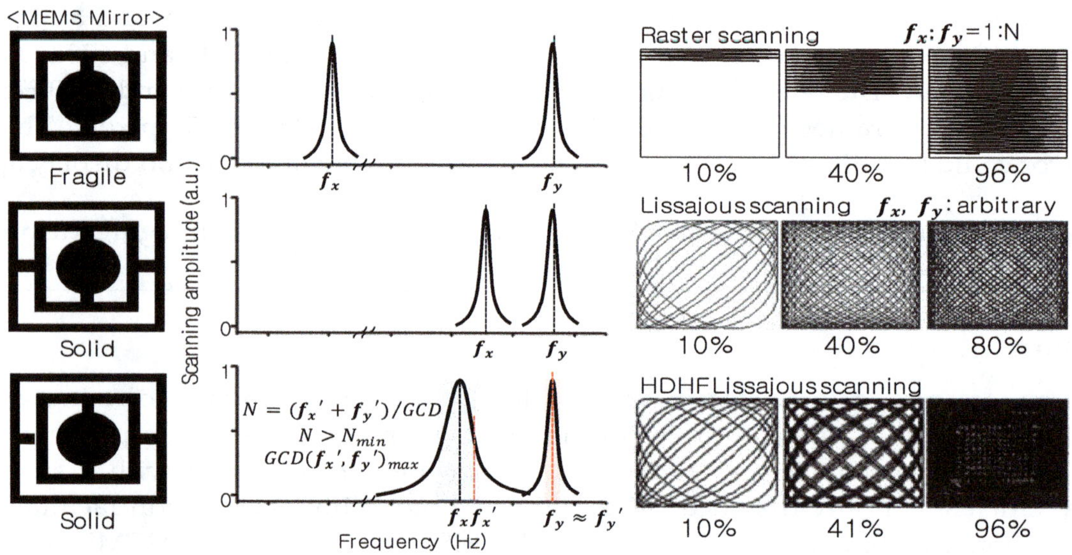

Figure 1. A schematic illustration of the high definition, high frame rate (HDHF) Lissajous MEMS mirror. A conventional raster MEMS mirror provides two-dimensional (2D) scanning with a ratio of two frequencies of 1:N and a torsional micromirror usually requires a flexible micro-spring. Unlike raster scanning MEMS mirrors, conventional Lissajous MEMS mirrors have high mechanical stability. Conventional Lissajous mirrors also have a high Q factor, which derives a substantial change of the scanning amplitude depending on the scanning frequency. In contrast, the HDHF Lissajous MEMS mirror features an inner mirror with a low Q-factor, which allowed a broad selection range of scanning frequencies. The selection of scanning frequencies at pseudo-resonance with a high greatest common divisor (GCD) and a high total lobe number (N, $(f_x + f_y)/\text{GCD}$), which is larger than the minimum total lobe number (N_{min}) for the targeted FF, enabled HDHF Lissajous scanning. Since the designed MEMS mirror is for 2D laser scanning, biaxial scanning frequencies had to be selected. Note that f_x and f_y infer the resonant frequencies of the inner mirror and the frame mirror, respectively. In addition, biaxial scanning frequencies are defined as f_x' and f_y', which infer the selected freque-ncies of the inner mirror and frame mirror, respectively, determined by the frequency selection rule.

2. Device Fabrication and Characterization

The microfabrication procedure of the Lissajous MEMS mirror is described in Figure 2a. A MEMS mirror was fabricated using a 6-inch SOI wafer (silicon-on-insulator wafer, top Si: 30 μm, buried oxide (BOX) layer: 2 μm, bottom Si: 400 μm) with high conductivity (resistivity: 0.01–0.02 Ω·cm). Firstly, the top silicon layer was defined by deep reactive ion etching (DRIE) and refilled with silicon dioxide through wet oxidation and poly-silicon by low pressure chemical vapor deposition (LPCVD). The front side was flattened using chemical mechanical polishing (CMP), followed by the thermal evaporation of a 200-Å-thick titanium and 1000-Å-thick gold film. The Au electrode pads were patterned with a wet-etch process. The top silicon layer and bottom silicon layers were etched down to define the MEMS mirrors with a backside opening using DRIE. A buried oxide layer of the opening area was removed in buffered oxide etchant (BOE) to release the MEMS mirror. The remaining photoresist layers were clearly stripped out by using oxygen plasma. Individual MEMS mirrors were completely detached from the SOI wafer using the fused-tether method with Y-shape tethers with a width of 4 μm [30]. Figure 2b shows a scheme of the electrical layout of the MEMS mirror. Gray, red, and blue indicate the driving voltage of the inner mirror, the driving voltage of the frame mirror, and the ground, respectively. Figure 2c indicates a top SEM image of the fabricated Lissajous MEMS mirror (scale bar: 200 μm). The physical dimensions of the MEMS mirror were 1.2 × 1.2 × 0.43 mm^3. Figure 2d,e show the perspective SEM images of the comb drives of the inner mirror and the frame mirror, respectively. The widths of the torsion bar were 2.8 μm and 8.8 μm in the inner mirror and the frame mirror, respectively. The Q-factor was determined by the flexure width, height, and length of the MEMS mirror. A thin torsion bar provided a low Q-factor for the inner mirror, which made a broad frequency tuning range [31]. The effective stiffness and the resonant frequencies of the Lissajous MEMS mirror were calculated using finite element analysis (COMSOL Multi-physics® ver. 5.3). The MEMS mirror provided a high yield (95% yield, 2000 mirrors in a 6-inch wafer).

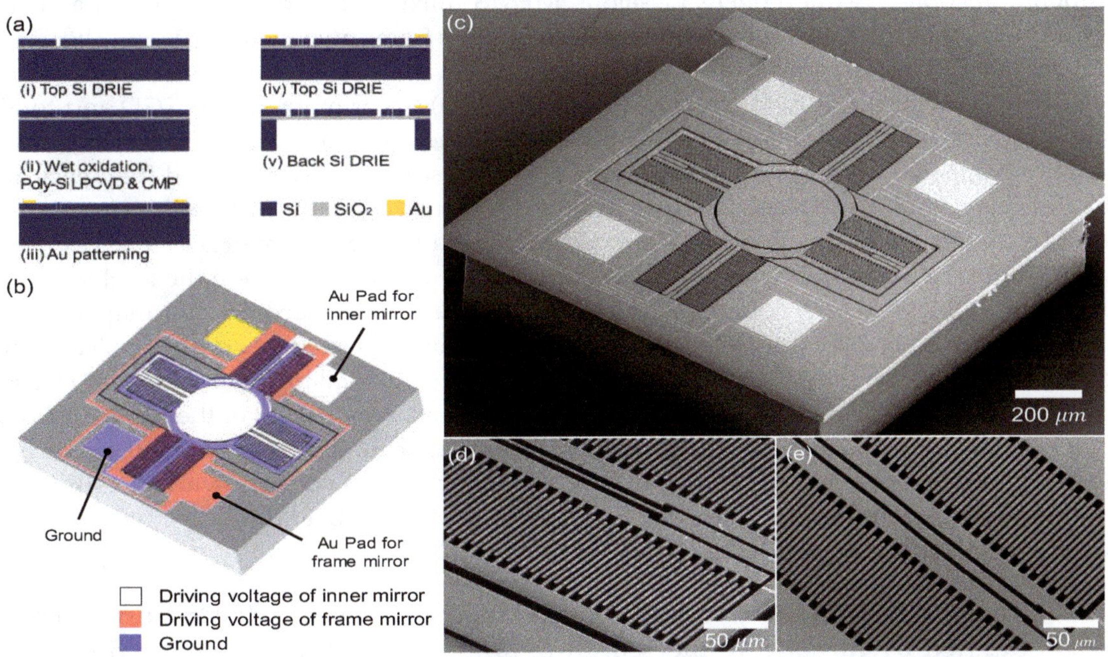

Figure 2. Microfabrication procedure and SEM images of HDHF Lissajous MEMS mirror. (**a**) Microfabrication procedure. The MEMS mirror was fabricated using a 6-inch SOI wafer with high conductivity. (**b**) A schematic of the electrical layout of the MEMS mirror. (**c**) Top SEM image of the microfabricated HDHF Lissajous MEMS mirror (scale bar: 200 μm). The physical dimensions of the MEMS mirror were 1.2 × 1.2 × 0.43 mm^3. (**d–e**) Perspective SEM images of the comb drives of the inner mirror and the frame mirror, respectively (scale bar: 50 μm). The widths of the torsion bar were 2.8 μm and 8.8 μm in the inner mirror and the frame mirror, respectively.

3. Scanning Frequency Selection for HDHF Lissajous Scanning

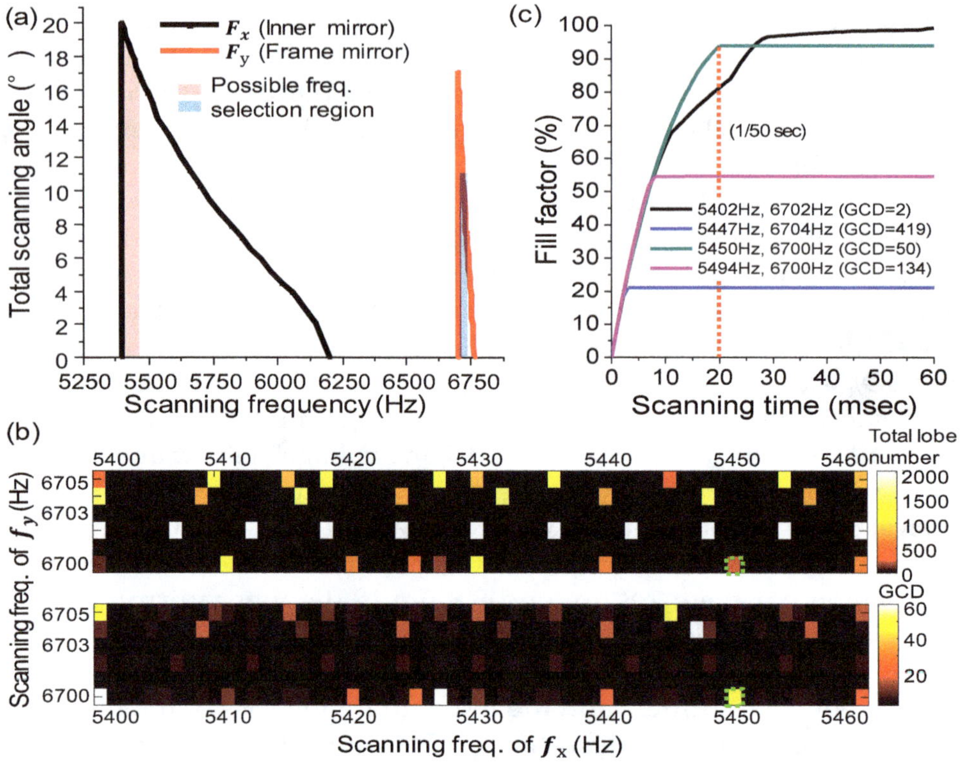

Figure 3. Scanning properties and scanning frequency selection for HDHF Lissajous scanning. (**a**) Frequency response of the HDHF Lissajous MEMS mirror. The MEMS mirror has resonant frequencies at 5402 Hz and 6702 Hz in the inner mirror and the frame mirror, respectively. The frequency tuning range should be larger than the greatest common divisor (GCD) frame rate. The inner mirror features a low Q-factor (Q = 18) for frequency selection. (**b**) Color maps of the GCD and total lobe number for selecting scanning frequency along biaxial frequency domain. High GCD and high total lobe number allow high definition and high frame rate Lissajous scanning. The selected frequency sets for HDHF Lissajous scanning should satisfy the requirements for both a high GCD and high lobe number. For instance, based on the frequency selection rule, the fill factor was over 85% at256 × 256 pixel resolution, while the total lobe number was 237 or more. Frequency sets where the total lobe number was greater than 237 in the first color map were selected. Next, in the second color map, a frequency set with the higher GCD value was selected from the previously selected frequency set. The scanning frequencies were determined as 5450 Hz and 6700 Hz (GCD = 50, total lobe number = 243) for HDHF Lissajous scanning. HDHF frequency set was selected within the range of 1% of the resonant frequency. (**c**) Calculated fill factor (FF) of the MEMS mirror along the scanning time. The fill factor initially increased with time; however, the maximum FF and the convergence time varied with the set of selected scanning frequencies. The scanning frequencies of 5450 Hz and 6700 Hz provide a single Lissajous figure of 94% in FF at every 1/50 s.

Figure 3a indicates the frequency response of the HDHF Lissajous MEMS mirror. The frequency response was obtained by measuring the scanning angle of the MEMS mirror depending on the operation frequency. The MEMS mirror had a resonant frequency at 5402 Hz and 6702 Hz in the inner mirror and the frame mirror, respectively. The total scanning angles were 20° and 18° with 40 V_{pp} operation voltages in the inner mirror and the frame mirror, respectively. The inner mirror featured a low Q-factor (Q = 18) for a broad band selection of scanning frequency. The Q-factor is calculated as $Q = f_r/\Delta f_{fwhm}$ (f_r: resonant frequency, Δf_{fwhm}: the full width at half maximum). The scanning frequencies were selected at the frequencies with a 0.7 dB bandwidth. Figure 3b shows the color maps of the GCD and the total lobe number with the different scanning frequencies. A high GCD and high lobe number play a significant role when selecting the frequency sets for HDHF Lissajous scanning. In order to acquire a fill factor over 85% at 256 × 256 pixel resolution, the required total lobe number based on the frequency selection rule should be greater than 237. The first color map in Figure 3b selects the frequency sets where the total lobe number is greater than 237. The second color map in Figure 3b selects the frequency set with the highest GCD value among the selected frequency sets in the first color map. The scanning frequencies were determined as 5450 Hz and 6700 Hz (GCD = 50, total lobe number = 243) for HDHF Lissajous scanning. Figure 3c shows a calculated fill factor (FF) along the scanning time. The convergence time and the maximum fill factor were apparently different as the scanning frequencies changed, while the FF increased with time. The selected scanning frequencies of 5450 Hz and 6700 Hz provided HDHF scanning (94% fill factor at 1/50 s).

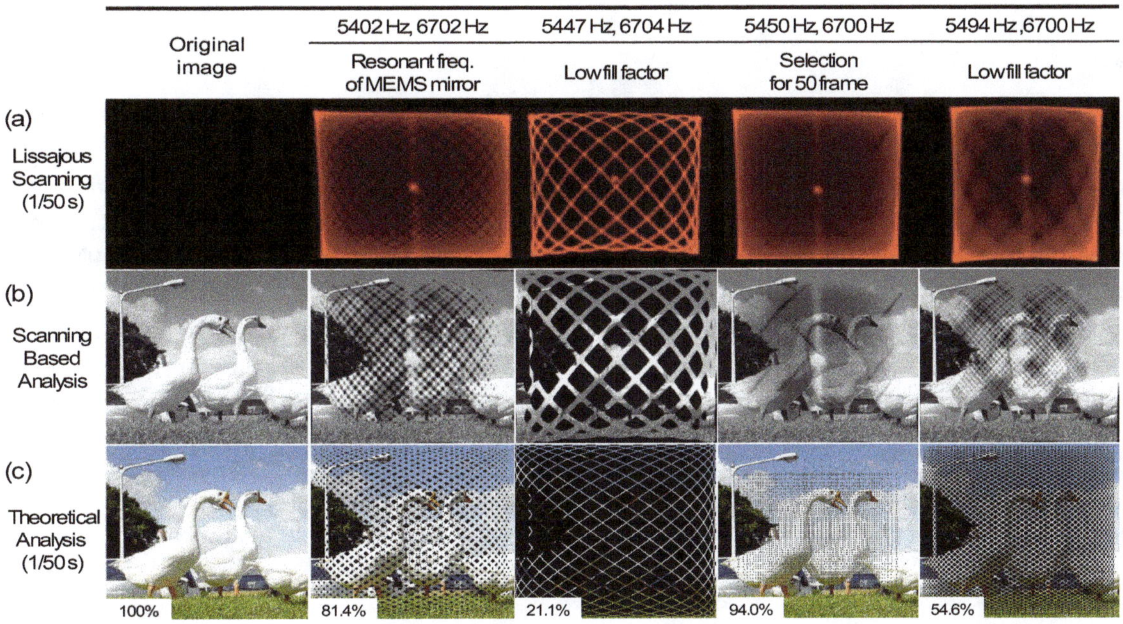

Figure 4. Lissajous scanning patterns and theoretical trajectory depending on different scanning frequencies. (**a**) Optical images of the Lissajous scanning patterns depending on different scanning frequencies (1/50 s). (**b**) Pattern-projected image of the geese. The Lissajous scanning pattern of (a) was projected onto the image of geese. (**c**) Theoretical analysis of Lissajous laser trajectory depending on different scanning frequencies at 1/50 s. Simulation was conducted using MATLAB R2017a and the source image had a 256 × 256 pixel resolution. Compared to resonance scanning, scanning at the selected frequencies of 5450 Hz and 6700 Hz provided a high fill factor with a high frame rate.

Figure 4a shows optical images of Lissajous scanning patterns at different sets of scanning frequencies (1/50 s). Scanning patterns were obtained at scanning frequencies of 5402 Hz/6702 Hz, 5447 Hz/6704 Hz, 5450 Hz/6700 Hz, and 5494 Hz/6700 Hz, respectively. Scanning at the selected frequencies of 5450 Hz and 6700 Hz provided a high fill factor, compared to other frequencies, including the resonant frequency. Figure 4b shows a pattern-projected image of the geese, wherein the Lissajous scanning pattern of Figure 4a was projected onto the image of geese. Figure 4c shows a theoretical analysis of the Lissajous laser projected image at 1/50 s. The simulation was conducted using MATLAB R2017a. The Lissajous pattern with two scanning frequencies was tracked through 256 × 256 pixels for 1/50 s and then overlapped with the image. The Lissajous scan trajectory gradually filled with time, and the fill factor at the selected frequencies of 5450 Hz and 6700 Hz reached up to 94% in 1/50 s. Compared to the resonance scanning, pseudo-resonant scanning at the selected frequencies provided a high fill factor with a high frame rate. In addition, Tables 1 and 2 show assorted sets of HDHF scanning for 256 × 256 and 1280 × 720 pixel resolutions, respectively. The HDHF MEMS mirror clearly provides a wide tuning range, as well as various frame rates with a high fill factor.

Table 1. A set of scanning frequencies with different frame rates and fill factors for 256 × 256 pixels.

Frequency (Hz)	5408/6704	5420/6700	5425/6700	5450/6700	5427/6700
Greatest common divisor (GCD) (frame rate (FR))	16	20	25	50	67
Fill factor (%)	100	98	100	94	84

Table 2. A set of scanning frequencies with different frame rates and fill factors for 1280 × 720 pixels.

Frequency (Hz)	5400/6702	5400/6708	5410/6700	5408/6704	5420/6700
GCD (FR)	6	8	10	16	20
Fill factor (%)	100	100	100	90	52

4. Summary

In summary, we have successfully demonstrated HDHF Lissajous MEMS mirrors. The Lissajous MEMS mirror had a low Q-factor for the inner mirror for a broad frequency tuning range, as well as similar resonant frequencies in the inner mirror and the frame mirror, with high mechanical stability. The MEMS mirror had resonant frequencies at 5402 Hz and 6702 Hz in the inner mirror and the frame mirror, respectively. The total scanning angles were 20° and 18° with 40 V_{pp} operation voltages in the inner mirror and the frame mirror, respectively. High definition and high frame rate (HDHF) Lissajous scanning was successfully realized by applying the scanning frequency selection. The controlled Lissajous MEMS mirror provided a 94% fill factor at 50 frames per second for 256 × 256 pixels. In addition, diverse sets of HDHF scanning were demonstrated for potential use in various applications. HDHF Lissajous MEMS mirrors can be utilized for assorted laser scanning-based imaging and display applications.

Author Contributions: Y.-H.S. and K.-H.J. designed the project, analyzed data, and wrote the manuscript. K.H. and H.K. analyzed the results. K.-H.J. supervised the project. All authors discussed the results and commented on the manuscript.

Acknowledgments: This work was supported by the Ministry of Science and ICT (2018029899), the Global Frontier Project (2011-0031848), and the Korea Health Industry Development Institute (KHIDI, HI13C2181) funded by the Ministry of Health and Welfare, Korea.

References

1. Hofmann, U.; Janes, J.; Quenzer, H.-J. High-Q MEMS Resonators for Laser Beam Scanning Displays. *Micromachines* **2012**, *3*, 509–528. [CrossRef]
2. Hofmann, U.; Senger, F.; Janes, J.; Mallas, C.; Stenchly, V.; von Wantoch, T.; Quenzer, H.-J.; Weiss, M. Wafer-level vacuum-packaged two-axis MEMS scanning mirror for pico-projector application. *Proc. SPIE* **2014**, *8977*, 89770A. [CrossRef]
3. Hung, A.C.L.; Lai, H.Y.H.; Lin, T.W.; Fu, S.G.; Lu, M.S.C. An electrostatically driven 2D micro-scanning mirror with capacitive sensing for projection display. *Sens. Actuators A Phys.* **2015**, *222*, 122–129. [CrossRef]
4. Yalcinkaya, A.D.; Urey, H.; Brown, D.; Montague, T.; Sprague, R. Two-axis electromagnetic microscanner for high resolution displays. *J. Microelectromech. Syst.* **2006**, *15*, 786–794. [CrossRef]
5. Wang, D.; Strassle, S.; Stainsby, A.; Bai, Y.; Koppal, S.; Xie, H. A compact 3D lidar based on an electrothermal two-axis MEMS scanner for small UAV. In Proceedings of the SPIE Defense + Security, Orlando, FL, USA, 17–19 April 2018; p. 7.
6. Zhang, X.; Koppal, S.J.; Zhang, R.; Zhou, L.; Butler, E.; Xie, H. Wide-angle structured light with a scanning MEMS mirror in liquid. *Opt. Express* **2016**, *24*, 3479–3487. [CrossRef] [PubMed]
7. Petitgrand, S.; Yahiaoui, R.; Danaie, K.; Bosseboeuf, A.; Gilles, J.P. 3D measurement of micromechanical devices vibration mode shapes with a stroboscopic interferometric microscope. *Opt. Lasers Eng.* **2001**, *36*, 77–101. [CrossRef]

8. Chudnovsky, A.; Golberg, A.; Linzon, Y. Monitoring complex monosaccharide mixtures derived from macroalgae biomass by combined optical and microelectromechanical techniques. *Proc. Biochem.* **2018**, *68*, 136–145. [CrossRef]
9. Seo, Y.-H.; Hwang, K.; Jeong, K.-H. 1.65 mm diameter forward-viewing confocal endomicroscopic catheter using a flip-chip bonded electrothermal MEMS fiber scanner. *Opt. Express* **2018**, *26*, 4780–4785. [CrossRef]
10. Hwang, K.; Seo, Y.-H.; Jeong, K.-H. Microscanners for optical endomicroscopic applications. *Micro Nano Syst. Lett.* **2017**, *5*, 1. [CrossRef]
11. Piyawattanametha, W.; Ra, H.; Qiu, Z.; Friedland, S.; Liu, J.T.C.; Loewke, K.; Kino, G.S.; Solgaard, O.; Wang, T.D.; Mandella, M.J.; et al. In vivo near-infrared dual-axis confocal microendoscopy in the human lower gastrointestinal tract. *J. Biomed. Opt.* **2012**, *17*, 021102. [CrossRef]
12. Jung, W.; Tang, S.; McCormic, D.T.; Xie, T.; Ahn, Y.-C.; Su, J.; Tomov, I.V.; Krasieva, T.B.; Tromberg, B.J.; Chen, Z. Miniaturized probe based on a microelectromechanical system mirror for multiphoton microscopy. *Opt. Lett.* **2008**, *33*, 1324–1326. [CrossRef] [PubMed]
13. Dickensheets, D.L.; Kino, G.S. Micromachined scanning confocal optical microscope. *Opt. Lett.* **1996**, *21*, 764–766. [CrossRef]
14. Rivera, D.R.; Brown, C.M.; Ouzounov, D.G.; Pavlova, I.; Kobat, D.; Webb, W.W.; Xu, C. Compact and flexible raster scanning multiphoton endoscope capable of imaging unstained tissue. *Proc. Natl. Acad. Sci. USA* **2011**, *108*, 17598–17603. [CrossRef] [PubMed]
15. Seo, Y.-H.; Hwang, K.; Park, H.-C.; Jeong, K.-H. Electrothermal MEMS fiber scanner for optical endomicroscopy. *Opt. Express* **2016**, *24*, 3903–3909. [CrossRef]
16. Park, H.-C.; Seo, Y.-H.; Jeong, K.-H. Lissajous fiber scanning for forward viewing optical endomicroscopy using asymmetric stiffness modulation. *Opt. Express* **2014**, *22*, 5818–5825. [CrossRef]
17. Holmström, S.T.S.; Baran, U.; Urey, H. MEMS Laser Scanners: A Review. *J. Microelectromech. Syst.* **2014**, *23*, 259–275. [CrossRef]
18. Morrison, J.; Imboden, M.; Little, T.D.; Bishop, D. Electrothermally actuated tip-tilt-piston micromirror with integrated varifocal capability. *Opt. Express* **2015**, *23*, 9555–9566. [CrossRef]
19. Hah, D.; Patterson, P.R.; Nguyen, H.D.; Toshiyoshi, H.; Wu, M.C. Theory and experiments of angular vertical comb-drive actuators for scanning micromirrors. *IEEE J. Sel. Top. Quantum Electron.* **2004**, *10*, 505–513. [CrossRef]
20. Urey, H. Torsional MEMS scanner design for high-resolution display systems. *Opt. Scanning II Proc. SPIE* **2002**, *4773*, 27–37. [CrossRef]
21. Schenk, H.; Dürr, P.; Kunze, D.; Lakner, H.; Kück, H. A Resonantly excited 2D-micro-scanning-mirror with large deflection. *Sens. Actuators A Phys.* **2001**, *89*, 104–111. [CrossRef]
22. Kim, J.; Christensen, D.; Lin, L. Monolithic 2-D scanning mirror using self-aligned angular vertical comb drives. *IEEE Photonics Technol. Lett.* **2005**, *17*, 2307–2309. [CrossRef]
23. Arslan, A.; Brown, D.; Davis, W.O.; Holmström, S.; Gokce, S.K.; Urey, H. Comb-actuated resonant torsional microscanner with mechanical amplification. *J. Microelectromech. Syst.* **2010**, *19*, 936–943. [CrossRef]
24. Cho, A.R.; Han, A.; Ju, S.; Jeong, H.; Park, J.-H.; Kim, I.; Bu, J.-U.; Ji, C.-H. Electromagnetic biaxial microscanner with mechanical amplification at resonance. *Opt. Express* **2015**, *23*, 16792–16802. [CrossRef] [PubMed]
25. Urey, H.; Wine, D.W.; Osborn, T.D. Optical performance requirements for MEMS-scanner-based microdisplays. *Proc. SPIE* **2000**, *4178*, 176–185. [CrossRef]
26. Hoy, C.L.; Durr, N.J.; Ben-Yakar, A. Fast-updating and nonrepeating Lissajous image reconstruction method for capturing increased dynamic information. *Appl. Opt.* **2011**, *50*, 2376–2382. [CrossRef]
27. Hwang, K.; Seo, Y.H.; Ahn, J.; Kim, P.; Jeong, K.H. Frequency selection rule for high definition and high frame rate Lissajous scanning. *Sci. Rep.* **2017**, *7*, 1–8. [CrossRef] [PubMed]
28. Liu, X.; Cobb, M.J.; Chen, Y.; Kimmey, M.B.; Li, X. Rapid-scanning forward-imaging miniature endoscope for real-time optical coherence tomography. *Opt. Lett.* **2004**, *29*, 1763–1765. [CrossRef] [PubMed]
29. Park, H.-C.; Seo, Y.-H.; Hwang, K.; Lim, J.-K.; Yoon, S.Z.; Jeong, K.-H. Micromachined tethered silicon oscillator for an endomicroscopic Lissajous fiber scanner. *Opt. Lett.* **2014**, *39*, 6675–6678. [CrossRef]

30. Chiu, Y.-S.S.; Chang, K.-S.J.; Johnstone, R.W.; Parameswaran, M. Fuse-tethers in MEMS. *J. Micromech. Microeng.* **2006**, *16*, 480. [CrossRef]
31. Jiunn-Horng, L.; Sheng-Ta, L.; Chih-Min, Y.; Weileun, F. Comments on the size effect on the microcantilever quality factor in free air space. *J. Micromech. Microeng.* **2007**, *17*, 139.

7

Micro-Optical Components for Bioimaging on Tissues, Cells and Subcellular Structures

Hui Yang [1,*], Yi Zhang [2], Sihui Chen [1] and Rui Hao [1,3]

1 Laboratory of Biomedical Microsystems and Nano Devices, Bionic Sensing and Intelligence Center, Institute of Biomedical and Health Engineering, Shenzhen Institutes of Advanced Technology, Chinese Academy of Sciences, Shenzhen 518055, China; sh.chen@siat.ac.cn (S.C.); rui.hao@siat.ac.cn (R.H.)
2 Institute of Biomedical Therapeutics, University of Southern California, Los Angeles, CA 90033, USA; zhangelliot@gmail.com
3 Pen-Tung Sah Institute of Micro-Nano Science and Technology, Xiamen University, Xiamen 361005, China
* Correspondence: hui.yang@siat.ac.cn

Abstract: Bioimaging generally indicates imaging techniques that acquire biological information from living forms. Among different imaging techniques, optical microscopy plays a predominant role in observing tissues, cells and biomolecules. Along with the fast development of microtechnology, developing miniaturized and integrated optical imaging systems has become essential to provide new imaging solutions for point-of-care applications. In this review, we will introduce the basic micro-optical components and their fabrication technologies first, and further emphasize the development of integrated optical systems for in vitro and in vivo bioimaging, respectively. We will conclude by giving our perspectives on micro-optical components for bioimaging applications in the near future.

Keywords: micro-optics; bioimaging; microtechnology; microelectromechanical systems (MEMS); in vitro; in vivo

1. Introduction

Nowadays, bioimaging has enabled us to dig out biological information from deep inside of our bodies, and also revolutionized the way we understand, detect, and treat diseases in different angles and dimensions. In the past couple of decades, the thriving of digital computing has paved the way for a wide variety of imaging techniques, including ultrasound, computed tomography (CT), magnetic resonance imaging (MRI), etc. [1]. Through different mediums other than light, these imaging modalities can harvest spatiotemporal parameters from living organisms such as concentration, tissue functionality, anatomical morphology. Modern clinics utilize these different imaging modalities to acquire metabolic and anatomical information from a patient. Against lung tumors and bone metastasis, CT has been extensively used given its short imaging time and high spatial resolution. The co-registration of microCT imaging and volumetric decomposition has proven valuable to study cell trafficking, tumor growth, trabecular bone microarchitecture, and response to therapy in vivo [2]. However, it is not often used in soft tissue scans since the X-ray absorption is rather low in soft tissue, fat, neurons, hence yielding low resolution and inaccuracy in diagnosis [3]. As a complementary method, MRI has its unique advantages in monitoring soft tissue abnormality, brain and neural activity. Specifically, different research objects are most well-fitted correspond to distinctive modalities. By functional MRI (fMRI), the metabolism of neural function can be revealed by mapping the contrast variation in blood flow in response to specific stimulus [4]. Magnetic resonance spectroscopy (MRS) has the ability to identify various biochemical markers of neoplasm in isolated voxels which are three-dimensional pixels, and therefore has been successfully employed in regard to brain, breast, and prostate cancer [5–7]. While the hazards of radiation and strong magnetic field are now well-controlled in most medical contexts, ultrasound imaging proposes a substitute with low health risks. Using acoustic pulses to reflect the contrast between different tissues and objects, ultrasound imaging has had a tremendous impact in hemodynamics and inflammatory study in the past decade [8]. Recent novel use of microbubbles or nanoparticles as indicators has allowed ultrasound to monitor and regulate on molecular level [9,10].

Besides these imaging techniques, as researchers further acquire enhanced resolution in both clinical and experimental imaging applications, optical microscopy plays a predominant role in observing tissues, cells and biomolecules, as this visualization technique has been able to literally and figuratively illuminate the inner workings of cells, for example by using fluorescent probes to light up proteins and subcellular structures. Leveraging the characteristic emissions of biological fluorophores, optical imaging technique is possible to gain insights on cell structures and functions [11]. Moreover, since the emission diffraction barrier, i.e., the conventional resolution limit, can be overcome by stimulated emission depletion (STED) microscopy etc., researchers can now image fluorophore-labelled systems with a resolution of 15 nm, i.e., 3000 times smaller than the width of a single human hair [12–14].

Along with the fast development of microtechnology, there is an intensive demand on developing miniaturized and integrated optical imaging systems. Over the last decade, a fast-growing interest was notice for developing microdevices that integrate one or several optical functionalities/components onto a single chip with size being of only millimeter-size up to a few square centimeters in size [15]. These optical microdevices have shown great potential on imaging living organisms, tissues, cells, as well as subcellular structures, both in vivo and in vitro. The in vivo imaging is usually achieved by integrating such microdevices into imaging instruments, e.g., endoscopy and optical coherence tomography (OCT) instruments. While the in vitro imaging can be performed by using microfluidic devices, the latter can provide prominent advantages on sample pre-treatment and handling. In these review, we focus on recent developments in the realization and use of micro-optical components for bioimaging applications. Typical micro-optical components used in bioimaging instruments are introduced at first, enabling us to sketch a blueprint of today's integrated imaging systems. Different technologies for the fabrication of micro-optical components are demonstrated. We further present the integration of these micro-optical components with instruments or devices for in vitro and in vivo bioimaging, respectively. We will conclude by giving our perspective on bioimaging with micro-optical components, especially on how this technology will impact modern biological/clinical study. We hope the review provides the reader with some orientation in the field and enables selecting platforms with appropriate characteristics for his/her application-specific requirement.

2. Micro-optical Components

Based on basic optical principles, one can classify micro-optical components into (i) refractive optical components that rely on the change of the refractive index at an interface, such as lenses, prisms and mirrors, (ii) diffractive optical structures that enable shaping of an optical beam by diffractive/interference effects, such as diffraction gratings, and (iii) hybrid (refractive/diffractive) structures. Refractive and diffractive optical components share many similarities when they are used to manipulate monochromatic light but their response to broadband light is very different. For a material with normal dispersion, refractive lenses have larger focal distances for red light than for blue light and prisms deflect longer wavelengths by a smaller angle; the contrary occurs for diffractive lenses and gratings. This contrasting behavior arises because two different principles are used to shape the light: refractive optics relies on the phase that is gradually accumulated through propagation, while diffractive optics operates by means of interference of light transmitted through an amplitude or phase mask. The decision to use diffractive or refractive optics for a specific optical problem depends on many parameters, e.g., the spectrum of the light source, the aimed optical application (beam shaping, imaging, etc.), the efficiency required, the acceptable straylight, etc. Arbitrary wavefronts can be generated very accurately by diffractive optics. A drawback for many applications is the strong wavelength-dependence. Diffractive optics is therefore mostly used with laser light and for non-conventional imaging tasks, like beam shaping, diffusers, filters and detectors. Refractive optical elements have in general higher efficiency and less stray light, even though in some cases it is more difficult to make refractive lenses with precise focal lengths or aspheric shapes. Moreover, for broadband applications, diffractive optical elements (DOEs) can be combined with refractive optics to correct for the chromatic aberration. This combination allows systems with low weight or which consist of only one material. In this section, we introduce in the following the most commonly used micro-optical components in bioimaging systems, categorized by their functionalities, including waveguides, mirrors and lenses.

2.1. Waveguides

An optical waveguide is a physical structure that transmits light along its axis, which is generally composed of a core with a cladding part. A planar optical waveguide is fabricated in a flat format and is particularly interesting to integrate into an imaging system. Recent research works have shown the great potential of optical waveguides in photonic integrated circuits based on high refractive index contrast (HIC) between the core and the cladding. Spiral waveguide geometries in HIC waveguides can be used to significantly increase the interaction length between the sample and the evanescent field of the waveguide [16], opening opportunities to develop, e.g., chip-based nanoscopy [17] and on-chip OCT [18]. Due to its suitable material properties and the compatibility of its fabrication process with standard complementary metal–oxide–semiconductor (CMOS) fabrication line, silicon nitride (Si_3N_4) has attracted the maximum attention. The suitable material property of Si_3N_4 includes transparency in visible wavelength, low absorption and high refractive index contrast to the cladding layer (typically SiO_2). Being transparent with low auto-fluorescence and low absorption in the visible range makes Si_3N_4 compatible with fluorescence techniques for bioimaging.

Tinguely et al. presented the usage of a Si_3N_4 waveguide platform for integrated optical microscopy for in vitro bioimaging applications [19]. A SiO_2 layer was first grown thermally on a silicon chip, followed by the deposition of Si_3N_4 layer using low-pressure chemical vapor deposition (LPCVD). Standard photolithography was employed to define the waveguide geometry using photoresist, and reactive ion etching (RIE) used to fabricate a waveguide rib of given height. The remaining photoresist was removed, and finally a top cladding layer was deposited by plasma-enhanced chemical vapor deposition (LPCVD). This low-loss Si_3N_4 waveguide platform was used to set up an evanescent field for total internal reflection fluorescence (TIRF) microscopy. The sample placed directly on top of the chip was illuminated by the evanescent field of the optical waveguide (Figure 1). In such waveguide chip-based microscopy, the illumination and collection light paths can be efficiently decoupled, opening several opportunities for bioimaging, e.g., on living cells [19] and on single molecules with super-resolution capability [17]. Besides, as the evanescent field is generated along the entire length of the waveguide, a low magnification objective lens can be employed to acquire TIRF images over a large field-of-view of even millimeter range. Moreover, as the evanescent field decays exponentially at the interface between the biological sample and the waveguide, only a thin, typically 100–200 nm section away from the surface can be illuminated, providing a high signal-to-noise ratio by reducing the background signal.

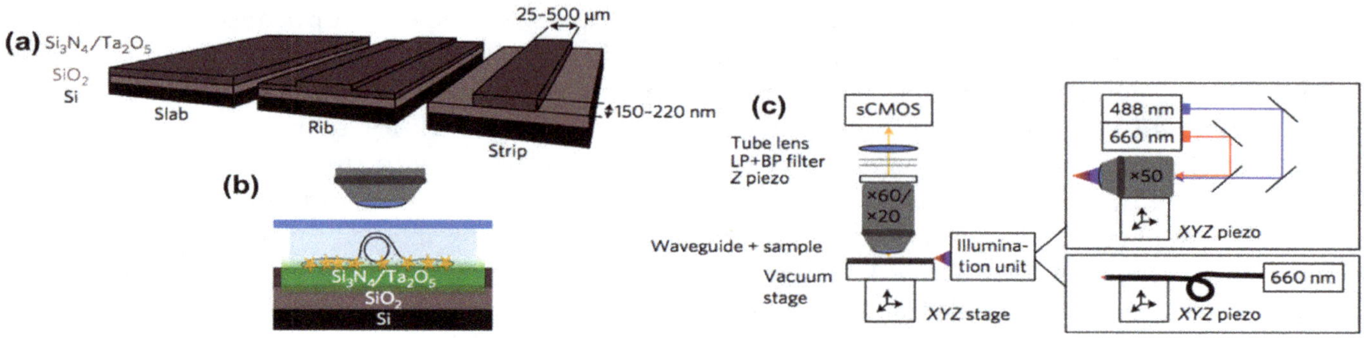

Figure 1. Schematic of the waveguide platform: (**a**) Channel-like waveguide geometries are realized by etching the SiO_2 slab waveguide either partially or completely; (**b**) Light guided inside the waveguide is the source of the evanescent field illuminating samples on top of the surface; (**c**) The optical set-up.

2.2. Mirrors

The effectiveness of microelectromechanical systems (MEMS) in biomedical imaging has been demonstrated in many research findings, where micromirrors used for beam deflection and shaping are one of the core components [20,21]. Commercially available deformable micromirrors that employ MEMS technology are now a common method of reducing astigmatisms and aberrations, increasing the resolution of the imaging system [22]. Micromirrors capable of dynamic focus as well as two-dimensional (2D) scanning have been fully integrated [21]. Such devices rely on electrostatic actuation for both focus and beam deflection. Imaging systems integrated with micromirrors can either work by scanning the micromirror in the form of a raster, or by using a Lissajous scan format. The raster scan uses a fast axis and perpendicular slow axis simultaneously to form a uniform projection area, while the Lissajous scan is performed by exciting a bi-directional mirror at resonance along two perpendicular axes. Comparing this two techniques, the Lissajous scan method is more prominent in imaging applications as such method can provide high-resolution images, but this method also requires more computational power [23].

As an example, Morrison et al. presented a MEMS micromirror using electrothermal actuation [24]. In this work, the fabrication process included three highly doped polysilicon layers, two sacrificial oxide layers, and a gold layer patterned using optical lithography. Residual compressive stresses in the polysilicon layer that were combined with residual tensile stresses in the gold layer due to the fabrication process provided a stress gradient along the boundary of the gold and polysilicon layers. Upon release, an initial curvature can be generated because of a bending strain due to the stress in the bimorph structures. The difference in coefficient of thermal expansion of the two layers can provide actuation, providing a temperature dependent curvature (Figure 2). Janak et al. proposed developing and integrating a three-dimensional (3D) micromirror for large deflection scanning in in vivo OCT [25]. A two-axes scanning micromirror was fabricated by using high-aspect-ratio deep reactive ion etching (DRIE) process instead of anisotropic etching of silicon in aqueous solution of potassium hydroxide (KOH), highly reducing the dead space on the chip and achieving a high-degree of integration. The micromirror was used to steer the scattered light from the tissue, and the steered signal was combined with a reference light beam at an optical coupler to produce interference patterns, which were collected at a detector to produce 2D cross-sectional image of the tissue structures.

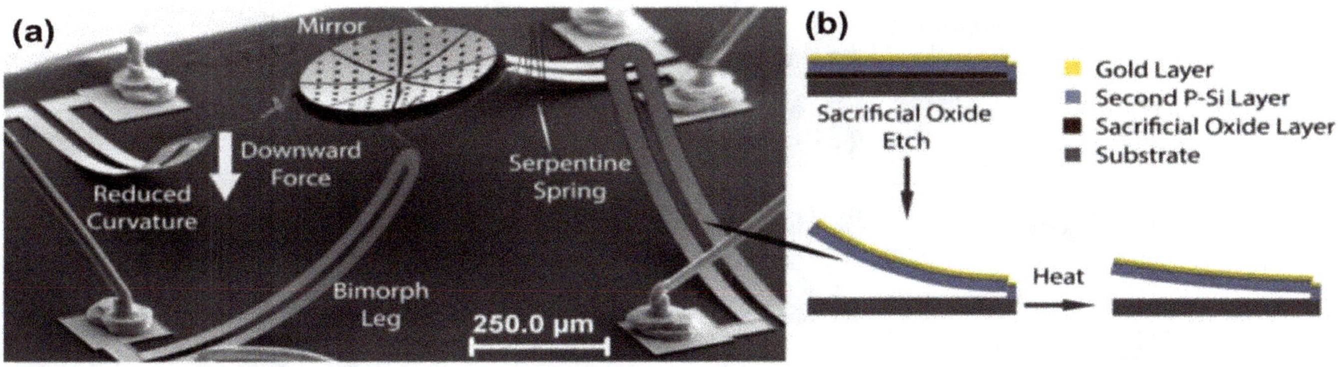

Figure 2. Pictures of a microelectromechanical systems (MEMS) micromirror using electrothermal actuation: (**a**) Scanning electron microscope (SEM) image of the micromirror device; (**b**) Illustration of bimorph layers before and after oxide etch and reduced curvature due to heating.

2.3. Lenses

The rapid growth of micro-opto-electro-mechanical systems (MOEMS or Optical MEMS) has attracted great interest in the field of microchip-based biophotonics for bio-sensing and high-resolution bioimaging [26]. One of the most important components in many optical micro-devices is a microlens, which can be integrated with emitters and detectors to improve the optical efficiency. In order to obtain high quality images for the application of some related fields in bio- and opto-electronics, high light focusing efficiency or high numerical aperture (NA) of the microlenses should be achieved. These two parameters are related to the geometry, particularly the curvature, of the microlenses. To date, many different fabrication technologies have been used for microlens fabrication, such as the photoresist reflow technique [27], photo- polymerization [28], LIGA (Lithographie, Galvanoformung, and Abformung, i.e., Lithography, Electroplating, and Molding) process [29], ink-jet printing [30], direct laser printing [31], and so on.

Although these methods are able to fabricate microlenses, they have drawbacks that result from the multiple process steps that are quite complex and sophisticated. Therefore, it is necessary to introduce a more efficient technique that allows easy variation in terms of the microlens curvature in order to obtain high numerical apertures, which result in increasing image quality in bioimaging systems. It has been demonstrated that dielectric microspheres can be used as solid immersion microlenses to explore the possibility of super-resolution capability in recent years. Wang et al. used silica microspheres with diameter ~2–9 µm for super-resolution imaging in the far field by generating a magnified virtual image underneath the specimen [32]. Later, microspheres with high refractive index (e.g., barium titanate glass) have been also used in optical nanoscopy [33–35]. In these works, the microspheres were simply placed on top of the sample object, where they collected the underlying sample's near-field nano-features and subsequently transformed the near-field evanescent waves into far-field propagating waves, creating a magnified image in the far-field, which is collected by a conventional optical microscope (shown in Figure 3). The super-resolution capability (imaging beyond the classical diffraction limit) of the microspheres, resulting from the enhanced optical field in the near field and the "photonic nanojet" phenomenon [35], has already been verified in bioimaging applications, such as molecular and subcellular structural characterizations [36,37].

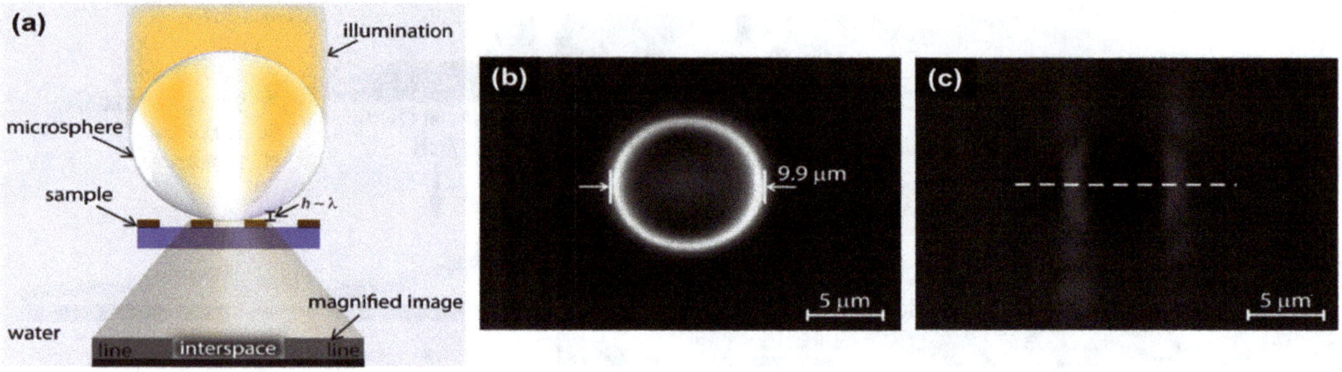

Figure 3. Microsphere lens used for super-resolution imaging: (**a**) A microsphere is positioned on a grating structure and illuminated from the front, the light reflected by the grating allows detecting a magnified image. When the distance h between the microsphere and the grating is small enough (of order of the illumination wavelength λ), the near-field evanescent wave carrying the fine details of the grating can become propagating in the high refractive index sphere, and later in the medium where it is to be collected by the microscope objective; (**b**,**c**) Optical microscopy images obtained by positioning a 9.9 μm microsphere on the grating. The image of (**b**) is focused on the microsphere's center plane, and the corresponding image (**c**) is focused on the image plane.

3. Fabrication Technologies of Micro-optical Components

Fabrication of micro-optical devices mainly relied on techniques transferred from the conventional two-dimensional (2D) integrated circuit (IC) and two- or three-dimensional (3D) MEMS processes. Semiconductor fabrication has been adopted to create several types of structures on chips, including waveguides, photonic circuits, and lenses. This includes photolithography, thin film deposition, and chemical etching. Silicon-, glass-, glass-silicon-, glass-polymer-based fabrication techniques were widely studied. However, silicon and glass are hampered from wider applications in micro-optics, because they possess micromachining difficulties and are relatively expensive; moreover, an inconvenience of silicon is the lack of optical transparency at ultraviolet (UV), visible and near-infrared (IR) wavelengths. Tremendous effort has been made to find alternative materials that are more cost-effective and easier machinable. With the development of related fabrication techniques, polymer/plastic-based devices have therefore gained increasing interest. Compared with silicon and glasses, polymer materials can avoid high-temperature annealing and stringent cleaning (if they are disposable), they are more cost-effective, easier in microfabrication, and there exists a wider range of materials to be chosen for characteristics that are required for each specific application, such as good optical transparency, biocompatibility, and chemical or mechanical properties. However, polymer materials usually do not result in strongly bonded layers like glass or silicon, and can exhibit structural deformation during device packaging processes. Each material has therefore both its advantages and disadvantages, and the choice of it will depend on the specific application. New technologies have also been developed in the meanwhile. This section reviews current fabrication methodologies to make optical structures on a chip, focusing on integrated waveguides, micromirrors and microlenses.

3.1. *Technologies for Waveguide Fabrication*

Waveguides that are integrated on-chip can be categorized as based on two working principles, namely total internal reflection (TIR) and interference. TIR-based waveguides require that the refractive index of the core n_c of the waveguide is bigger than that of the cladding n_s. Interference-based waveguides are conceptually different. In these structures, light is multiple times reflected from a periodic dielectric cladding layer by wave interference, therefore, they do not require a cladding material with a lower index than that of the core material [15]. Integrated waveguides can be constructed using a variety of micromachining procedures.

Common processes include lithographic patterning, thin-film deposition, and etching, these techniques can be used to fabricate a ridged waveguide, i.e., a solid-core waveguide. Usually, a thin layer of the core material is deposited on a planar substrate first. The substrate is coated with photoresist, the latter is then exposed to UV light or X-rays through a lithography mask that defines the waveguide shape, and developed to form a pattern on the surface of the substrate. With the remaining photoresist as a mask for either wet-chemical or dry etching to define the ridge waveguide structures. Dry etching methods, for example ion-beam etching, produce smooth edges, particularly on curved sections, but it also causes some lattice damage, which must be removed by annealing if minimum optical losses are desired. Wet chemical etching on the other hand produces less lattice damage, but it is very difficult to control the etch depth and profile. Most chemical etchants are preferential regarding crystal orientation, thus leading to ragged edges on curved sections of waveguides when using Si substrates. After the photolithography and etching procedures to process the core, a cladding layer is deposited. As an example, silicon oxynitride waveguides were fabricated in a standard silicon fabrication line by PECVD and LPCVD deposition processes in combination with 1100 °C annealing treatments to remove light-absorbing hydrogen bonds; and optical lithography for pattern definition and dry RIE for the pattern transfer process [38]. As shown in Figure 4, a 2 μm thick SiO_2 buffer layer (n = 1.45) and a 1 μm thick SiO_xN_y core layer (n = 1.85) were both deposited by LPCVD; a ~ 0.5 μm thick borophosphosilicate glass (BPSG) layer (n = 1.45) was grown by LPCVD in order to optimize the surface planarity after RIE. Finally, the whole system was coated with a thin SiNx film (50 nm of thickness). This waveguide system was applied to detect low surface concentration (10^{-11} mol·cm^{-2}) of a green light-emitting organic dye.

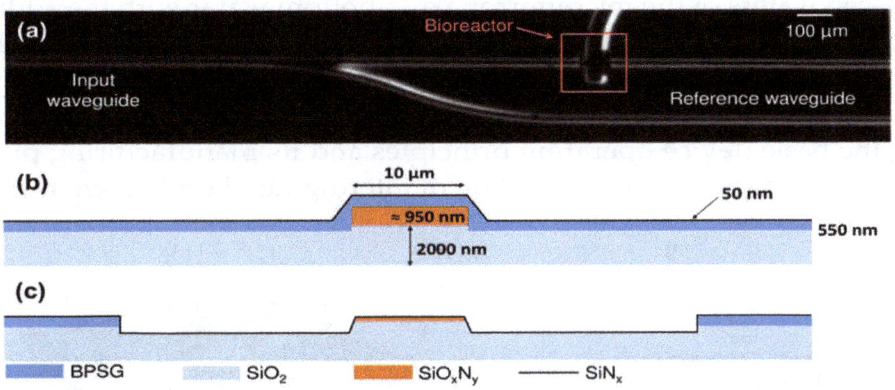

Figure 4. Fabrication procedure of silicon oxynitride waveguides: (**a**) Optical image of the top view of the waveguide; (**b**,**c**) Schematic cross-sections of the waveguide structure before (**b**) and at the bioreactor well (**c**).

Focused-beam direct writing can also be used to define a solid-core waveguide, rather than using lithography and etching. Either electron beam or proton beam can work, the former was used to densify doped silica on a silicon substrate for fabricating a silica waveguide on a chip [39], and the latter was used to selectively slow down the rate of porous silicon formation during subsequent anodization [40]. When the doped silica was exposed to the electron beam, an appropriate change in the refractive index was generated, and the surface kept planar and was suitable for further integration, without the need for cladding layers [39]. The proton bombardment reduced the free-carrier density and increased the local resistivity of the material. During the subsequent electrochemical etching process, these defects acted as traps for holes and thereby avoided their migration to the silicon/electrolyte surface, reducing the rate of porous silicon formation in the exposed regions. This method generated a silicon core surrounded by a region of porous silicon that has a lower index of refraction [40]. Besides the solid-state waveguides, liquid medium can also be used as the core material of the waveguide. Many different formats of the liquid-core waveguide have been proposed, however, their applications in integrated bioimaging system are still limited and mainly stay in the research phase.

3.2. *Technologies for Micromirror Fabrication*

MOEMS (micro-optical-electro-mechanical-systems) are one of promising techniques for developing optical switching connection devices [41]. A micromachined mirror is well known to be an optical key component. The advantages of using an optical micromirror include its low sensitivity to polarization and functionality in broadband optical applications. The micromirrors have been widely used in optical communication, for example, in optical scanners, projection display systems, variable optical attenuators, and other specific applications.

Prior works on micromirror fabrication have shown the feasibility of bulk or surface micromachining techniques, through silicon deep etching or using expensive silicon-on-insulator (SOI) wafers [42]. However, issues considered in the literature include high process complexity, high operation voltage or power consumption, etc. The standard CMOS process offers good opportunities for creating much smaller devices and more intelligent optical cross-connect devices with driving circuits on the same chip, based on a micromirror switch array, for optical telecommunication, steering light beams and communication applications. In such devices, the micromirrors are usually electrostatically actuated with a planar bottom drive that can steer a light beam in a continuous and controllable fashion [43]. Yoo et al. proposed an electrostatically actuated torsional micromirror [44]. The micromirror membrane was suspended by a pair of torsional springs, and an aluminum film, deposited by thermal evaporation, was used as a reflective material on the micromirror. A buried oxide (BOX) played the role of an insulating layer with a thickness of 1 μm and amorphous silicon was deposited on a glass substrate as the material for the electrodes, electrical lines and grounding shields. Figure 5 illustrates the two individually processed wafers of the micromirror, i.e., a bottom wafer with the addressing electrodes and a top wafer with the micromirror. Usually, the electrostatically actuated micromirror has a high fill factor, i.e., the ratio of the active reflecting micromirror area to the device area. Due to the high fill factor of the electrostatic micromirror, the discrete structure can be easily expanded to an array system without changing the basic device operating principles and its manufacturing process, such as the micromirror array based on the bending actuation of interdigitated cantilevers that was proposed by Kim et al. [45].

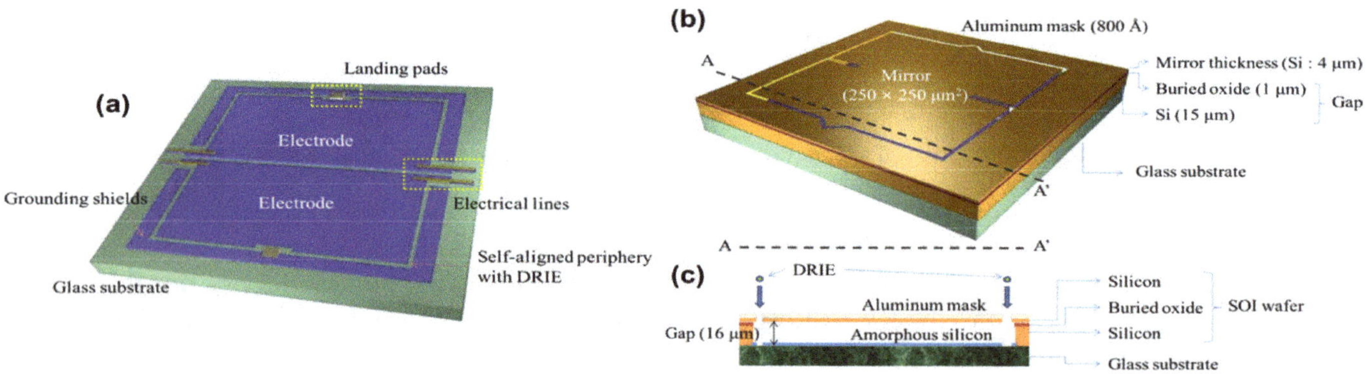

Figure 5. Schematic of a micromirror: (**a**) The electrodes on the glass substrate; (**b**) The micromirror structure; (**c**) Cross-section view of the device and its deep reactive-ion etching (DRIE) process.

Besides the torsional micromirrors, a simple format with a 45° or an angular facet can be used as vertical optical interconnecting structure. These structures are relatively easy to fabricate, and their performances are generally acceptable. Performances of the devices using curved-shape mirrors are known better than the flat mirror devices, but curved mirrors are hard to fabricate. A variety of fabrication techniques have been utilized, such as excimer laser ablation, use of V-shaped 90° diamond blades to create a 45° cut, anisotropic etching of (100) silicon in potassium hydroxide solutions, modified reactive ion etch techniques relying on angular bombardment of ions, and so on [46]. Lee et al. proposed using silicon deep etch process and photoresist reflow process to fabricate a silicon structure which has curved structures that made of reflowed photoresist [47]. The fabricated structure can be used as a master structure for subsequent embossing process to produce a 12-channel waveguide device with curved-shape micromirror for vertical optical interconnection. Koh et al. presented a right-angle micromirror integrated into a polydimethylsiloxane (PDMS) microfluidic device for measurement of particles [48]. The micromirror with precise 45° reflection angle was fabricated using conventional microfabrication techniques including wet etch and soft lithography. A 90° V-groove was generated on a (100) silicon wafer by anisotropic etching first. After two steps of PDMS replication, commercial UV photopolymer was filled in the V-grooved PDMS channels and cured, followed by a metal layer deposition step on the hypotenuse of the polymer micromirror (as shown in Figure 6).

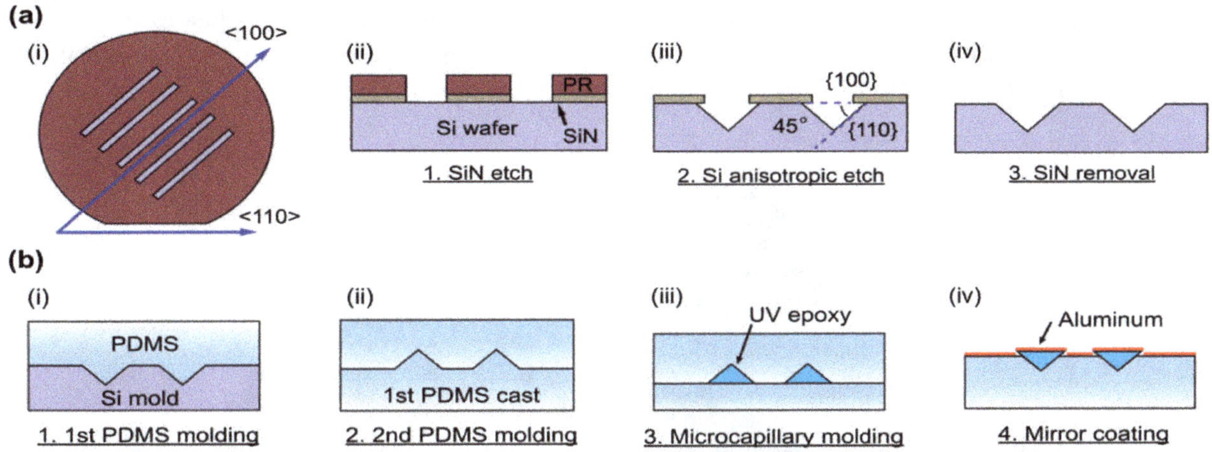

Figure 6. Micromirror fabrication process: (**a**) Line patterns with 45° alignment to (110) wafer flat were formed on a SiN wafer. Anisotropic Si etch leads to cross-section of right angle isosceles triangle. RIE etch of remaining SiN gives final Si master mold; (**b**) Polydimethylsiloxane (PDMS) microchannels were made by two step replica molding from the Si master mold. UV curable photopolymer was filled and cured in the micro- channels. The released structure was coated with aluminum using sputtering.

3.3. Technologies for Microlens Fabrication

A microlens is an important key component for focusing and collimating light. It can be made up as a solid curved surface or as a tunable interface between two deformable materials/media. On-chip hard solid-state lenses usually are fixed-focus lenses, similar to miniaturized traditional lenses that are used in a free-space detection system. Different methods have been developed for building solid microlenses, including photoresist thermal reflow, direct writing, soft replica molding, ink-jet printing, etc.

Thermal reflow processes have been widely used for the fabrication of large arrays of hemispherical microlenses. In this technique, a glass substrate is first coated with a layer of photoresist. Photolithography technique is then used to pattern the photoresist layer and generate a series of cylindrical islands, which are heated above the glass transition temperature of the photoresist. Due to surface tension, the shape of the photoresist cylinders changes to minimize the surface energy and becomes hemispherical, therefore generating a microlens array on the substrate. As the surface tension governs the contact angle of the photoresist and the shape of the microlens eventually, a thin layer of additives can be deposited on the substrate to influence the surface tension between the substrate and the photoresist, tuning the focal length and numerical aperture of the fabricated lenses. Yang et al. utilized a bottom polyimide layer to form a pedestal to sustain the upper photoresist lens after the heat reflow process [49]. The interactive force between two material interfaces causes the upper photoresist to form a spherical profile and transform the polyimide pedestal into a trapezoid with arc sides (as shown in Figure 7a). Advantages of the thermal reflow technique include a low material consumption, low manufacturing costs, the intrinsic simplicity of the technique, and an easy process control. Microlens arrays can be produced over large surface areas. However, the low transparency and thermal instability of photoresist features during the reflow process limit its widespread application [15].

Another widely used technique to fabricate microlens is direct writing, including electron beam lithography [50], direct laser writing [51], focused ion beam writing [52], and laser ablation [53]. With the direct writing technique, the material is exposed and processed in a way that the local thickness of the material is a continuous and preferably linear function of the energy deposited by the beam. The major advantage of this technique is its potential to fabricate microlenses with characteristics that can be tailored for every lens individually. Typically, electron beam lithography and direct laser writing methods correlate the surface profile data of the desired microlens to the beam intensity values, the latter being synchronously modulated to write a continuous pattern in the material to generate a microlens (as shown in Figure 7b). Alternatively, focused ion beam writing and laser ablation methods rely on the principle of precision removal of substrate materials. The depth of cut is controlled by the dwell time at each step and the number of times that the area is scanned.

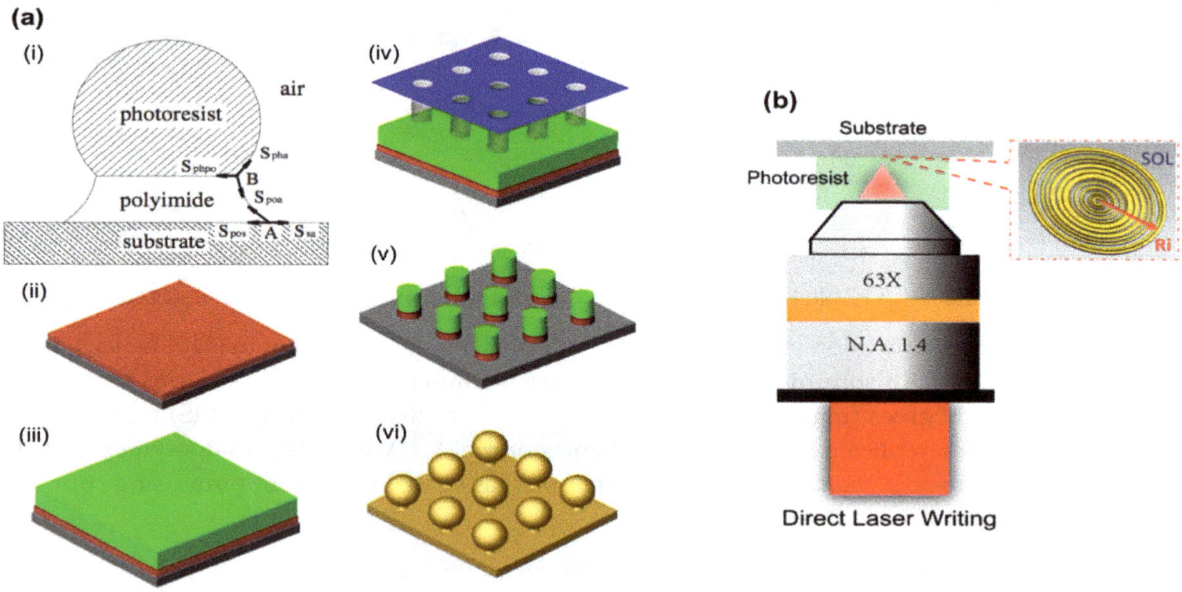

Figure 7. Fabrication methods for microlenses: (**a**) Illustration of a micro-ball lens formation in the thermal reflow process. A polyimide layer is coated on a Si wafer beneath a photoresist layer. Photolithography process is used to pattern these two materials through a mask. Micro-ball lens array with a pedestal can be generated after heat reflow; (**b**) Schematic diagrams of direct laser writing to form a super-oscillatory lens. ((**a**) Reproduced with permission [49], Copyright 2004, Institute of Physics; (**b**).

Besides, micromolding methods, such as compression molding, injection molding and soft replica molding, are most suitable for low-cost mass-production. Compression molding, including hot embossing, is a simple process with relatively low initial cost to replicate microlenses. The final height and radius of curvature of hot-embossed microlenses are determined by the combination of processing parameters, such as pressure, temperature and time. In the injection molding, sub-micron features in the mold are difficult to be filled because the solidified layer or solidified shell in a glassy state has very high viscosity. Therefore, the surface temperature of the mold can be maintained above the glass transition temperature of the polymer and then the micro/nanopatterns in the mold can be fully filled [54]. One can also use UV polymerization of a polymer in the mold. Soft replica molding based on soft lithography technology is widely used in molding PDMS and UV-curable materials and suitable to duplicate 3D topography in a single step. Convex and concave PDMS molds which define the microlens geometry can be fabricated first. Then both concave and convex microlenses can be fabricated by casting the polymeric liquid, for example polymethyl methacrylate (PMMA), in the corresponding convex and concave molds, respectively.

4. Micro-optics Integrated within Bioimaging Systems

This section will review the main applications of micro-optical components for bioimaging on tissues, cells and subcellular structures. We will consecutively discuss in vitro and in vivo imaging applications.

4.1. Micro-optical Components for in vitro Bioimaging

Recent advances in photonics and imaging techniques offer new possibilities for optical imaging systems and sensor devices for fundamental studies and future biomedical applications. Ongoing developments suggest that an impressive diversity of biological and medical questions can be answered using optical microscopy. Advanced optical techniques have been proposed for achieving high-resolution imaging of sample of interest. For example, multi-photon microscopes can investigate cortical micro-architecture in animals' brain with single cell resolution [55]. Also in regard to detecting levels of the tumor suppressing protein p53 in cells, fluorescence microscopy has been used to image cancerous tissues that were stained by specially designed oncolytic adenoviruses, the latter being programmed to replicate if the cellular p53 level is low [56,57]. However, these techniques are frequently accompanied by the need for high-end, bulky and expensive optical set-ups that are rather cumbersome to operate and to maintain, especially for untrained users. Such drawbacks have motivated researchers to minimize and integrate optical components in imaging systems for in situ analysis and observation of bio-samples under *in vitro* environment. MOEMS or Optical MEMS technology has recently demonstrated a strong potential in biomedical imaging applications due to its outstanding advantages including, for instance, low cost, high operating frequency and convenience of batch fabrication.

Integrating micro-optical components with optical imaging setups for *in vitro* observation and analysis has been demonstrated by many researchers. Here, we will review several works as examples, showing the capability and potential of the miniaturized optical components. Diekmann et al. demonstrated the use of a waveguide-integrated optical chip, which hosts the biological sample and utilizes the waveguide as the illumination source, and a standard low-cost microscope to acquire super-resolved images of single molecules via two different approaches [17]. The waveguides composed of a material with high refractive-index contrast can provide a strong evanescent field that is used for single-molecule switching and fluorescence excitation, thus enabling chip-based single-molecule localization microscopy. Additionally, multimode interference patterns can induce spatial fluorescence intensity variations that enable fluctuation-based super-resolution imaging [17]. The waveguides on the chip are used for total-internal-reflection fluorescence excitation, and the detection signal are collected and recorded by conventional optical microscope. By achieving visualization of fenestrations in liver sinusoidal endothelial cells with feature size smaller than the diffraction limit, the setup shows its great potential on upgrading standard optical microscopes to super-resolution microscopic tools [17]. Yokokawa et al. reported a micro-device that is equipped with an optical fiber, a microlens and a micro-prism for in situ observation and analysis of cells [58]. The optical components were used to compose a TIR-based chip to perform TIR fluorescence microscopy on adherent cells. The cells were cultured under continuous medium perfusion in a microfluidic channel that is located on top of the TIR-based chip (Figure 8a,b). The device was evaluated by monitoring the location of insulin granules in mouse pancreatic cells. The system allowed a higher imaging signal-to-noise ratio than obtained with epifluorescence microscopy.

Advanced microelectronics and emerging computational microscopy techniques have provided another scheme to bypass various limitations of conventional optical microscopy. Typically, bioimaging is performed at the microscopic scale and this usually requires lenses integrated in a microscopic system. Conventional optical microscope can be downsized to a portable device by utilizing commercial electronic devices. Breslauer et al. developed a microscope attachment for cell-phones that is capable of both bright-field and fluorescent imaging [59]. This microscope utilizes trans-illumination configuration with standard microscope eyepieces and objectives; magnification and resolution can be adjusted using different objectives. This cellphone microscope shows promising results for clinical use by imaging *P. falciparum*-infected and sickled red blood cells in bright-field mode, and *M. tuberculosis*-infected sputum samples in fluorescent mode with light-emitting diode (LED) excitation.

Furthermore, lens-free imaging has matured as a modality competitive with traditional lens-based microscopy. By placing an image sensor (CMOS/CCD) beneath a biological sample and using it to record light transmission pixel by pixel, a diffraction pattern resulting from the sample is recorded directly on the image sensor without being optically imaged or magnified by any lens elements, traditional lens components in a microscopic system can be abandoned [60]. Such lens-free (or lensless) scheme shows great flexibility on the integration format, and offers great possibilities to provide a compact and non-diffraction-limited imaging technique with large field-of-view, of the same size as the sensor size and a numerical aperture close to 1, since the large-area detector is placed very close to the sample. In the last decade, multiple lens-free on-chip microscope modus have been proposed to perform imaging on microorganisms [61] and cells [62] etc., showing exciting breakthroughs in point-of-care applications.

Yang's group demonstrated an optofluidic microscope (OFM) for lens-free contact imaging on *Caenorhabditis elegans* [61]. The OFM mobilizes the specimen along a microfluidic channel by laminar flow, and the channel is positioned directly over the image sensor. A tilted array of metallic apertures is patterned directly over the image sensor. Each aperture is carefully positioned at the center of a pixel of the image sensor, so that shadows of the specimens can be sampled by these sub-micron apertures as they flow along the microfluidic channel. By using OFM, automated phenotype characterization of different *Caenorhabditis elegans* mutant strains, as well as imaging of spores and single cellular entities, have been demonstrated [61]. The same group later on presented the implementation of color OFM prototypes color imaging of red blood cells infected with *Plasmodium falciparum*, a particularly harmful type of malaria parasites and one of the major causes of death in the developing world [62].

Ozcan's research group has developed different lens-free holographic imaging platforms for on-chip cytometry and diagnostics, with either fluorescent imaging format [63] or shadow imaging format [64]. Zhu et al. demonstrated a compact platform that integrated imaging cytometry and fluorescent microscopy and could be attached to a cell phone [65]. The resulting device could be used to rapidly image bodily fluids for cell counts or cell analysis (Figure 8c). Wei et al. proposed using gold and silver nanobeads as specific labels to identify and count the number of CD4 and CD8 cells in a cell suspension [66]. CD4 and CD8 cells are specific types of T lymphocytes, and their relative populations are important for evaluating the stage of human immunodeficiency virus (HIV) infection or acquired immune deficiency syndrome (AIDS), as well as for evaluating the efficacy of antiretroviral treatment. Counting the relative populations of these cells can be challenging, however, because the only significant difference between these cells is in the types of proteins expressed on their membranes.

Under a conventional optical microscope, both types of cells look virtually identical. However, by using gold nanoparticles functionalized with anti-CD4 antibodies to label CD4 cells and silver nanoparticles functionalized with anti-CD8 to label CD8 cells, the different spectral response of the labelled cells can be used to discriminate these two types of cells with greater than 95% accuracy using a machine learning algorithm.

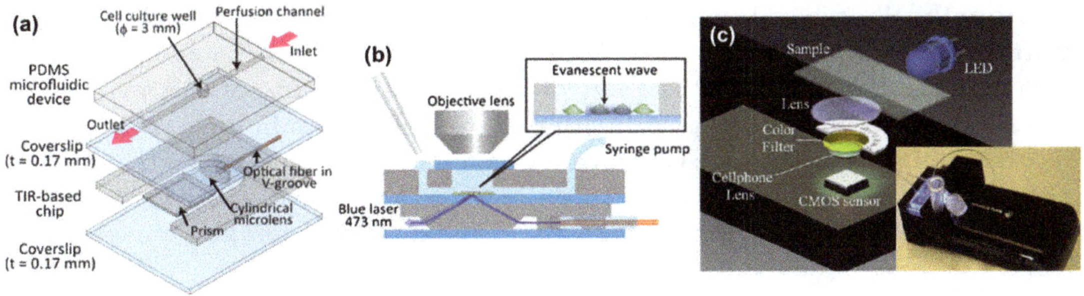

Figure 8. Microsystems used for in vitro imaging: (**a**) Schematic of a microdevice that is equipped with an optical fiber, a microlens and a micro-prism; (**b**) The integrated device for *in situ* observation and analysis of cells; (**c**) Schematic of an optofluidic device used for fluorescent imaging cytometry on a cellphone, the insert is a picture of the setup.

4.2. Micro-optical Components for in vivo Bioimaging

In vitro imaging of biological samples remains as one of the main tools for diagnosis of disease. However, it typically requires invasive sample collection (e.g., biopsy) steps as well as time consuming sample preparation protocols (e.g., fixation and staining) [67]. On the other hand, in vivo optical imaging techniques enable real-time visualization and might provide accurate information for diagnostics, making them highly desirable for diagnostics. In this section, we will briefly review two main in vivo optical imaging techniques, i.e., microendoscopy and OCT, that hold various integration format with the micro-optical components.

Microendoscopy is a promising approach for *in vivo* imaging. It combines conventional intravital microscopy and miniature endoscopy, using a narrow-diameter optical probe that provides minimally invasive access to internal organs that are otherwise difficult to reach with conventional instruments [68]. Optical microendoscopy provides spatial resolution that can approach that of a conventional water-immersion objective lens [69]; is compatible for use with multiple contrast modalities including epifluorescence, two-photon excited fluorescence, and second-harmonic generation; and has been used in both live animals and humans [70]. Kim et al. developed an *in vivo* confocal and multiphoton microendoscopic imaging system which integrated with gradient index lenses [68]. The cellular resolution of the system was demonstrated by imaging the micrometer-scale structures of the fluorescence labelled pollen grains. Besides, the boundaries of spherical starch granules in a sliced fresh potato were acquired with the second-harmonic generation imaging mode. Individual dendritic cells in the epidermis and dermis, blood vessels, as well as collagen fibrillar structure in live mice, were clearly imaged [68]. By using high-end micro-optical structures, such as high-resolution microlenses [69], the performance of the imaging system can be further improved. Barretto et al. demonstrated two-photon imaging of dendritic spines on hippocampal neurons and dual-color nonlinear optical imaging of neuromuscular junctions in live mice [69].

Many advances in microendoscopy have been reported in the last decade. Most endoscope designs involve three key components: optical fibers used for efficient laser pulse delivery and signal collection, micro-optics used for imaging, such as microlenses, and miniaturized scanning devices, such as micromirrors [71]. Rogers et al. demonstrated an integrated microendoscope and presented images of fixed biological samples acquired by the microendoscope to demonstrate its ability to image the cellular structure of tissue [72]. To be useful as an endoscopic device, the instrument should be no more than a few millimeters in diameter. As shown in Figure 9, the objective includes a 1-mm plano-spherical glass lens mounted in a custom precision micromount and three aspheric microlenses printed via grayscale lithography in hybrid sol-gel glass. The device incorporates a MEMS scanning grating, and the grating actuator is an electrostatic comb-drive actuator designed to scan the grating in resonance. The illumination is provided by a light-emitting diode (LED) that is coupled to a multimode fiber. The light from the fiber is collected by a 2-mm plano-spherical glass condenser lens mounted in a precision micromount. The device has a 250-μm-diameter field of view (FOV) and a working distance of 300 μm. The working distance allows for optical sectioning of epithelial cells below the tissue surface [72]. To verify the imaging ability of this optical system in relevant biological samples, such as cervix, oral epithelial cells and tissues were imaged by the system due to their structural and biomolecular similarity between the oral cavity and cervix. Human oral carcinoma cells were labelled and imaged, cell membranes were clearly visible and the results were comparable with a Zeiss optical microscope [72].

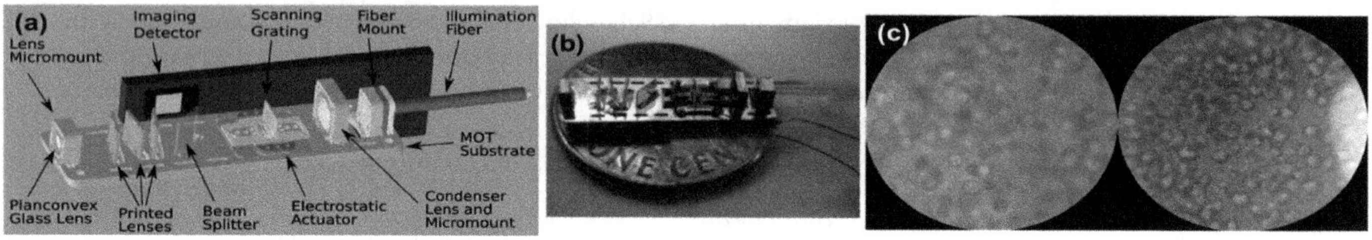

Figure 9. A microendoscope used for in vivo imaging: (**a**) Optical components mounted on the substrate; (**b**) The integrated device shown above a United States penny for scale; (**c**) Widefield image of cells labeled with gold nanoparticles, the image taken with the microendoscope is on the right, and a similar image taken with a Zeiss Axiovert 100 M is shown on the left for comparison.

OCT is a 3D microscopic imaging technique that is especially suitable for *in vivo* imaging applications, such as biomedical tissue cross-sectional analysis. With an axial resolution of less than 15 μm and cross-sectional imaging to a depth of ~1–3 mm, it has significant potential in ophthalmology, cardiology, gastroenterology and oncology applications, etc. OCT is an interferometric imaging technique that employs light sources (typically in the near-infrared) with relatively large spectral bandwidths (e.g., ~10–300 nm), to achieve cross-sectional biomedical imaging. OCT systems in general employ a fiber-based Michelson interferometer to measure the backscattered light from an object. This back-scattered light is used to calculate the reflectivity or scattering potential profile of the biological sample along the probe beam direction. By scanning the probe beam in the transverse direction, 3D images of the object can be reconstructed [67]. With the increasing availability of micro-optical components, OCT becomes a promising non-invasive imaging technique that lends itself to a compact, relatively cost- effective and portable architecture for diagnostic imaging applications. Aljasem et al. presented a membrane-based microfluidic tunable microlens and an electrostatic 2D scanning micromirror which were fabricated using silicon and polymer-based MEMS technologies [73]. These components were assembled inside a 4.5 mm diameter probe of an endoscopic OCT system for beam focus and steering, and the system was used to test a slide of wood with a surface layer of varnish and a leek skin [73]. Mu et al. demonstrated a prototype of an OCT bioimaging endoscopic probe utilizing a MEMS micromirror as the light beam manipulator [74]. To exert a large mirror platform tilt angle, electrothermal bimorph actuator was selected as the micromirror structure for its large deflection and low driving voltage, of which the latter is of particular importance for clinical applications. The MEMS micromirror and the silicon optical bench (SiOB) assembly were enclosed within a biocompatible, transparent and waterproof polycarbonate tube equipped with toroidal-lens for in vivo diagnostic applications. The muscle and skin next to the hind leg of a 6-week-old male mouse was tested by the OCT probe, epimysium, perimysium and endomysium layers were observed, and even the blood vessels that enclosed within the underneath layer of the epimysium can be easily distinguished from perimysium. Similarly, the superficial epidermis of the mouse leg skin tissue and the dermis layer were also successfully detected [74].

5. Conclusions

We have briefly introduced basic features of several imaging techniques that permit harvesting spatiotemporal information from living organisms, such as CT, MRI, etc. In particular, we have pointed out that optical microscopy plays a predominant role in observing tissues, cells and biomolecules. Over the last decade, a fast-growing interest was notice for developing micro-optical components and miniaturized optical imaging tools, these optical microdevices have shown great potential on imaging living organisms, tissues, cells, as well as subcellular structures, both *in vivo* and *in vitro*. We introduced several typical micro-optical components and their fabrication technologies, followed by the integration of these components with instruments or devices for in vivo and in vitro bioimaging, respectively.

We hope this review has made clear that micro-optical components can advantageously contribute to the bioimaging applications and the integration of such components with microscopic instruments is key to the improvement of the performance of an optical imaging system and to the miniaturization of the system. Aiming to bring effective medical diagnostic tools to patients, the continued development of optical bioimaging instruments that are cost-effective, sensitive and accurate is essential. In this quest, the advances in optical microdevices/microsystems can transform the field of biomedical optics, therefore playing an increasing important role. Conventional optical imaging techniques, such as optical microscope, endoscopes and OCT systems can be redesigned to provide highly integrated and miniaturized imaging tools, as described in this review. It is probable that the miniaturization of the imaging instruments can compromise their imaging performances, such as low spatial and temporal resolution. Therefore, further developments have to be performed so as to improve the performance of these tools up to, or even beyond, the level of their respective gold standards. We believe that the technical eruptions in the aspect of micro-optics will play a prominent role in the new bioimaging techniques development.

Author Contributions: H.Y. and Y.Z. designed the structure of the review; H.Y. wrote the Sections 2–5. S.C. wrote the Section 1. Y.Z and R.H. organized all the references.

Acknowledgments: The authors would like to thank the National Natural Science Foundation of China (61805271); the Guangdong Province Introduction of Innovative and Entrepreneurial Teams (2016ZT06D631); and the Shenzhen Science and Technology Innovation Commission (JCYJ20170818154035069 and JCYJ20170413153034718) for providing funding of this work.

References

1. Kherlopian, A.R.; Song, T.; Duan, Q.; Neimark, M.A.; Po, M.J.; Gohagan, J.K.; Laine, A.F. A review of imaging techniques for systems biology. *BMC Syst. Biol.* **2008**, *2*, 74. [CrossRef] [PubMed]
2. Liu, X.S.; Sajda, P.; Saha, P.K.; Wehrli, F.W.; Guo, X.E. Quantification of the roles of trabecular microarchitecture and trabecular type in determining the elastic modulus of human trabecular bone. *J. Bone Miner. Res.* **2006**, *21*, 1608–1617. [CrossRef] [PubMed]
3. Mizutani, R.; Suzuki, Y. X-ray microtomography in biology. *Micron* **2012**, *43*, 104–115. [CrossRef] [PubMed]
4. Parrish, T.B.; Gitelman, D.R.; LaBar, K.S.; Mesulam, M.-M. Impact of signal-to-noise on functional MRI. *Magn. Reson. Med.* **2000**, *44*, 925–932. [CrossRef]
5. Arias-Mendoza, F.; Brown, T.R. In vivo measurement of phosphorous markers of disease. *Dis. Markers* **2004**, *19*, 49–68. [CrossRef] [PubMed]
6. Bolan, P.J.; Nelson, M.T.; Yee, D.; Garwood, M. Imaging in breast cancer: Magnetic resonance spectroscopy. *Breast Cancer Res.* **2005**, *7*, 149–152. [CrossRef]
7. Karam, J.A.; Mason, R.P.; Koeneman, K.S.; Antich, P.P.; Benaim, E.A.; Hsieh, J.-T. Molecular imaging in prostate cancer. *J. Cell. Biochem.* **2003**, *90*, 473–483. [CrossRef]
8. Jensen, J.A. Medical ultrasound imaging. *Prog. Biophys. Mol. Biol.* **2007**, *93*, 153–165. [CrossRef]
9. Christiansen, J.P.; Lindner, J.R. Molecular and cellular imaging with targeted contrast ultrasound. *Proc. IEEE* **2005**, *93*, 809–818. [CrossRef]

10. Lanza, G.M.; Wickline, S.A. Targeted ultrasonic contrast agents for molecular imaging and therapy. *Prog. Cardiovasc. Dis.* **2001**, *44*, 13–31. [CrossRef]
11. König, K. Multiphoton microscopy in life sciences. *J. Microsc.* **2000**, *200*, 83–104. [CrossRef] [PubMed]
12. Hell, S.W.; Wichmann, J. Breaking the diffraction resolution limit by stimulated emission: Stimulated-emission-depletion fluorescence microscopy. *Opt. Lett.* **1994**, *19*, 780–782. [CrossRef] [PubMed]
13. Klar, T.A.; Jakobs, S.; Dyba, M.; Egner, A.; Hell, S.W. Fluorescence microscopy with diffraction resolution barrier broken by stimulated emission. *Proc. Natl. Acad. Sci. USA* **2000**, *97*, 8206–8210. [CrossRef] [PubMed]
14. Fölling, J.; Belov, V.; Riedel, D.; Schönle, A.; Egner, A.; Eggeling, C.; Bossi, M.; Hell, S.W. Fluorescence nanoscopy with optical sectioning by two-photon induced molecular switching using continuous-wave lasers. *ChemPhysChem* **2008**, *9*, 321–326. [CrossRef] [PubMed]
15. Yang, H.; Gijs, M.A.M. Micro-optics for microfluidic analytical applications. *Chem. Soc. Rev.* **2018**, *47*, 1391–1458. [CrossRef] [PubMed]
16. Moss, D.J.; Morandotti, R.; Gaeta, A.L.; Lipson, M. New CMOS-compatible platforms based on silicon nitride and Hydex for nonlinear optics. *Nat. Photonics* **2013**, *7*, 597–607. [CrossRef]
17. Diekmann, R.; Helle, Ø.I.; Øie, C.I.; McCourt, P.; Huser, T.R.; Schüttpelz, M.; Ahluwalia, B.S. Chip-based wide field-of-view nanoscopy. *Nat. Photonics* **2017**, *11*, 322–328. [CrossRef]
18. Yurtsever, G.; Dumon, P.; Bogaerts, W.; Baets, R. Integrated photonic circuit in silicon on insulator for Fourier domain optical coherence tomography. *Proc. SPIE* **2010**, *7554*, 75514B.
19. Tinguely, J.-C.; Helle, Ø.I.; Ahluwalia, B.S. Silicon nitride waveguide platform for fluorescence microscopy of living cells. *Opt. Express* **2017**, *25*, 27678–27690. [CrossRef] [PubMed]
20. Pan, Y.; Xie, H.; Fedder, G.K. Endoscopic optical coherence tomography based on a microelectromechanical mirror. *Opt. Lett.* **2001**, *26*, 1966–1968. [CrossRef]
21. Strahman, M.; Liu, Y.; Li, X.; Lin, L.Y. Dynamic focus-tracking MEMS scanning micromirror with low actuation voltages for endoscopic imaging. *Opt. Express* **2013**, *21*, 23934–23941. [CrossRef] [PubMed]
22. Booth, M.J. Adaptive optical microscopy: The ongoing quest for a perfect image. *Light Sci. Appl.* **2014**, *3*, e165. [CrossRef]
23. Morrison, J.; Imboden, M.; Bishop, D.J. Tuning the resonance frequencies and mode shapes in a large range multi-degree of freedom micromirror. *Opt. Express* **2017**, *25*, 7895–7906. [CrossRef] [PubMed]
24. Morrison, J.; Imboden, M.; Little, T.D.C.; Bishop, D.J. Electrothermally actuated tip-tilt-piston micromirror with integrated varifocal capability. *Opt. Express* **2015**, *23*, 9555–9566. [CrossRef]
25. Janak, S.; Xu, Y.; Premachandran, C.S.; Jason, T.H.S.; Chen, N. Novel 3D micromirror for miniature optical bio-probe SiOB assembly. *Proc. SPIE* **2008**, *6886*, 688608.
26. Kuo, J.-N.; Hsieh, C.-C.; Yang, S.-Y.; Lee, G.-B. An SU-8 microlens array fabricated by soft replica molding for cell counting applications. *J. Micromech. Microeng.* **2007**, *17*, 693–699. [CrossRef]
27. Oder, T.N.; Shakya, J.; Lin, J.Y.; Jiang, H.X. Nitride microlens arrays for blue and ultraviolet wavelength applications. *Appl. Phys. Lett.* **2003**, *82*, 3692–3694. [CrossRef]
28. Malinauskas, M.; Gilbergs, H.; Zukauskas, A.; Purlys, V.; Paipulas, D.; Gadonas, R. A femtosecond laser-induced two-photon photopolymerization technique for structuring microlenses. *J. Opt.* **2010**, *12*, 035204. [CrossRef]
29. Kim, D.S.; Lee, H.S.; Lee, B.-K.; Yang, S.S.; Kwon, T.H.; Lee, S.S. Replications and analysis of microlens array fabricated by a modified LIGA process. *Polym. Eng. Sci.* **2006**, *46*, 416–425. [CrossRef]
30. Kim, J.Y.; Martin-Olmos, C.; Baek, N.S.; Brugger, J. Simple and easily controllable parabolic-shaped microlenses printed on polymeric mesas. *J. Mater. Chem. C* **2013**, *1*, 2152–2157. [CrossRef]
31. Florian, C.; Piazza, S.; Diaspro, A.; Serra, P.; Duocastella, M. Direct laser printing of tailored polymeric microlenses. *ACS Appl. Mater. Interfaces* **2016**, *8*, 17028–17032. [CrossRef] [PubMed]
32. Wang, Z.; Guo, W.; Li, L.; Luk'yanchuk, B.; Khan, A.; Liu, Z.; Chen, Z.; Hong, M. Optical virtual imaging at 50 nm lateral resolution with a white-light nanoscope. *Nat. Commun.* **2011**, *2*, 218. [CrossRef]
33. Yang, H.; Gijs, M.A.M. Optical microscopy using a glass microsphere for metrology of sub-wavelength nanostructures. *Microelectron. Eng.* **2015**, *143*, 86–90. [CrossRef]
34. Darafsheh, A.; Guardiola, C.; Palovcak, A.; Finlay, J.C.; Cárabe, A. Optical super-resolution imaging by high-index microspheres embedded in elastomers. *Opt. Lett.* **2015**, *40*, 5–8. [CrossRef] [PubMed]
35. Yang, H.; Trouillon, R.; Huszka, G.; Gijs, M.A.M. Super-resolution imaging of a dielectric microsphere is governed by the waist of its photonic nanojet. *Nano Lett.* **2016**, *16*, 4862–4870. [CrossRef] [PubMed]

36. Li, L.; Guo, W.; Yan, Y.; Lee, S.; Wang, R. Label-free super-resolution imaging of adenoviruses by submerged microsphere optical nanoscopy. *Light Sci. Appl.* **2013**, *2*, e104. [CrossRef]
37. Yang, H.; Moullan, N.; Auwerx, J.; Gijs, M.A.M. Super-resolution biological microscopy using virtual imaging by a microsphere nanoscope. *Small* **2014**, *10*, 1712–1718. [CrossRef] [PubMed]
38. Aparicio, F.J.; Froner, E.; Rigo, E.; Gandolfi, D.; Scarpa, M.; Han, B.; Ghulinyan, M.; Pucker, G.; Pavesi, L. Silicon oxynitride waveguides as evanescent-field-based fluorescent biosensors. *J. Phys. D Appl. Phys.* **2014**, *47*, 405401. [CrossRef]
39. Cleary, A.; Glidle, A.; Laybourn, P.J.R.; García-Blanco, S.; Pellegrini, S.; Helfter, C.; Buller, G.S.; Aitchison, J.S.; Cooper, J.M. Integrating optics and microfluidics for time-correlated single-photon counting in lab-on-a-chip devices. *Appl. Phys. Lett.* **2007**, *91*, 071123. [CrossRef]
40. Teo, E.J.; Bettiol, A.A.; Breese, M.B.H.; Yang, P.; Mashanovich, G.Z.; Headley, W.R.; Reed, G.T.; Blackwood, D.J. Three-dimensional control of optical waveguide fabrication in silicon. *Opt. Express* **2008**, *16*, 573–578. [CrossRef]
41. Cheng, Y.-C.; Dai, C.-L.; Lee, C.-Y.; Chen, P.-H.; Chang, P.-Z. A circular micromirror array fabricated by a maskless post-CMOS process. *Microsyst. Technol.* **2005**, *11*, 444–451. [CrossRef]
42. Houlet, L.; Helin, P.; Bourouina, T.; Reyne, G.; Dufour-Gergam, E.; Fujita, H. Movable vertical mirror arrays for optical microswitch matrixes and their electromagnetic actuation. *IEEE J.* **2002**, *8*, 58–63. [CrossRef]
43. Ma, Y.; Islam, S.; Pan, Y.-J. Electrostatic torsional micromirror with enhanced tilting angle using active control methods. *IEEE ASME Trans. Mechatron.* **2011**, *16*, 994–1001. [CrossRef]
44. Yoo, B.-W.; Park, J.-H.; Jin, J.-Y.; Jang, Y.-H.; Kim, Y.-K. Design and fabrication of a self-aligned parallel-plate-type silicon micromirror minimizing the effect of misalignment. *J. Micromech. Microeng.* **2009**, *19*, 055004. [CrossRef]
45. Kim, D.-H.; Kim, M.-W.; Jeon, J.-W.; Lim, K.S.; Yoon, J.-B. Modeling, design, fabrication, and demonstration of a digital micromirror with interdigitated cantilevers. *J. Microelectromech. Syst.* **2009**, *18*, 1382–1395.
46. Ponoth, S.S.; Agarwal, N.T.; Persans, P.D.; Plawsky, J.L. Fabrication of micromirrors with self-aligned metallization using silicon back-end-of-the-line processes. *Thin Solid Films* **2005**, *472*, 169–179. [CrossRef]
47. Lee, M.-W.; Choi, C.H.; Lim, K.J.; Beom-Hoan, O.; Lee, S.G.; Park, S.-G.; Lee, E.H. Novel fabrication of a curved micro-mirror for optical interconnection. *Microelectron. Eng.* **2006**, *83*, 1343–1346. [CrossRef]
48. Koh, J.; Kim, J.; Shin, J.H.; Lee, W. Fabrication and integration of microprism mirrors for high-speed three-dimensional measurement in inertial microfluidic system. *Appl. Phys. Lett.* **2014**, *105*, 114103. [CrossRef]
49. Yang, H.; Chao, C.-K.; Lin, C.-P.; Shen, S.-C. Micro-ball lens array modeling and fabrication using thermal reflow in two polymer layers. *J. Micromech. Microeng.* **2004**, *14*, 277–282. [CrossRef]
50. Fujita, T.; Nishihara, H.; Koyama, J. Fabrication of micro lenses using electron-beam lithography. *Opt. Lett.* **1981**, *6*, 613–615. [CrossRef]
51. Ni, H.; Yuan, G.; Sun, L.; Chang, N.; Zhang, D.; Chen, R.; Jiang, L.; Chen, H.; Gu, Z.; Zhao, X. Large-scale high-numerical-aperture super-oscillatory lens fabricated by direct laser writing lithography. *RSC Adv.* **2018**, *8*, 20117–20123. [CrossRef]
52. Harriott, L.R.; Scotti, R.E.; Cummings, K.D.; Ambrose, A.F. Micromachining of integrated optical structures. *Appl. Phys. Lett.* **1986**, *48*, 1704–1706. [CrossRef]
53. Naessens, K.; Ottevaere, H.; Baets, R.; Van Daele, P.; Thienpont, H. Direct writing of microlenses in polycarbonate with excimer laser ablation. *Appl. Opt.* **2003**, *42*, 6349–6359. [CrossRef] [PubMed]
54. Lee, B.-K.; Kim, D.S.; Kwon, T.H. Replication of microlens arrays by injection molding. *Microsyst. Technol.* **2004**, *10*, 531–535. [CrossRef]
55. Ohki, K.; Chung, S.; Ch'ng, Y.H.; Kara, P.; Reid, R.C. Functional imaging with cellular resolution reveals precise micro-architecture in visual cortex. *Nature* **2005**, *433*, 597–603. [CrossRef] [PubMed]
56. Woo, Y.; Adusumilli, P.S.; Fong, Y. Advances in oncolytic viral therapy. *Curr. Opin. Investig. Drugs* **2006**, *7*, 549–559. [PubMed]
57. Ramachandra, M.; Rahman, A.; Zou, A.; Vaillancourt, M.; Howe, J.A.; Antel-man, D.; Sugarman, B.; Demers, G.W.; Engler, H.; Johnson, D.; et al. Re-engineering adenovirus regulatory pathways to enhance oncolytic specificity and efficacy. *Nat. Biotechnol.* **2001**, *19*, 1035–1041. [CrossRef]
58. Yokokawa, R.; Kitazawa, Y.; Terao, K.; Okonogi, A.; Kanno, I.; Kotera, H. A perfusable microfluidic device with on-chip total internal reflection fluorescence microscopy (TIRFM) for *in situ* and real-time monitoring of live cells. *Biomed. Microdevices* **2012**, *14*, 791–797. [CrossRef]

59. Breslauer, D.N.; Maamari, R.N.; Switz, N.A.; Lam, W.A.; Fletcher, D.A. Mobile phone based clinical microscopy for global health applications. *PLoS ONE* **2009**, *4*, e6320. [CrossRef]
60. Ozcan, A.; McLeod, E. Lensless imaging and sensing. *Annu. Rev. Biomed. Eng.* **2016**, *18*, 77–102. [CrossRef]
61. Cui, X.; Lee, L.M.; Heng, X.; Zhong, W.; Sternberg, P.W.; Psaltis, D.; Yang, C. Lensless high-resolution on-chip optofluidic microscopes for *Caenorhabditis elegans* and cell imaging. *Proc. Natl. Acad. Sci. USA* **2008**, *105*, 10670–10675. [CrossRef] [PubMed]
62. Lee, S.A.; Leitao, R.; Zheng, G.; Yang, S.; Rodriguez, A.; Yang, C. Color capable sub-pixel resolving optofluidic microscope and its application to blood cell imaging for Malaria diagnosis. *PLoS ONE* **2011**, *6*, e26127. [CrossRef] [PubMed]
63. Arpali, S.A.; Arpali, C.; Coskun, A.F.; Chiang, H.-H.; Ozcan, A. High-throughput screening of large volumes of whole blood using structured illumination and fluorescent on-chip imaging. *Lab Chip* **2012**, *12*, 4968–4971. [CrossRef]
64. Seo, S.; Su, T.-W.; Tseng, D.K.; Erlinger, A.; Ozcan, A. Lensfree holographic imaging for on-chip cytometry and diagnostics. *Lab Chip* **2009**, *9*, 777–787. [CrossRef] [PubMed]
65. Zhu, H.; Mavandadi, S.; Coskun, A.F.; Yaglidere, O.; Ozcan, A. Optofluidic fluorescent imaging cytometry on a cell phone. *Anal. Chem.* **2011**, *83*, 6641–6647. [CrossRef]
66. Wei, Q.; McLeod, E.; Qi, H.; Wan, Z.; Sun, R.; Ozcan, A. On-chip cytometry using plasmonic nanoparticle enhanced lensfree holography. *Sci. Rep.* **2013**, *3*, 1699. [CrossRef] [PubMed]
67. Zhu, H.; Isikman, S.O.; Mudanyali, O.; Greenbaum, A.; Ozcan, A. Optical imaging techniques for point-of-care diagnostics. *Lab Chip* **2013**, *13*, 51–67. [CrossRef] [PubMed]
68. Kim, P.; Puoris'haag, M.; Côté, D.; Lin, C.P.; Yun, S.H. *In vivo* confocal and multiphoton microendoscopy. *J. Biomed. Opt.* **2008**, *13*, 010501. [CrossRef] [PubMed]
69. Barretto, R.P.J.; Messerschmidt, B.; Schnitzer, M.J. *In vivo* fluorescence imaging with high-resolution microlenses. *Nat. Methods* **2009**, *6*, 511–512. [CrossRef]
70. Llewellyn, M.E.; Barretto, R.P.J.; Delp, S.L.; Schnitzer, M.J. Minimally invasive high-speed imaging of sarcomere contractile dynamics in mice and humans. *Nature* **2008**, *454*, 784–788. [CrossRef]
71. Zhao, Y.; Nakamura, H.; Gordon, R.J. Development of a versatile two-photon endoscope for biological imaging. *Biomed. Opt. Express* **2010**, *1*, 1159–1172. [CrossRef] [PubMed]
72. Rogers, J.D.; Landau, S.; Tkaczyk, T.S.; Descour, M.R.; Rahman, M.S.; Richards-Kortum, R.; Kärkäinen, A.H.O. Imaging performance of a miniature integrated microendoscope. *J. Biomed. Opt.* **2008**, *13*, 054020. [CrossRef] [PubMed]
73. Aljasem, K.; Froehly, L.; Seifert, A.; Zappe, H. Scanning and tunable micro-optics for endoscopic optical coherence tomography. *J. Microelectromech. Syst.* **2011**, *20*, 1462–1472. [CrossRef]
74. Mu, X.; Sun, W.; Feng, H.; Yu, A.; Chen, K.W.S.; Fu, C.Y.; Olivo, M. MEMS micromirror integrated endoscopic probe for optical coherence tomography bioimaging. *Sens. Actuator A Phys.* **2011**, *168*, 202–212. [CrossRef]

8

Remote Microwave and Field-Effect Sensing Techniques for Monitoring Hydrogel Sensor Response

Olutosin Charles Fawole [1], Subhashish Dolai [2], Hsuan-Yu Leu [3], Jules Magda [3] and Massood Tabib-Azar [2,4,*]

[1] Livanova Inc., 100 Cyberonics Blvd, Houston, TX 77058, USA; olutosin.fawole@gmail.com
[2] Electrical and Computer Engineering Department, University of Utah, Salt Lake City, UT 84112, USA; subhashish.dolai@utah.edu
[3] Chemical Engineering Department, University of Utah, Salt Lake City, UT 84112, USA; u1011614@utah.edu (H.-Y.L.); magda@chemeng.utah.edu (J.M.)
[4] Bio Engineering Department, University of Utah, Salt Lake City, UT 84112, USA
* Correspondence: azar.m@utah.edu

Abstract: This paper presents two novel techniques for monitoring the response of smart hydrogels composed of synthetic organic materials that can be engineered to respond (swell or shrink, change conductivity and optical properties) to specific chemicals, biomolecules or external stimuli. The first technique uses microwaves both in contact and remote monitoring of the hydrogel as it responds to chemicals. This method is of great interest because it can be used to non-invasively monitor the response of subcutaneously implanted hydrogels to blood chemicals such as oxygen and glucose. The second technique uses a metal-oxide-hydrogel field-effect transistor (MOHFET) and its associated current-voltage characteristics to monitor the hydrogel's response to different chemicals. MOHFET can be easily integrated with on-board telemetry electronics for applications in implantable biosensors or it can be used as a transistor in an oscillator circuit where the oscillation frequency of the circuit depends on the analyte concentration.

Keywords: smart hydrogels; bio-sensors; chemo-sensor; electrochemical sensors; transduction techniques; near-field microwave; microwave resonator; microwave remote sensing; potentiometric sensor; gold nanoparticles; metal oxide field-effect transistor; chemo-FET; bio-FET

1. Introduction

Chemical, biological, and gas sensors usually rely on sensing materials that change their electromagnetic and physical properties in response to molecules and chemicals of interest (analytes). These changes are then measured with electric, magnetic, optical, thermal, or mechanical techniques to identify and quantify the analytes. Hydrogels and aerogels are nearly ideal sensing materials because they contain large voids and open regions (cages) in their structures. These voids allow liquid and gas molecules to diffuse in/out of the hydrogel interior thereby resulting in physical, chemical, electromagnetic, and mechanical changes in the hydrogel. Hydrogels' cage-like structures comprise cross-linked polymer networks that can be manipulated to interact with molecules with different shapes, ionic content, and pH [1,2]. Moreover, at the microscopic and nanoscopic level, the hydrogel structure can be modified with functional groups for sensitive and selective interactions with specific molecules. Figure 1 schematically shows a hydrogel functionalized with pendant negatively charged molecules that attract a target positively-charged analyte. The combination of these two oppositely-charged molecules results in dimensional, electrochemical, and physical changes in the hydrogel.

Interesting applications of hydrogels include the sensing of important biological analytes such as glucose. Hydrogels respond to stimuli by gradually absorbing/releasing water as shown in Figure 1. The absorption of water by these hydrogels results in an increase in hydrogel volume (swelling) while the release of water results in the decrease (de-swelling) of hydrogel volume. Hydrogel swelling and de-swelling also result in electrical, chemical, and optical changes in the hydrogel.

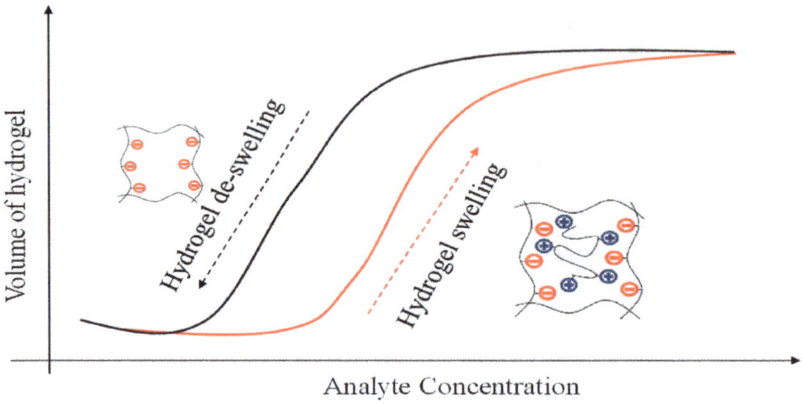

Figure 1. Schematic of a hydrogel functionalized with pendant negatively-charged molecules that attract or release positively-charged target analytes, resulting in physical, electrical, and chemical changes in the hydrogel.

Various transduction techniques, such as optical, electrical, and mechanical techniques, have been developed in the past to monitor hydrogel response to chemicals and biomolecules [3–12]. The optical transduction technique measure changes in optical and dimensional properties of the hydrogels with optical methods. This technique can detect small dimensional changes (at a nanometer scale) of hydrogel, as well as small refractive index changes of the hydrogel when the hydrogel responds to chemicals and stimuli. However, the major drawback of the optical technique is the bulkiness of the readout instrumentation needed to capture the optical response of the hydrogel. The electrical technique for measuring the hydrogel's response to chemicals and stimuli relies on measuring hydrogel conductance [11], resistance or impedance [12]. This electrical technique has the advantage of high sensitivity and it can be used with compact read-out instrumentation. However, the technique requires the hydrogel to be physically connected to an electronic circuit in applications where it is to be applied. Mechanical techniques use strain gauges to measure changes in the hydrogel's Young's modulus or volume/density. The main advantage of the mechanical technique is its simplicity. However, a major disadvantage of this technique is that the output signal from the mechanical transducers is prone to drift.

Microwave techniques have been used to measure and monitor changes in the electromagnetic properties of materials [13–23]. Microwave measurements can be very sensitive and can be used remotely through many different media to non-invasively monitor the sensing material's response to its environment. The intervening media can be air, dielectric layers, and biological tissues (skin, fat, etc.) without the probe making physical contact with the hydrogel or the enclosing media. Microwave wavelengths can vary over a wide range from 100 cm (300 MHz) down to 30 μm (10 THz) providing a powerful monitoring technique with a wide range of spatial resolutions and penetration depth. We are in the process of performing terahertz reflectometry [24,25] and high-spatial resolution measurements of hydrogels, and these results will be reported in the near future.

This paper demonstrates for the first time the remote microwave monitoring of hydrogels in real time. In order to verify that the hydrogel that was synthesized for this study is responsive to analytes and to check the feasibility and accuracy of the microwave technique, we measured the impedance of the hydrogel sample in contact mode. Impedance spectroscopy is a well-known method for the electrical characterization of materials and is extensively used in hydrogels [8,10,12]. Subsequently, we developed "in contact" and remote microwave methods for hydrogel monitoring.

We also developed a potentiometric (measured the potential across the hydrogel with current ~0) technique to monitor the changes in ionic content of the hydrogel. The potentiometric approach was used in the past to construct hydrogel-based batteries and piezoelectric transducers [26,27] but was not used as a transduction technique for hydrogel sensors. Here, the electric potential across the hydrogel was used to detect the ionic concentration gradient across the hydrogel due to an analyte. This phenomenon was then exploited to design a novel metal-oxide-hydrogel field-effect transistor (MOHFET) whose channel material is a smart hydrogel. The MOHFET [28] design was based on an open-face Field-Effect Transistor (FET) structure reported before [28–31]. Here, drop-casting was used for depositing the hydrogel channel. The MOHFET characteristics changed as a function of the hydrogel's ionic content. Furthermore, a MOHFET with gold nanoparticles, (AuNP)-embedded, was developed [32]. This gold-doped hydrogel channel increases the conductivity of the MOHFET channel compared to the undoped MOHFET channel. MOHFETs are of great interest because they can be used to detect the microscopic biomolecules in media with high ionic concentrations without the limits imposed by the double electrical layer shielding the effect of the ionic medium (Debye-length free sensing) [33]. The threshold voltage of the MOHFET reported in this paper varied reproducibly with the concentration of the analyte that was measured.

2. Materials and Methods

2.1. Hydrogel Synthesis

2.1.1. Reagent Materials for Hydrogel Synthesis

For the synthesis [2,32] of the hydrogel, acrylamide (AAM) was obtained from Fluka Analytical. *N*-[3 (dimethylamino)propyl]acrylamide (DMA) was purchased from Polysciences Inc. (Warrington, PA, USA), and 3-acrylamidophenylboronic acid (3-APB) was purchased from Frontier Scientific (Logan, UT, USA). *N,N*-methylenebisacrylamide (BIS), 4-(2-Hydroxyethyl)-1-piperazineethanesulfonic acid (HEPES), dimethyl sulfoxide (DMSO), ammonium persulfate (APS), and *N,N,N′,N′*-tetramethylethylenediamine (TEMED) were purchased from Sigma-Aldrich (St. Louis, MO, USA). For hydrogel testing in a medium with high ionic concentrations, 1X-PBS was prepared from Dulbecco's phosphate buffered saline powder with pH and ionic strength adjusted to 7.4 and 155 mM, respectively. For hydrogel testing of an analyte with low ionic concentration, deionized (DI) water was used for testing.

2.1.2. Synthesis of Stimulus-Responsive Hydrogel

The hydrogel was a polyampholytic copolymer with a nominal monomer composition of 80 mole% AAM, 10 mole% DMA, 8 mole% 3-APB, and 2 mole% BIS. The resulting hydrogel had a composition optimized for measuring blood glucose levels in diabetic patients and it also had a large sensitivity to ionic concentrations [34]. This hydrogel was synthesized by the free-radical crosslinking copolymerization method using APS/TEMED as the free radical initiator [35]. Pre-gel solutions were made by dissolving 19.1 mg of 3-APB powder in 85 μL DMSO in a 1.5 mL centrifuge tube, then adding appropriate amounts of AAM and BIS stock solutions followed by DMA. Monomer mixtures were diluted with additional HEPES to obtain 13 wt% (monomer/solvent) pre-gel solutions. TEMED was added to pre-gel mixtures right before polymerization. Pre-gel mixtures were mixed well using a vortex mixer and purged with Nitrogen gas for 5–10 min. After that, APS was added in an amount equal to 0.2% of the total molar concentration of monomers. The mixtures were mixed for 10 s and then quickly injected into the mold. Molds for hydrogels were constructed from two 8 cm × 8 cm hydrophobic glass slides separated by a 400 μm Teflon spacer. Hydrogel mixtures were left in the mold for 12 h at room temperature. After polymerization, the hydrogels were removed from molds and washed with deionized (DI) water in order to remove excess monomers. The hydrogels were cut into cylindrical disks of diameter 5 mm. The thickness of each hydrogel disc was 400 μm. Next, the hydrogels were alternatively washed in 1X-PBS solutions and 0.5X-PBS solutions (three cycles), and then stored in 1X-PBS at ambient conditions in a dark place until experimental testing.

The gold nanoparticle-doped (AuNP) hydrogel used in the MOHFET was made by polymerized acrylamide gel as backbones and bis-acrylamide as crosslinks with the gel thickness of the channel being approximately 50 μm. The gold nanoparticle diameter was 50.7 ± 7.1 nm as measured with a transmission electron microscope. Figure 2 shows a picture of the synthesized undoped and AuNP-doped hydrogel.

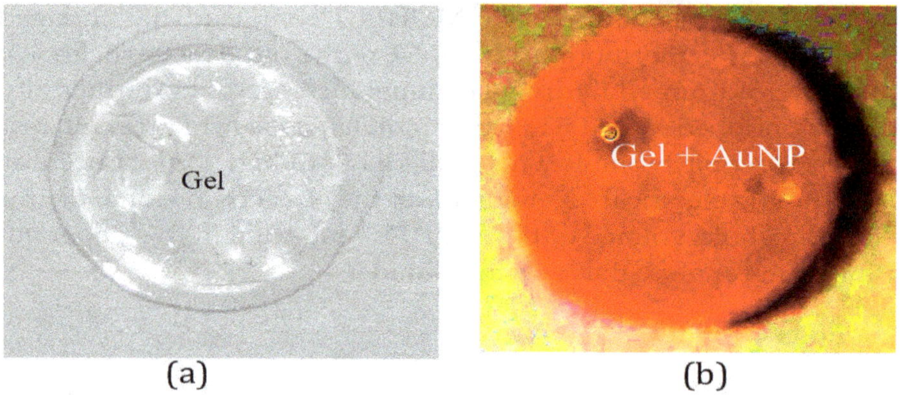

Figure 2. Photograph of the synthesized hydrogel. (**a**) Undoped hydrogel. (**b**) AuNP-doped hydrogel.

2.2. Impedance Spectroscopy of Hydrogel

Impedance spectroscopy is a well-established electrochemical technique for measuring hydrogel response to different analytes [8,10,12]. In this paper, impedance spectroscopy was used to measure the impedance change of the synthesized hydrogel as a function of its ionic content. As shown in Figure 3, the hydrogel was placed inside a fluidic cell (volume of 472 μL) centered over the 1 mm wide inter-electrode gap of two planar triangular 35 μm-thick copper electrodes. The substrate for the copper electrodes was a Roger RO4003C hydrocarbon/ceramic material of thickness 1.524 mm from Rogers Corporation (Chandler, AZ, USA). The fluidic cell was glued to the substrate/copper electrodes with epoxy. The sensor terminals were connected to the terminals of a 4284A Hewlett Packard Precision LCR meter (Hewlett Packard, Palo Alto, CA, USA). An analyte was introduced into the sensor cell, and the series capacitance and series resistance of the hydrogel sensor were monitored from 20 Hz to 1 MHz in 25 logarithmic steps.

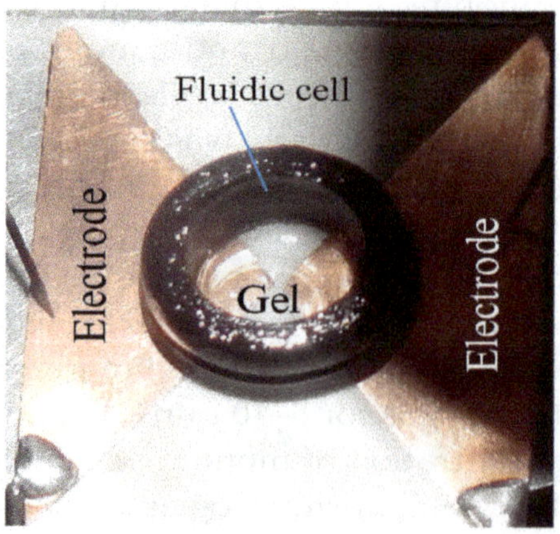

Figure 3. The device used for monitoring impedance changes of the hydrogel as the hydrogel responds to chemical concentrations.

2.3. Contact-Mode Microwave Hydrogel Measurements

Resonator-based microwave sensors have been used in the past in material-assisted sensors because resonant microwave circuits are most sensitive at or around their resonance frequencies [19–23]. To demonstrate the use of microwaves for hydrogel response monitoring, a hydrogel-integrated microwave resonator sensor was developed. This sensor consisted of a planar 1.3412 GHz half-wavelength copper microstrip resonator on a Rogers TMM13i grounded ceramic substrate (Rogers Corporation, Chandler, AZ, USA). The TMM13i ceramic was used in the sensor design because it has a low dielectric loss (loss tangent 0.0019) and was not very porous to the analytes that were used in this study. The relative dielectric constant of the ceramic substrate was 13. A fluidic cell was glued to the open circuit end of a half-wavelength microstrip resonator, and the hydrogel was placed inside the fluidic cell, as shown in Figure 4. The half-wavelength microwave resonator of this sensor was 35.5 mm long and 1.8 mm wide. The other end of the sensor resonator was critically coupled [14–16,36] to a 58.5 mm-long microstrip transmission line through a 100 μm coupling gap (Figure 4). The TMM13i dielectric substrate of the resonator was 2.54 mm thick and it has an area of 53 mm × 94 mm. A SubMiniature version A (SMA) connector (Amphenol Corp., Wallingford, CT, USA) was used to connect the resonator to an 8720C HP Vector Network Analyzer (VNA) (Hewlett Packard, CA, USA). The power, number of points, and the intermidate frequency (IF) bandwidth of the VNA were set to 0 dBm, 201, and 3.7 kHz, respectively. A LabVIEW program (LabVIEW version 2016, National Instruments, Austin, TX, USA) was used to automatically monitor the change in probe's S11 due to the hydrogel response to the DI water and 1× PBS.

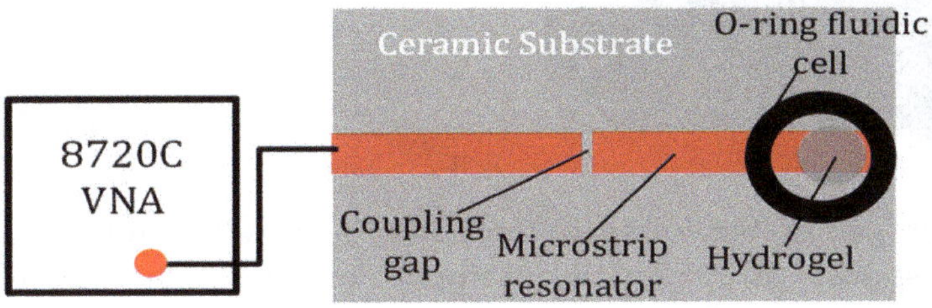

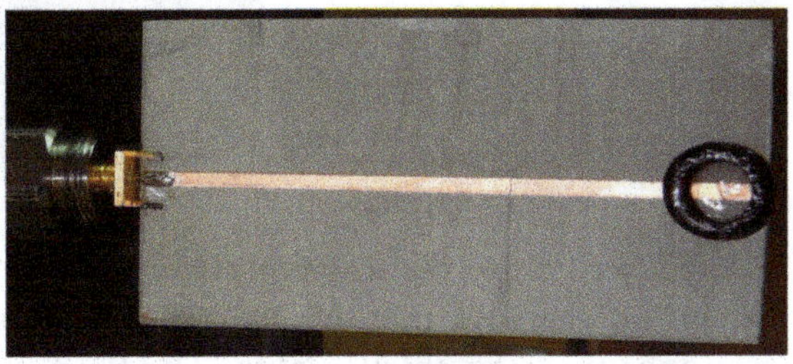

Figure 4. Sensor for monitoring hydrogel response with microwaves in the contact mode. (**a**) Schematic of the sensor. (**b**) Photograph of the sensor.

2.4. Contactless (Remote) Microwave Monitoring of Hyrogel Response

Microwave coaxial probes have been used in the past to remotely monitor the dielectric properties of materials [37]. The setup for non-contact monitoring of the hydrogel response via remote microwave sensing of hydrogel response is shown in Figure 5. The setup employs a coaxial microwave probe. The probe consists of a Teflon cylinder coupled to a RG 58U coaxial cable of length 50 cm. The Teflon cylinder has a diameter of 8.5 mm and length 5 mm. A brass ring was used to secure a copper back plate to one of the flat surfaces of the Teflon cylinder, as shown in Figure 5a. To transfer the microwave signals from the coaxial cable to the Teflon block, 1 mm length of the center conductor of the coaxial cable was force-fitted into the Teflon cylinder and the outer conductor of the coaxial was soldered to the copper back plate. The coaxial cable of the probe was connected to the 8720C HP Vector Network Analyzer (Hewlett Packard, CA, USA). The power, number of points, and IF bandwidth of the VNA were set to 0 dBm, 201 and 3.7 kHz, respectively.

To remotely monitor the hydrogel response through animal skin, the hydrogel was implanted under the skin of a chicken drumstick. The probe was positioned at a standoff distance of 0.5 mm from the chicken-skin surface over the embedded hydrogel (Figure 5b,c). A syringe and needle were then used to inject water or 1× PBS into the chicken thigh and the microwave probe was used to remotely monitor hydrogel response through the chicken skin. This measurement was done inside a protective Plexiglass box to prevent the chicken thigh sample from drying up. A 0.5 mm standoff distance was chosen in these measurements because 0.5 mm is the resolution of the positioning system used in the test setup. However, the closer the probe is to the container, the stronger the interaction of the microwave with the hydrogel. The manner in which the E-field of the microwaves decay can be seen in the E-field plot in Figure 5b.

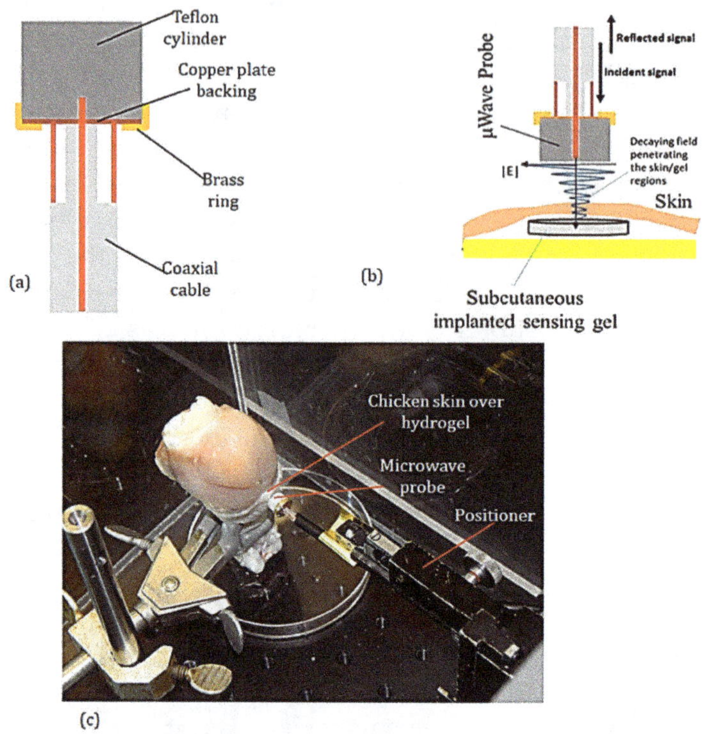

Figure 5. Remote microwave probing of hydrogel. (**a**) Schematic of the Teflon microwave probe for remote microwave monitoring of hydrogel response. (**b**) Schematic of setup for monitoring hydrogel response through chicken skin. The field distribution of the decaying microwave fields is perturbed when hydrogel swells or de-swells. This results in changes in the S_{11} of the probe. (**c**) Photograph of setup for monitoring hydrogel response through the skin of a chicken drumstick.

2.5. Potentiometric Method for Monitoring Hydrogel Response

A potentiometric method for monitoring hydrogel response is a desirable method because it will enable the hydrogel sensor to be integrated with inexpensive voltage readout electronics. Furthermore, it opens up the possibility of using the hydrogel in novel electronic circuits for highly sensitive detection. In the potentiometric method for monitoring hydrogel response, the hydrogel was placed asymmetrically at the inter-electrode gap of the two planar triangular electrodes, as shown in Figure 3, and the electric potential difference across the hydrogel (due to the difference in the ionic concentrations between the two regions where the electrodes make contact with the hydrogel) was measured with a 175A Keithley Multimeter (Keithley Instruments, Cleveland, OH, USA) every 0.02 min over 1× PBS and DI water cycles.

2.6. Monitoring Hydrogel Response with MOHFET Current-Voltage Characteristics

Based on the observed potentiometric responses of the hydrogel to analytes from the measurement of the previous section, the hydrogel was used to develop a field-effect transistor (FET) sensor. This hydrogel sensor with FET was designed by using undoped and gold nanoparticle-doped hydrogel as the channel material in an open-channel FET structure. In earlier publications, we have reported the fabrication and characterization of this device, used as a platform for experimenting with different post-deposited channel materials [30,31]. The FET consisted of a bottom-embedded gate with hafnium oxide gate dielectric [30,31] and surface-exposed platinum drain and source electrodes with effective channel length of 1 μm. The drop-cast hydrogel thickness was 50 μm. The schematic and photograph of this FET sensor is shown in Figure 6. The electrodes of the sensor were connected to a 4156A HP Precision Semiconductor Current-Voltage Parameter Analyzer (Hewlett Packard, CA, USA) through a probe station. The experiment with this FET was carried out with various concentrations of PBS (percentage by volume). The IV Characteristics curve of the FET were recorded for gate-source voltage (V_{gs}) of −3 V, 0 V and +3 V for drain-source voltage (V_{ds}) from −6 Volt to +6 Volt.

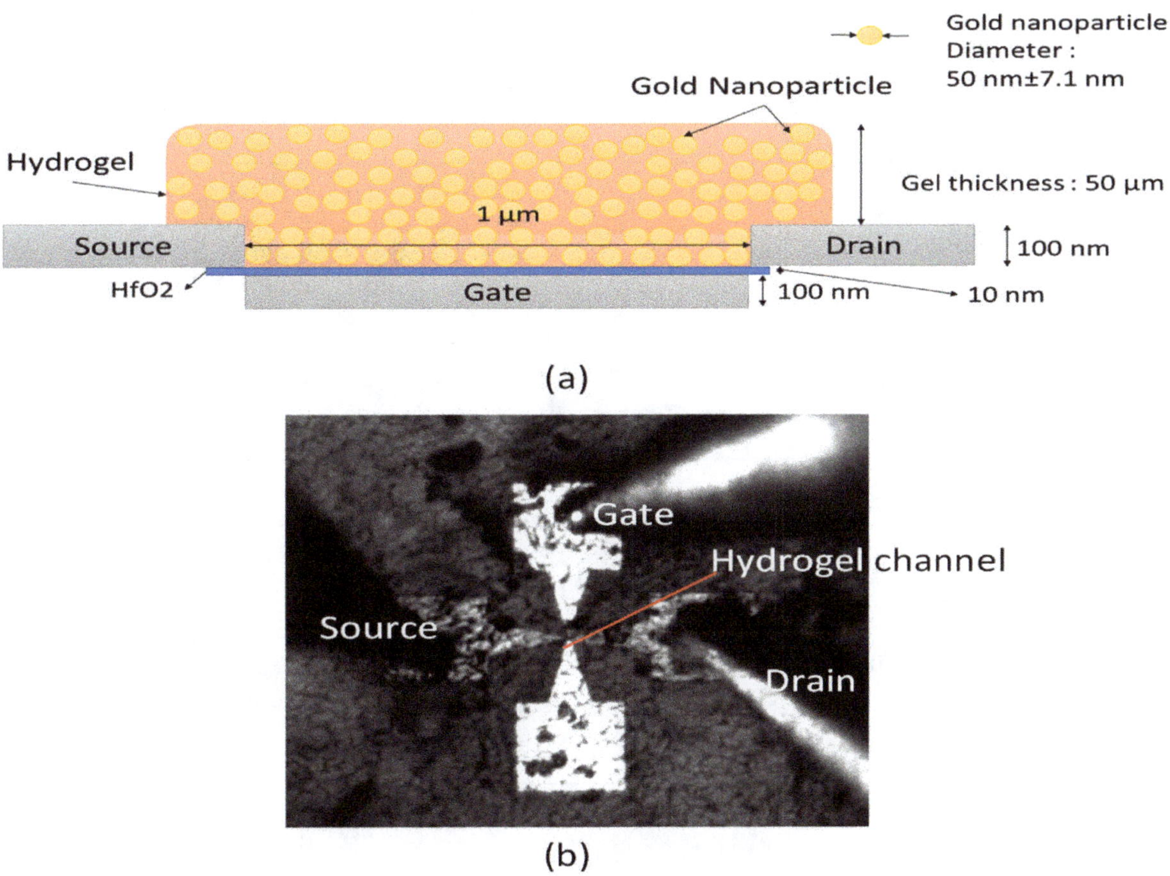

Figure 6. Hydrogel field-effect transistor (FET) sensor. (**a**) Schematic of the sensor. (**b**) Photograph of sensor. The fabricated devices consisted of four electrodes but only three of the electrodes were probed in the actual FET sensor.

3. Results

3.1. Impedance Spectroscopy for Monitoring Hydrogel Response

Figure 7a,b show the measured impedance (capacitance and resistance) of the DI water and 1× PBS of the hydrogel sensor (sensor shown in Figure 3) as a function frequency at different times. The measurements were taken over a frequency range of 20 Hz to 1 MHz at 4 different times. Time t = 0 was when the hydrogel was taken from its original 1× PBS medium, placed at the inter-electrode gap of the fluidic cell, and DI water added to the fluidic cell; time t = 60 min was at 60 min and this was the time when the DI water was siphoned out of the fluidic cell and replaced with 1× PBS and so on, as indicated in the insets of Figure 7. Figure 8a,b shows the result of the continuous monitoring of hydrogel capacitance and resistance over cycles of adding 1× PBS and DI water to the fluidic cell at a single frequency. The single frequency for the continuous monitoring (every 1.28 min) of the hydrogel was 638 kHz. It can be seen from these results that the signature of the hydrogel response to DI water is a decrease in sensor capacitance, while the signature of hydrogel response to 1× PBS is an increase in sensor capacitance. The reverse is the case for sensor resistance.

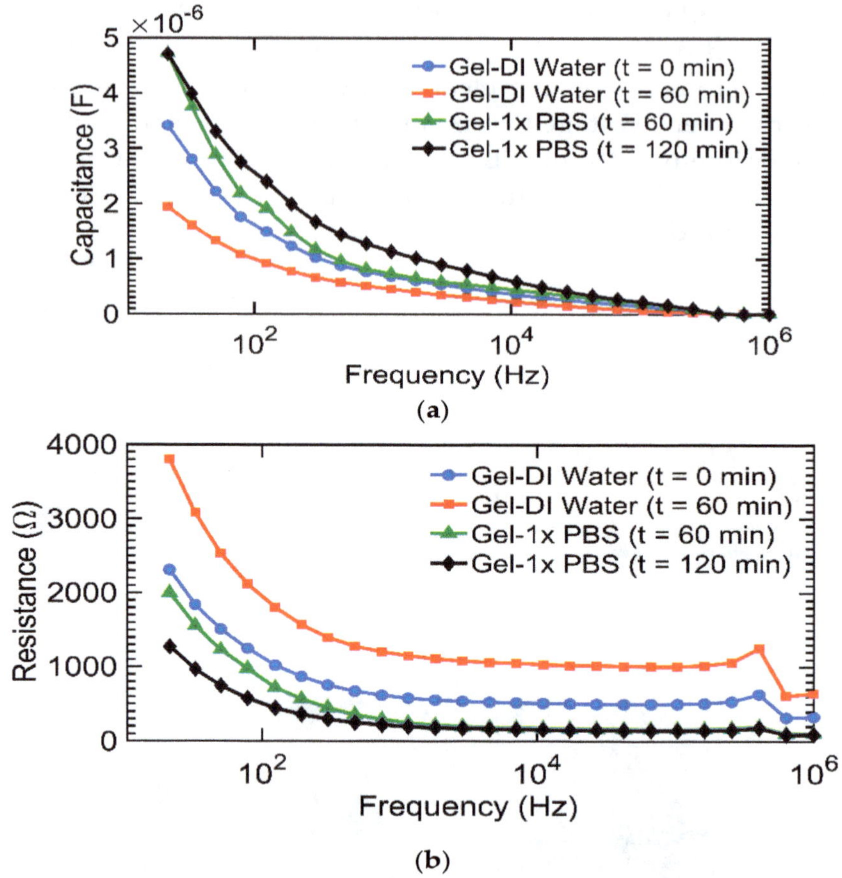

Figure 7. Impedance of the hydrogel-integrated sensor. (**a**) Time-dependent change in capacitance of the hydrogel sensor. (**b**) Time-dependent change in resistance of the hydrogel sensor. It can be seen that phosphate buffered saline (PBS) reduces the hydrogel sensor's electric resistance and increases hydrogel's response capacitance.

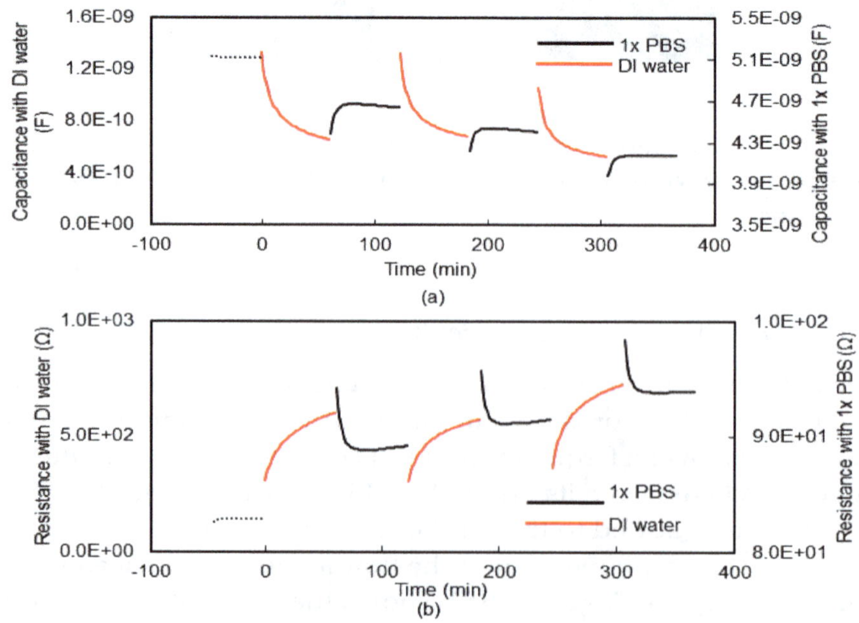

Figure 8. Impedance of the hydrogel sensor as a function of time as solutions with different ionic concentrations were introduced. (**a**) Hydrogel sensor capacitance in response to deionized (DI) water or 1× PBS. (**b**) Hydrogel sensor resistance in response to DI water or 1× PBS.

3.2. Contact-Mode Microwave Measurements of Hydrogels

The hydrogel from impedance spectroscopy measurements was used in the contact-microwave hydrogel sensor device shown in Figure 4. The S_{11} spectrum of the microwave resonator probe and fluidic cell assembly before loading the hydrogel and the analyte into the fluidic cell is shown in Figure 9a. Figure 9b shows the S_{11} of the probe assembly when the fluidic cell of the probe was loaded with DI water or with 1× PBS, without hydrogel integration with the resonator. With only the analyte present in the fluidic cell, the S_{11} spectra of the sensor did not change significantly with time. Figure 9c shows the S_{11} of the probe loaded with DI water and 1× PBS, now with the hydrogel at the tip of the resonator inside the fluidic cell. This measurement was done over a frequency band of 1.175 GHz to 1.2 GHz at 4 different times. At time t = 0 the hydrogel was taken from its original 1× PBS medium, placed in the fluidic cell at the tip of the microstrip resonator, and DI water added to the fluidic cell. At time t = 60 min, the DI water was siphoned out of the fluidic cell and replaced with 1× PBS; and so on. Figure 10 shows the result of continuously monitoring (every 6 s) the S_{11} of the hydrogel sensor over cycles of 1× PBS and DI water at a chosen frequency within the 1.175 GHz to 1.2 GHz band. The chosen single frequency for this S_{11} monitoring was 1.1917 GHz. This frequency was chosen because it is the frequency where the S_{11} change of the sensors was maximum when the analyte was changed from DI water to 1× PBS.

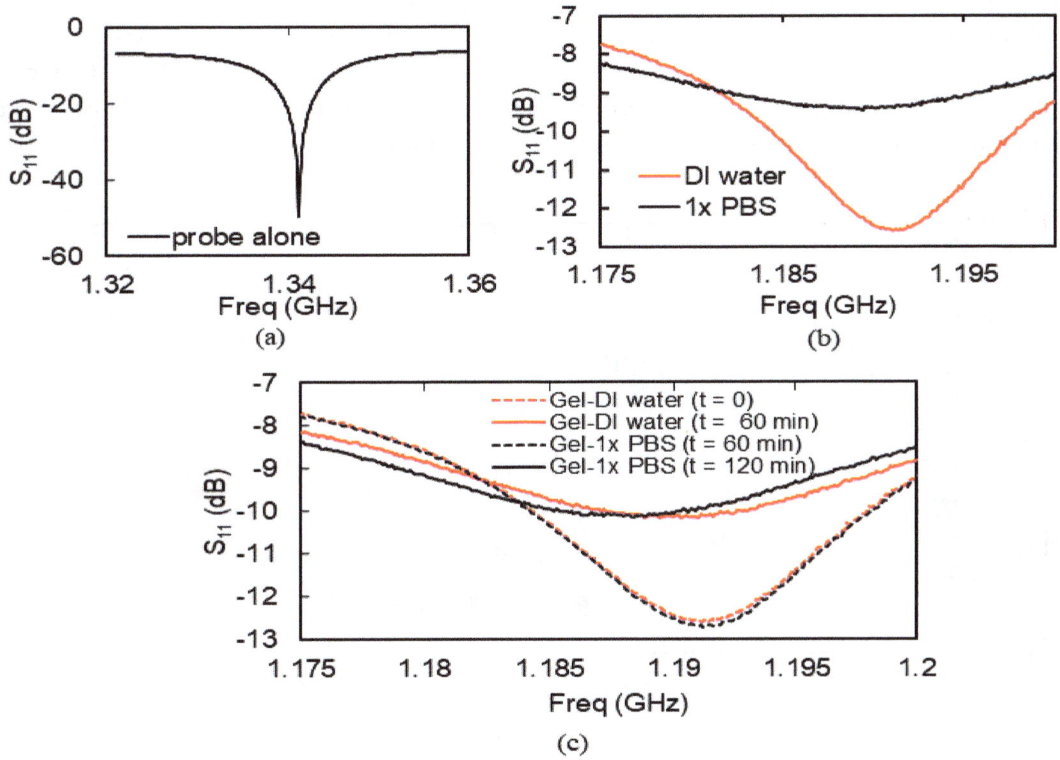

Figure 9. Microwave reflection spectra of the microwave probe. (**a**) Spectrum of the microwave probe with no hydrogel or analyte; (**b**) Spectrum of the microwave probe with analyte but no hydrogel; (**c**) Spectra of the microwave probe with hydrogel for different analytes at different times.

It should be noted that the smaller resistance of the PBS + hydrogel loads down the microwave resonator resulting in a shallow S_{11} around the resonance frequency as can be seen in Figure 9b. With the water analyte, however, the hydrogel resistance increases and the S_{11} at resonance becomes much smaller. These observations are corroborated by the impedance measurement results shown in Figure 7.

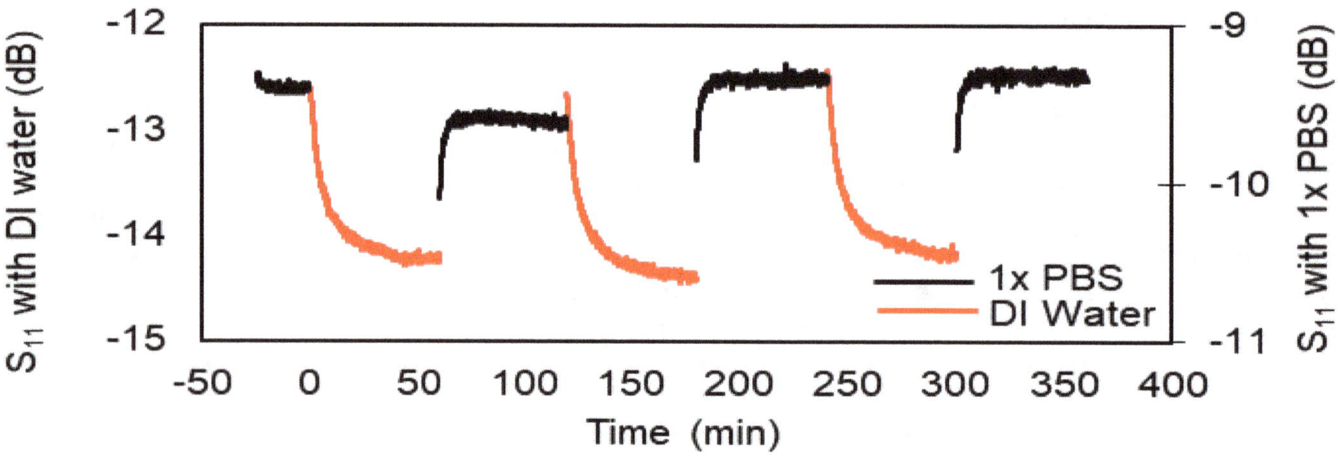

Figure 10. S_{11} of microwave resonator/probe with hydrogel at 1.1917 GHz as a function time with different analytes.

3.3. *Remote Microwave Monitoring of Hydrogel Response*

Figure 11 shows the result of using the probe to continuously monitor the hydrogel implanted under the skin of a chicken drumstick. The frequency for the remote monitoring was 3.726 GHz. The probe response is more complex than before because of other ionic species inside the chicken. However, the change in the S_{11} is consistent with the results obtained in the contact-mode measurements (Figure 9). In this measurement, at probe resonance, the injection of PBS solution reduces the magnitude of S_{11} while the injection of water increases S_{11} magnitude.

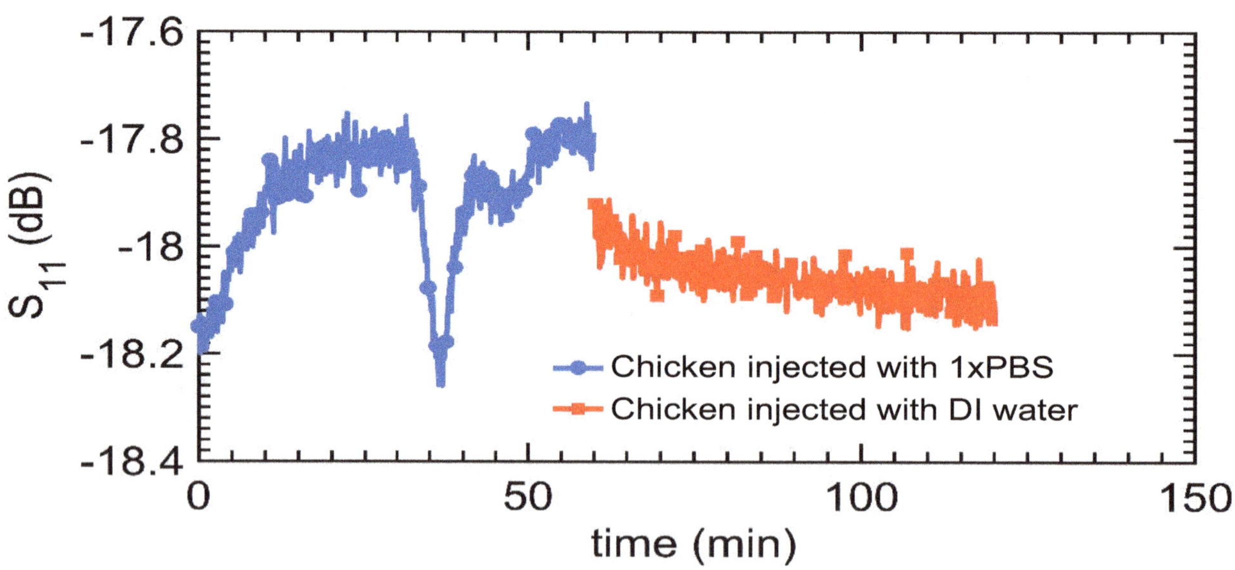

Figure 11. Remote monitoring of the swelling/de-swelling of hydrogel sensor implanted under the skin of a chicken drumstick with the Teflon-protected microwave probe.

3.4. *Potentiometric Method for Monitoring Hydrogel Response*

The voltage difference across the hydrogel in response to different analytes was measured as a function of time. As shown in Figure 12, the potentiometric response to the hydrogel to DI water and 1× PBS was measured. The interesting aspect of this measurement is that it can be accomplished using a simple digital voltmeter. It does not require any additional signal source or sensitive detection equipment Moreover, it can be used as the basis of a voltage-controlled hydrogel oscillator for wireless telemetry of hydrogel response to chemicals. The normalized change in the voltage ($\Delta V/V$) is very large, at around 500%.

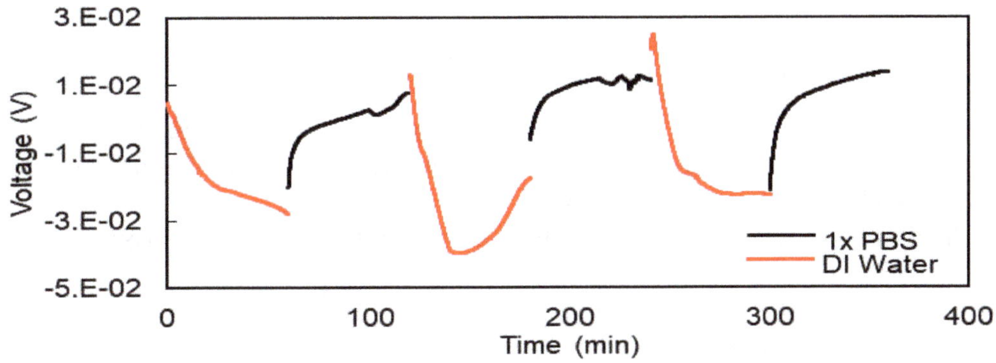

Figure 12. Potential generated across the hydrogel sensor as a function of time in response to 1× PBS and DI water.

3.5. *Montioring Hydrogel Response with Metal-Oxide-Hydrogel Field-Effect Transistor (MOHFET) Current-Voltage (IV) Characteristics*

The hydrogel FET sensor was characterized with various concentrations of phosphate buffer solution (PBS). The Current-Voltage (IV) characteristics were measured for gate voltage $V_{gs} = -3$, 0 and +3 V for drain to source voltage V_{ds} from −6 Volt to +6 Volt as shown in Figure 13. The percentage changes in the channel conductance with and without PBS was around 120%, which is similar to the resistance changes discussed in the potentiometric measurements.

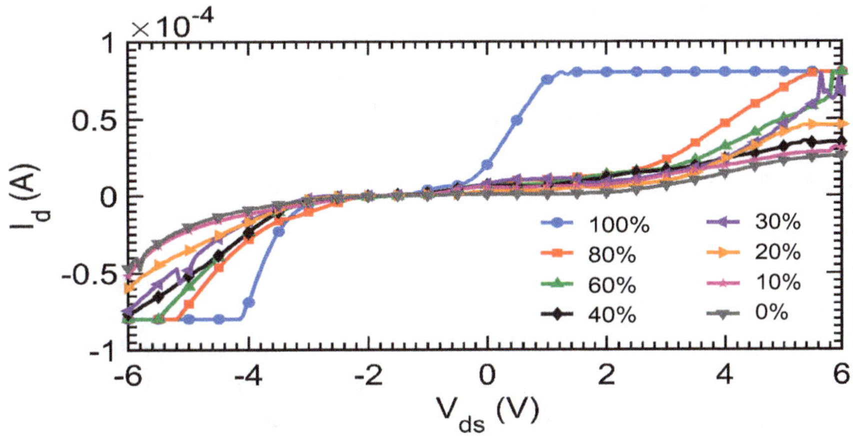

(a)

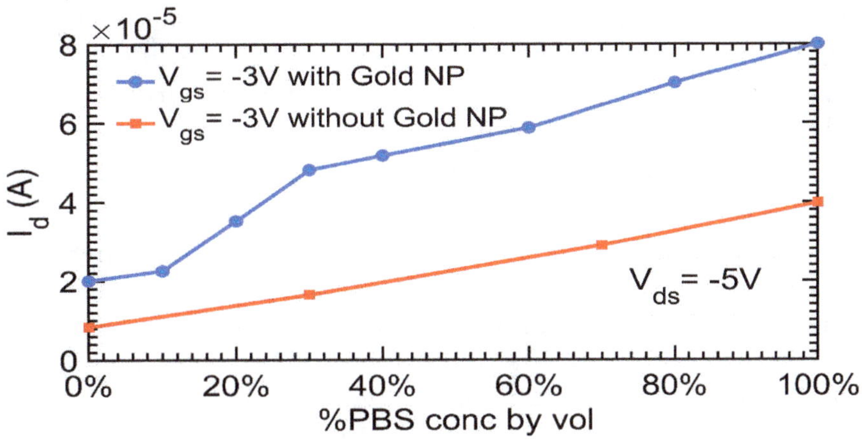

(b)

Figure 13. Chemical sensing with the hydrogel FET (**a**) I_d-V_{ds} plot of the hydrogel with Au-NP device with various concentrations of PBS in DI water by volume at $V_{gs} = -3$ V and $V_{ds} = -6$ V to +6 V (**b**) I_d at $V_{ds} = -5$ V for different concentrations of PBS by volume for $V_{gs} = -3$ V.

4. Discussion

4.1. Microwave Monitoring of Hydrogel Response

As mentioned earlier, hydrogel responds to changes in ionic concentration by absorbing or releasing water (swelling or de-swelling). In the hydrogel integrated with the contact-mode microwave hydrogel sensors, the absorption/release of water leads to changes in the dielectric constant of the hydrogel, and this change can be computed with the Maxwell–Garnett approximation [38]:

$$\varepsilon_{eff} = \varepsilon_m \frac{(2\delta_i(\varepsilon_i - \varepsilon_m) + \varepsilon_i + 2\varepsilon_m)}{2\varepsilon_m + \varepsilon_i + \delta_i(\varepsilon_m - \varepsilon_i)} \tag{1}$$

where ε_{eff} is the dielectric constant of the swollen or de-swollen hydrogel, ε_m is the dielectric constant of the hydrogel matrix, ε_i is the dielectric constant of the water contained in the hydrogel, and δ_i is the volume fraction of water contained in the hydrogel. Since the hydrogel is in close proximity with the microwave probe, changes in hydrogel dielectric property result in changes in the probe's response. In the hydrogel sensor with contact-mode microwave readout, the hydrogel was placed at the tip of the microstrip resonator. This tip is where the electric field of the resonator is maximum and where slight changes in the hydrogel's complex permittivity result in big changes in the microwave impedance of the probe.

The open-circuit half-wavelength resonator of the hydrogel probe can be modeled as a parallel resonant resistor-capacitor-inductor (RCL) circuit [36] as shown in the model of Figure 14. In this model, the hydrogel and the analyte are modeled as an RC circuit [39]. The microwave resonator and the analyte are modeled with constant circuit parameters because their properties do not change over time in the measurements. However, the hydrogel's electrical parameters change in a time-dependent manner since the hydrogel respond slowly to changes in the concentration of an analyte in contact with the hydrogel (as the hydrogel gradually swells or de-swells). In addition to the hydrogel, the background analyte also loads the resonator. However, the analyte loads the hydrogel instantaneously and the loading effect is stationary.

The hydrogel response sensing with remote microwave probe can be modeled in a similar way as the contact-mode sensor. However, the dielectric layers (air, plastic, or skin) between the hydrogel and the microwave probe are modeled by a coupling capacitor as shown in Figure 14c. In the subcutaneously implanted hydrogel, due to the low coupling capacitance between the probe and the implanted hydrogel, the observable change in probe S_{11} due to the swelling/de-swelling of the hydrogel is low. This is seen by the small variation in the S_{11} in Figure 11 as the hydrogel swells/de-swells. Furthermore, the environment of the hydrogel when the hydrogel was implanted under the chicken skin differs significantly from the controlled fluidic cell of the hydrogel in the contact-mode microwave measurement. Hence, there is a noticeable artifact in Figure 11 of the S_{11} of the probe in response to the swelling/de-swelling of the hydrogel under the skin of the chicken.

From the results presented in Sections 3.2 and 3.3 and from the analysis above, it can be concluded that the hydrogel responds to the analyte because it is a water encapsulation medium whose encapsulation property is time-dependent. When the hydrogel swells by absorbing water, it brings more water closer to the microwave probe. Therefore, the S_{11} measured by the probe varies in a time-dependent manner towards the S_{11} of the probe when the probe is sensing only water (without the hydrogel present). The reverse occurs when the hydrogel de-swells. The schematic illustrating the hydrogel as a transient encapsulation medium for the hydrogel sensors with contact-mode microwave is shown in Figure 15. The degree to which the fields of the probe interact with the hydrogel/analytes can be seen in the figure. This illustration is easily extended to the remote microwave readout case. This illustration also applies to the results of the hydrogel impedance sensor of Section 3.1.

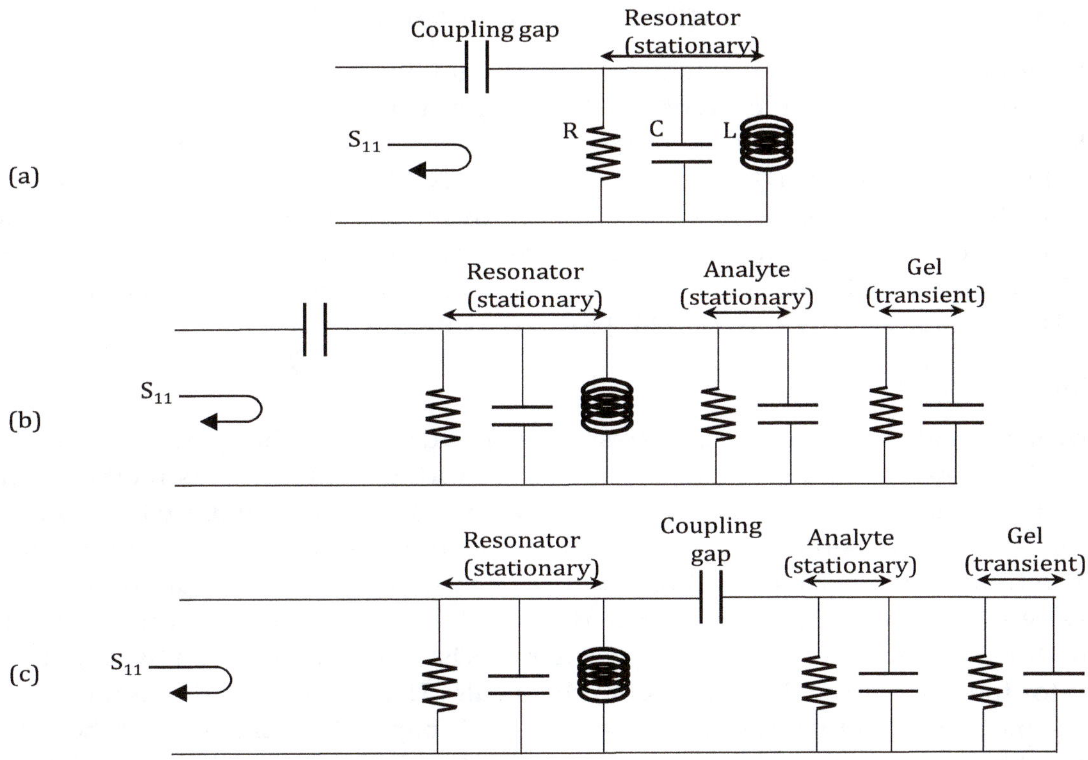

Figure 14. Circuit model of hydrogel sensing with microwave. (**a**) Circuit model of the microstrip microwave resonator; (**b**) Circuit model of the resonator, analyte and hydrogel of the hydrogel sensor with contact-mode microwave readout; (**c**) Circuit model of the probe, analyte and hydrogel of hydrogel sensing with remote microwave readout.

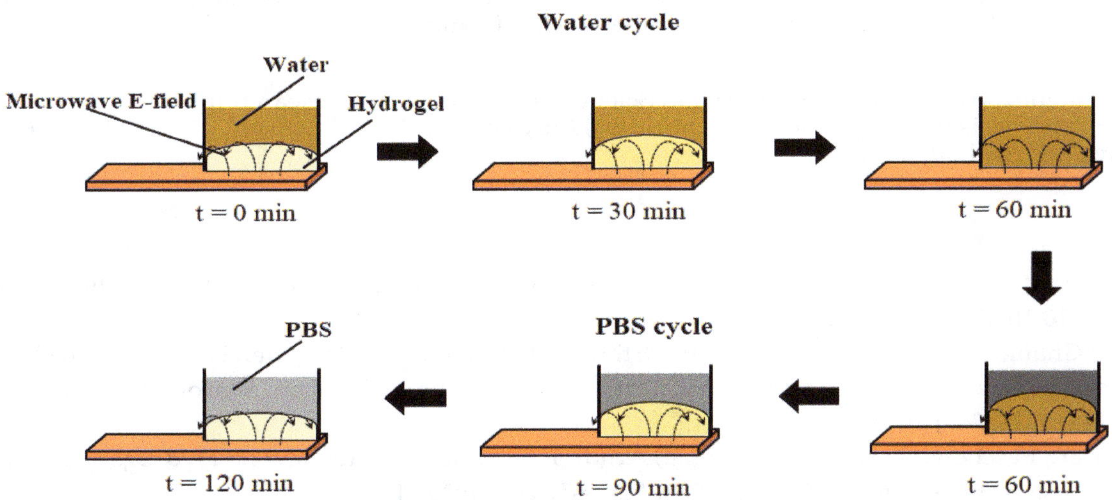

Figure 15. Schematic illustrating the behavior of a hydrogel as an encapsulation medium for water.

In future studies, the contact and remote microwave probes will be calibrated to different chemicals, including glucose, in order to compare their sensitivities to that of other transduction techniques for hydrogel sensing. It should be mentioned that the microwave transduction technique has the advantage that its sensitivity can be easily amplified with innovative detection techniques such as the heterodyne detection technique [33]. Developing a highly-sensitive transduction technique for hydrogel sensing will allow researchers to focus more on synthesizing hydrogels for chemical and biomolecule selectivity rather than focusing on synthesizing for both sensitivity and selectivity at the same time.

4.2. *Montioring Hydrogel Response with MOHFET IV Characteristics*

The predominant conduction mechanism in hydrogel film is ionic conduction [40]. A hydrogel doped with Au-NP increases the current conduction limit due to additional conductivity of gold nanoparticles and possible current tunneling between them. The channel conductivity increased as a function of PBS concentration in both hydrogel and AuNP-hydrogel channels but the change was larger in AuNP-hydrogel channel. At zero PBS concentrations the channel conductivities of both devices were low and similar, indicating that the hydrogel was swollen and any additional conductivity due to AuNP was lost. The MOHFET data will be used to design an implantable oscillator that can wirelessly [41] send glucose concentration [42] to an outside reader unit.

5. Conclusions

Two novel methods for monitoring the response of hydrogels to chemicals have been developed in this paper. The first method is the microwave-monitoring method. This method measures the perturbation of the fields of a microwave probe by swelling/de-swelling hydrogel to monitor hydrogel response. This allows both contact (invasive) and remote (non-invasive) monitoring of the hydrogel response. The remote microwave sensing is of greater interest because it can be used for sensing the response of subcutaneously implanted hydrogels. The other novel method is the field-effect transistor method in which the current-voltage characteristics of a FET with a hydrogel channel was used to monitor the response of the hydrogel to chemicals. The FET monitoring is an extension of the potentiometric measurement that was also presented in this paper. The sensitivity of the potentiometric technique was 3 times larger than the resistance and MOHFET changes (Figure 7) and 35 times larger than the S_{11} changes (Figure 10). The FET sensing technique has the advantage that it can be used in an oscillator for wireless telemetry of hydrogel response to chemicals.

Author Contributions: Supervision and the original ideas, M.T.-A.; Writing—original draft, O.C.F.; Writing—review and editing, S.D.; Hydrogel synthesis, H.-Y.L. and J.M.

Acknowledgments: We wish to thank the Utah Science Technology and Research Initiative (USTAR) program. The hydrogel synthesis was supported by Sentiomed, Inc., The Joe W. and Dorothy Dorsett Brown Foundation, and the Olive Tupper Foundation.

References

1. Guenther, M.; Gerlach, G. Hydrogels for Chemical Sensors. Available online: https://link.springer.com/chapter/10.1007/978-3-540-75645-3_5 (accessed on 11 August 2009).
2. Lin, G.; Chang, S.; Hao, H.; Tathireddy, P.; Orthner, M.; Magda, J.; Solzbacher, F. Osmotic Swelling Pressure Response of Smart Hydrogels Suitable for Chronically-Implantable Glucose Sensors. *Sens. Actuators B Chem.* **2010**, *144*, 332–336. [CrossRef] [PubMed]
3. Richter, A.; Paschew, G.; Klatt, S.; Lienig, J.; Arndt, K.F.; Adler, H.P. Review on Hydrogel-based pH Sensors and microsensors. *Sensors* **2008**, *8*, 561–581. [CrossRef] [PubMed]
4. Cong, J.; Zhang, X.; Chen, K.; Xu, J. Fiber optic Bragg grating sensor based on hydrogels for measuring salinity. *Sens. Actuators B Chem.* **2002**, *87*, 487–490. [CrossRef]
5. Kuzimenkova, M.V.; Ivanov, A.E.; Thammakhet, C.; Mikhalovska, L.I.; Galaev, I.Y.; Thavarungkul, P.; Kanatharana, P.; Mattiasson, B. Optical responses, permeability and diol-specific reactivity of thin polyacrylamide gels containing immobilized phenylboronic acid. *Polymer* **2008**, *49*, 1444–1454. [CrossRef]
6. Tierney, S.; Volden, S.; Stokke, B.T. Glucose sensors based on a responsive gel incorporated as a Fabry-Perot cavity on a fiber-optic readout platform. *Biosens. Bioelectron.* **2009**, *24*, 2034–2039. [CrossRef] [PubMed]
7. Tierney, S.; Hjelme, D.R.; Stokke, B.T. Determination of swelling of responsive gels with nanometer resolution. Fiber-optic based platform for hydrogels as signal transducers. *Anal. Chem.* **2008**, *80*, 5086–5093. [CrossRef] [PubMed]

8. Sheppard, N.F., Jr.; Salehi-Had, S.; Tucker, R.C. Design of a conductimetric microsensor based on pH-sensitive polymer hydrogels. *Proc. Annu. Conf. Eng. Med. Biol.* **1991**, *13*, 1581–1582.
9. Huang, H.M.; Liu, C.H.; Lee, V.; Lee, C.; Wang, M.J. Highly sensitive glucose biosensor based on CF4-plasma-modified interdigital transducer array (IDA) microelectrode. *Sens. Actuators B Chem.* **2010**, *149*, 59–66. [CrossRef]
10. Guan, T.; Ceyssens, F.; Puers, R. Fabrication and testing of a MEMS platform for characterization of stimuli-sensitive hydrogels. *J. Micromech. Microeng.* **2012**, *22*, 087001. [CrossRef]
11. Kikuchi, A.; Suzuki, K.; Okabayashi, O.; Hoshino, H.; Kataoka, K.; Sakurai, Y.; Okano, T. Glucose-sensing electrode coated with polymer complex gel containing phenylboronic acid. *Anal. Chem.* **1996**, *68*, 823–828. [CrossRef] [PubMed]
12. Mac Kenna, N.; Calvert, P.; Morrin, A. Impedimetric transduction of swelling in pH-responsive hydrogels. *Analyst* **2015**, *140*, 3003–3011. [CrossRef] [PubMed]
13. Tabib-Azar, M.; Leclair, S.R. Applications of evanescent microwave probes in gas and chemical sensors. *Sens. Actuators B Chem.* **2000**, *67*, 112–121. [CrossRef]
14. Tabib-Azar, M.; Wang, R. Planar evanescent microwave imaging probes for nondestructive evaluation of materials with very high spatial resolutions and scan rates. *AIP Conf. Proc.* **2001**, *557*, 446.
15. Tabib-Azar, M. Microwave microscopy and its applications. *AIP Conf. Proc.* **2001**, *557*, 400–413.
16. Tabib-Azar, M. Evanescent Microwave Microscope: A New Nondestructive Material Evaluation Tool with Very High Resolutions-Part 2. *CSNDT J.* **2001**, *22*, 14–21.
17. Sinha, K.; Fawole, O.C.; Tabib-Azar, M. Non-invasive monitoring of electrical parameters of Schefflera arboricola leaf. In Proceedings of the 2015 IEEE SENSORS, Busan, South Korea, 1–4 November 2015.
18. García-Valenzuela, A.; Tabib-Azar, M. Evanescent microwave probes and microscopy. *Rev. Mex. Fis.* **1999**, *45*, 539–550.
19. Jones, T.R.; Member, G.S.; Zarifi, M.H.; Member, S. Miniaturized Quarter-Mode Substrate Integrated Cavity Resonators for Humidity Sensing Miniaturized Quarter-Mode Substrate Integrated Cavity Resonators for Humidity Sensing. *IEEE Microw. Wireless Compon. Lett.* **2017**, *27*, 612–614. [CrossRef]
20. Bogner, A.; Steiner, C.; Walter, S.; Kita, J.; Hagen, G.; Sensors, R.M. Planar Microstrip Ring Resonators for Microwave-Based Gas Sensing: Design Aspects and Initial Transducers for Humidity and Ammonia Sensing. *Sensors* **2017**, *17*, 2422. [CrossRef] [PubMed]
21. Rydosz, A.; Maciak, E.; Wincza, K.; Gruszczynski, S. Microwave-based sensors with phthalocyanine films for acetone, ethanol and methanol detection. *Sens. Actuators B Chem.* **2016**, *237*, 876–886. [CrossRef]
22. Zarifi, M.H.; Gholidoust, A.; Abdolrazzaghi, M.; Shariaty, P.; Hashisho, Z.; Daneshmand, M. Sensitivity enhancement in planar microwave active-resonator using metal organic framework for CO_2 detection. *Sens. Actuators B Chem.* **2018**, *255*, 1561–1568. [CrossRef]
23. Li, H.; Chen, Z.; Borodinov, N.; Luzinov, L.; Yu, G.J.; Wang, P.S. Multi-frequency measurement of volatile organic compounds with a radio-frequency interferometer. *IEEE Sens. J.* **2017**, *17*, 3323–3331. [CrossRef]
24. Fawole, O.; Sinha, K.; Tabib-Azar, M. Monitoring yeast activation with sugar and zero-calorie sweetener using terahertz waves. In Proceedings of the 2015 IEEE SENSORS, Busan, South Korea, 1–4 November 2015.
25. Fawole, O.C.; Tabib-Azar, M. Terahertz Near-Field Imaging of Biological Samples with Horn Antenna-Excited Probes. *IEEE Sens. J.* **2016**, *16*, 8752–8760. [CrossRef]
26. Wu, H.; Yu, G.; Pan, L.; Liu, N.; McDowell, M.T.; Bao, Z.; Cui, Y. Stable Li-ion battery anodes by in-situ polymerization of conducting hydrogel to conformally coat silicon nanoparticles. *Nat. Commun.* **2013**, *4*, 1943. [CrossRef] [PubMed]
27. Shi, Z.; Zhao, W.; Li, S.; Yang, G. Self-Powered Hydrogel Induced by Ion Transport. *Nanoscale* **2017**, *9*, 17080–17090. [CrossRef] [PubMed]
28. Dolai, S.; Leu, H.Y.; Magda, J.; Tabib-Azar, M. Hydrogel Gold Nanoparticle Switch. *IEEE Electron Device Lett.* **2018**, *39*, 1421–1424. [CrossRef]
29. Dolai, S.; Leu, H.Y.; Magda, J.; Tabib-Azar, M. Metal-Oxide-Hydrogel Field-Effect Sensor. *IEEE Electron Device Lett.* **2018**, *39*, 1421–1424. [CrossRef]
30. Pai, P.; Chowdhury, F.K.; Dang-Tran, T.V.; Tabib-Azar, M. TiOx memristors with variable turn-on voltage using field-effect for non-volatile memory. In Proceedings of the 2013 IEEE SENSORS, Baltimore, MD, USA, 3–6 November 2013.

31. Mou, N.I.; Zhang, Y.; Pai, P.; Tabib-Azar, M. Steep sub-threshold current slope ($\sim$2 mV/dec) Pt/Cu2S/Pt gated memristor with Ion/Ioff> 100. *Solid State Electron.* **2017**, *127*, 20–25. [CrossRef]
32. Thoniyot, P.; Tan, M.J.; Karim, A.A.; Young, D.J.; Loh, X.J. Nanoparticle–Hydrogel Composites: Concept, Design, and Applications of These Promising, Multi-Functional Materials. *Adv. Sci.* **2015**, *2*, 1400010. [CrossRef] [PubMed]
33. Matsumoto, A.; Sato, N.; Sakata, T.; Yoshida, R.; Kataoka, K.; Miyahara, Y. Chemical-to-electrical-signal transduction synchronized with smart gel volume phase transition. *Adv. Mater.* **2009**, *21*, 4372–4378. [CrossRef] [PubMed]
34. Orthner, M.P.; Lin, G.; Avula, M.; Buetefisch, S.; Magda, J.; Rieth, L.W.; Solzbacher, F. Hydrogel based sensor arrays (2 $\times$ 2) with perforated piezoresistive diaphragms for metabolic monitoring (in vitro). *Sens. Actuators B Chem.* **2010**, *145*, 807–816. [CrossRef] [PubMed]
35. Flory, P.J. *Principles of Polymer Chemistry*; Cornell University Press: New York, NY, USA, 1953.
36. Pozar, D.M. *Microwave Engineering*; John Wiley & Sons: Hoboken, NJ, USA, 2009.
37. Meaney, P.M.; Gregory, A.P.; Epstein, N.R.; Paulsen, K.D. Microwave open-ended coaxial dielectric probe: Interpretation of the sensing volume re-visited. *BMC Med. Phys.* **2014**, *14*, 3. [CrossRef] [PubMed]
38. Garnett, J.M. VII. Colours in metal glasses, in metallic films, and in metallic solutions.—II. *Phil. Trans. R. Soc. Lond. A* **1906**, *205*, 237–288. [CrossRef]
39. Jilani, M.; Wen, W.; Cheong, L.Y.; Zakariya, M.A.; Rehman, M.Z. Equivalent circuit modeling of the dielectric loaded microwave biosensor. *Radioengineering* **2014**, *23*, 1038–1047.
40. Kataoka, H.; Saito, Y.; Sakai, T.; Quartarone, E.; Mustarelli, P. Conduction Mechanisms of PVDF-Type Gel Polymer Electrolytes of Lithium Prepared by a Phase Inversion Process. *J. Phys. Chem. B* **2000**, *104*, 11460–11464. [CrossRef]
41. Salsbery, G.; Tabib-Azar, M. Wireless sensor for determining the impedance of human skin. In Proceedings of the 2016 IEEE SENSORS, Orlando, FL, USA, 30 October–3 November 2016.
42. Salsbery, G.; Tabib-Azar, M. Optical sensor for determining concentration of glucose in water. In Proceedings of the 2016 IEEE SENSORS, Orlando, FL, USA, 30 October–3 November 2016.

9

Miniaturized Optical Resolution Photoacoustic Microscope Based on a Microelectromechanical Systems Scanning Mirror

Weizhi Qi [1,2,†], Qian Chen [1,2,†], Heng Guo [1,2], Huikai Xie [3] and Lei Xi [1,2,*]

1 Department of Biomedical Engineering, Southern University of Science and Technology, Shenzhen 518055, China; qiweizhi@std.uestc.edu.cn (W.Q.); QianChen@std.uestc.edu.cn (Q.C.); guoheng95@std.uestc.edu.cn (H.G.)

2 School of Physics, University of Electronic Science and Technology of China, Chengdu 610054, China

3 Department of Electrical and Computer Engineering, University of Florida, Gainesville, FL 32611, USA; hkxie@ece.ufl.edu

* Correspondence: xilei@sustc.edu.cn

† These authors contributed equally to this work.

Abstract: In this paper, we report a miniaturized optical resolution photoacoustic microscopy system based on a microelectromechanical system (MEMS) scanning mirror. A two-dimensional MEMS scanning mirror was used to achieve raster scanning of the excitation optical focus. The wideband photoacoustic signals were detected by a flat ultrasound transducer with a center frequency of 10 MHz and an active area of 2 mm in diameter. The size and weight of this device were 60 mm × 30 mm × 20 mm and 40 g, respectively. We evaluated this system using sharp blades, carbon fibers, and a silver strip target. In vivo experiments of imaging vasculatures in the mouse ear, brain, and human lip were completed to demonstrate its potential for biological and clinical applications.

Keywords: photoacoustic; microelectromechanical systems (MEMS); miniaturized microscope

---

1. Introduction

Optical resolution photoacoustic microscopy (ORPAM) is one of the fastest evolving microscopic imaging techniques [1–4]. ORPAM uses a highly converging laser beam with an ultrashort pulse duration to generate wideband acoustic waves that can be detected by acoustic transducers [5,6]. It uses intrinsic biological contrast and has a comparative lateral resolution with a deeper penetration depth compared with conventional pure optical microscopic imaging modalities [7]. In a conventional ORPAM, a two-dimensional (2D) motorized mechanical scanner is required to perform raster scanning of the overlapped optical and acoustic focuses to form a three-dimensional (3D) image [8–10]. However, improving the temporal resolution and realizing miniaturization of these mechanical-scanning-based ORPAMs are difficult due to the limited moving velocity and bulky size of the scanners. To achieve high-speed imaging and compact configuration, several new scanning mechanisms and scanners have been proposed. Xi et al. developed an intraoperative photoacoustic tomography system with a lateral resolution of up to 0.2 mm based on a microelectromechanical systems (MEMS) scanning mirror and a ring-shaped ultrasound transducer [11]. In addition, a rotary-scanning-based portable ORPAM (pORPAM) has been reported and applied to various biomedical and clinical applications [12,13]. Wang and colleagues used a water-immersible magnetic MEMS mirror with a plate size of 9 mm × 9 mm to simultaneously scan both optical and acoustic focuses for fast brain and single circulating melanoma cells imaging [14–16]. As an improvement on previous systems, they reported a handheld ORPAM using a newly developed two-axis magnetic MEMS mirror with an active imaging area of 2.5 mm × 2.5 mm, and dimensions of 80 mm × 115 mm × 150 mm [17]. Wang et al. also reported magnetic MEMS-based all-optical photoacoustic microscopy [18]. Kim et al. introduced a high-speed and high-signal to noise ratio (SNR) photoacoustic microscopy immerged in non-conducting liquid [19], and a polydimethylsiloxane (PDMS)-based two axis MEMS scanner with a size of 15 mm × 15 mm × 15 mm for developing a handheld ORPAM [20–22]. Use of a graded-index (GRIN) lens integrated with an image-guided optical fiber bundle, Zemp et al. developed a 500 g, 40 mm × 60 mm portable ORPAM probe with an imaging area of 800 μm [23]. Although these attempts are encouraging, the systems' inherent limitations are still challenging for clinical applications.

In this study, we used an electrothermal-bimorph-actuation-based MEMS mirror to develop a miniaturized ORPAM probe. The MEMS mirror had a diameter of 2 mm, a resonant frequency of 800 Hz, and a 7° optical scanning angle [24]. The entire probe was 60 mm × 30 mm × 20 mm with a weight of 40 g. Phantom experiments showed that the system has a lateral resolution of 10.4 μm and an active imaging area of 0.9 mm × 0.9 mm. In vivo imaging of a mouse ear, brain, and human lip were performed to highlight the potential biological and clinical applications.

2. Materials and Methods

2.1. Configurations of the Imaging System and Probe

The illumination of the MEMS-based ORPAM is presented in Figure 1. Laser pulses with a pulse energy of 20 μJ, a 5 ns duration, and a repetition rate of 10 kHz were emitted from a 532 nm Nd:YAG laser (FQS-Y-1-532, Elforlight, Daventry, UK) that was split into two parts through a cover glass. The reflected part was delivered to a photodiode (PD818-BB-21, Newport Corp., Irvine, CA, USA), which was used as the trigger and synchronization signals for MEMS scanning and data acquisition. The transmission part was spatially filtered through a customized spatial filter with a 10× objective (GCO-2112, Daheng Optics, Beijing, China), a 15 μm pinhole, and a Plano-convex lens, and then coupled into a single-mode optical fiber via a space-to-fiber coupler built by an objective (GCO-2112, Daheng Optics) and a customized five-dimensional single mode optical fiber manipulator. The output beam from the optic fiber was collimated by a fiber-compatible collimator (F240FC-532, Thorlabs Inc., Newton, NJ, USA) and then scanned by the MEMS mirror (WM-LS_5, WiO TECH, Wuxi, China).

The MEMS was driven by a multifunctional data acquisition card (PCI-6731, National Instrument, Austin, TX, USA) to achieve raster scanning on the surface of an imaging lens (AC080-010-A, Thorlabs Inc., Newton, NJ, USA), using triangle waves for the fast axis and saw-tooth waves for the slow axis. To allow full transmission of the laser pulses and reflection of the generated photoacoustic signals, a water cube including two isosceles right-angle water prisms using a tilted 0.1 mm cover glass was used. The photoacoustic signals were recorded by a small ultrasound transducer (center frequency: 10 MHz, active area: 2 mm in diameter, bandwidth: 60%), amplified by a homemade low noise pre-amplifier at ~66 dB, acquired by a high-speed data acquisition card (PXI-5124, NI, Austin, TX, USA) and stored in a computer for image reconstruction.

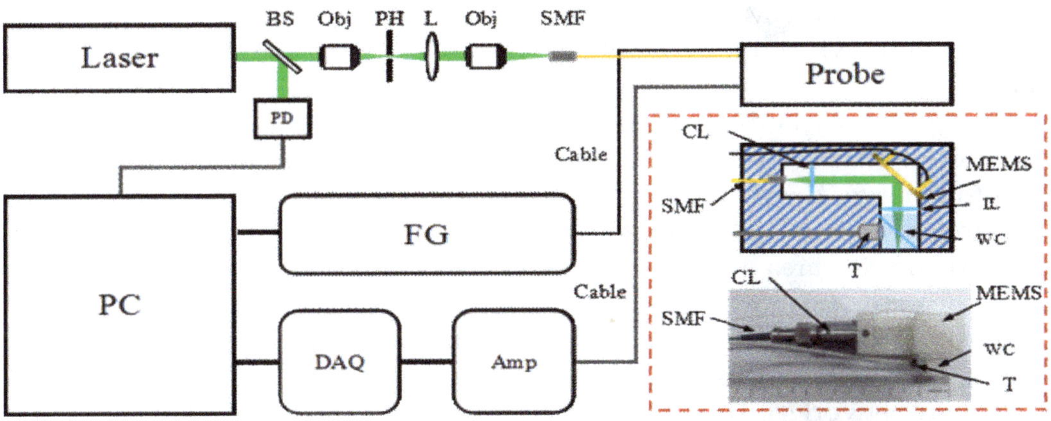

Figure 1. The schematic of the system and imaging probe. The detailed design and photograph of the imaging probe are provided in the dashed red box. The dimensions of the probe were roughly 60 mm × 30 mm × 20 mm. PD: photodiode, Obj: Objective, SMF: single mode fiber, FG: function generator, DAQ: data acquisition card, AMP: amplifier, CL: collimator, T: transducer, L: convex lens, BS: beam splitter, PH: pinhole, PC: personal computer, IL: imaging lens, and WC: water cube.

2.2. *Phantom and Animal Experiments*

To measure the field of view (FOV) and spatial resolution of the system, a metal strip target with a strip width of 0.1 mm and the edge of a shape surgical blade were imaged. We also performed phantom experiments and in vivo experiments to further assess the system. Multiple 7 μm diameter carbon fibers embedded in a tissue mimicking agarose phantom mixed with India ink and intralipid were imaged to simulate the vasculature in biological tissues. Then mouse ears and brains were imaged to evaluate the system performance for in vivo animals. During the experiment, mice were kept motionless using an isoflurane inhalation anesthetic system and the body temperature was maintained at 37 °C using a temperature control pad (17673, Lankai Inc., Changzhou, China). The ears were gently depilated, then tightly attached to the sealing membrane. For brain imaging, scalps were carefully removed with a sharp blade and skulls remained intact. All mice were kept 24 h after the experiments and no obvious damage were observed in the imaging area. The frame size for the phantom and animal experiments was 500 × 500 pixels. Considering the maximal repetition rate of the laser source, each experiment lasted 28 s. All procedures were approved by the Southern University of Science and Technology.

2.3. *In Vivo Human Experiments*

To demonstrate the clinical potential of this probe, we performed in vivo human oral imaging. During the experiments, the male volunteer sat on a chair and wore protective goggles to avoid potential laser damage to the eyes. The image probe was held and attached to the volunteer's lower lip. Due to insufficient repetition rate of the laser source and involuntary movement of the human lip, we reduced the frame size (250 × 250 pixels) to improve the imaging speed. A total of 8 s were required to acquire each volume data. After the experiments, the dentist inspected the imaging area and no obvious damage was observed. We obtained consent from the volunteer and all procedures were approved by the Southern University of Science and Technology.

3. Results

Figure 2a shows the maximum amplitude projection (MAP) image of the sharp blade. To estimate the lateral resolution, a profile along the red dashed line was fitted to obtain the edge spread function (ESF), which was used to derive the line spread function (LSF), as shown in Figure 2b. By calculating the full width-at-half-maximum (FWHM) of the LSF, the lateral resolution was measured as 10.4 μm.

As shown in Figure 2c, the FWHM of the Gaussian-fitted axial profile of a typical depth-resolved PA signal was about 150 μm, which represents the axial resolution of the system. Considering that the diameter of the optical focus was 10.4 μm and the energy of the laser pulse after the imaging lenses was 80 nJ, the energy density at the focal plane in the air was 94 mJ/cm^2. When we assembled the probe, the optical focal plane was adjusted to be approximately 10.25 mm outside the imaging window, leading to a photon energy density of 1 mJ/cm^2 on the tissue surface during in vivo experiments. Figure 2d shows the MAP image of the silver strip target. There were five strips in the entire imaging area, resulting in an effective area of 0.9 mm × 0.9 mm. In addition, no obvious distortion of the strips was evident over the entire imaging domain.

Figure 3a shows the MAP image of carbon fibers buried in an agarose phantom. We could clearly distinguish each carbon fiber with sufficient contrast and resolution. Figure 3b,c present the MAP images of the vascular networks inside a mouse ear and brain, respectively. Large, medium, and small blood vessels are clearly identified. However, we noticed that the SNR and resolution in Figure 3b is better than in Figure 3c. The major reason for this observation is that the skull of the brain significantly reduces the photoacoustic signals and slightly distorts the optical focus due to optical scattering. Figure 3d shows the MAP image of the human lower lip, in which we observed vasculatures with acceptable image quality. The animal and human experiments suggest that the proposed miniaturized ORPAM probe is applicable for both fundamental and clinical applications.

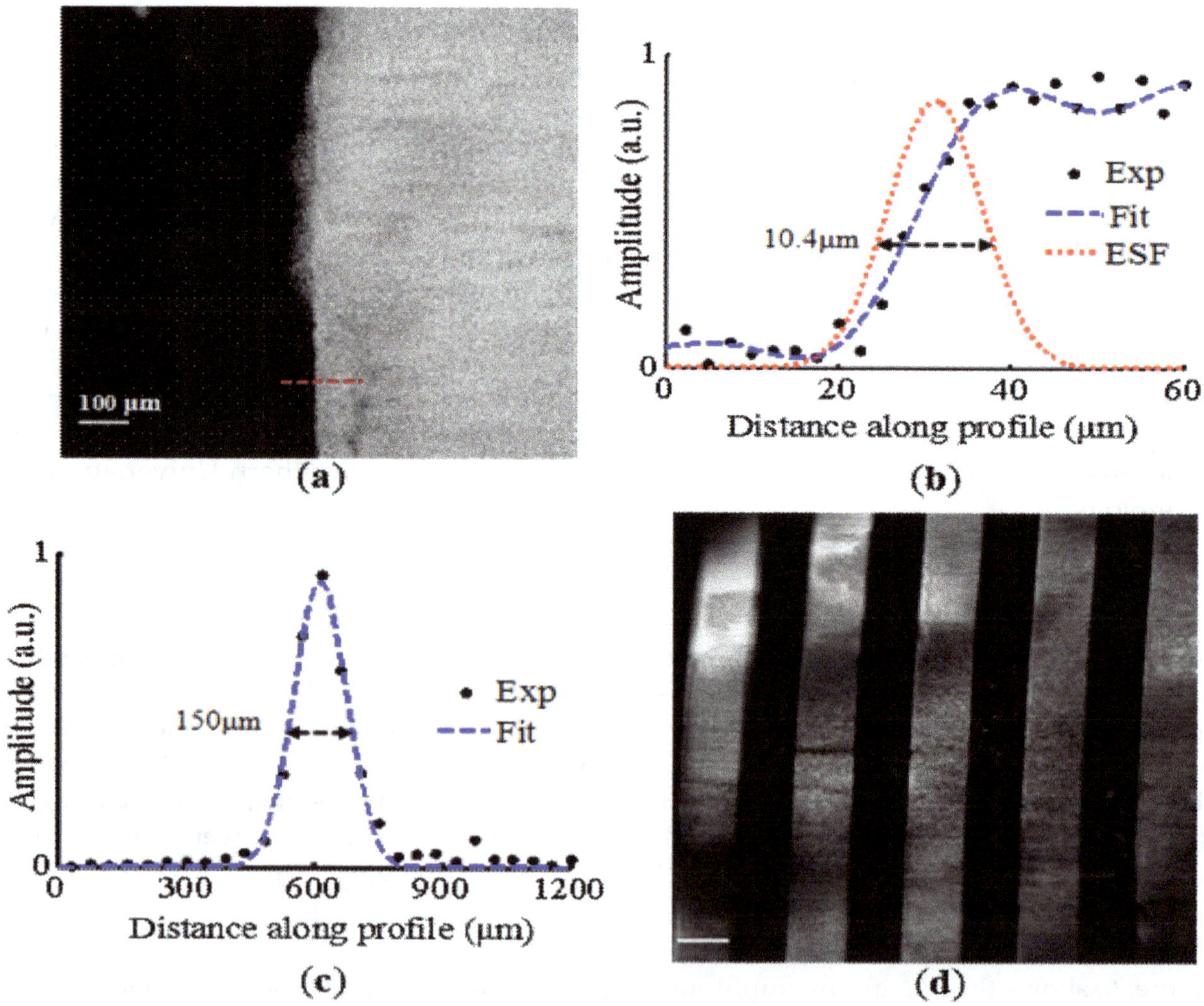

Figure 2. Evaluation of the system performance. (**a**) The maximum amplitude projection (MAP) image of the sharp blade. Estimation of the (**b**) lateral and (**c**) axial resolutions of the system. (**d**) The MAP image of the silver strip target to measure the effective field of view (FOV). Scale bar: 100 μm.

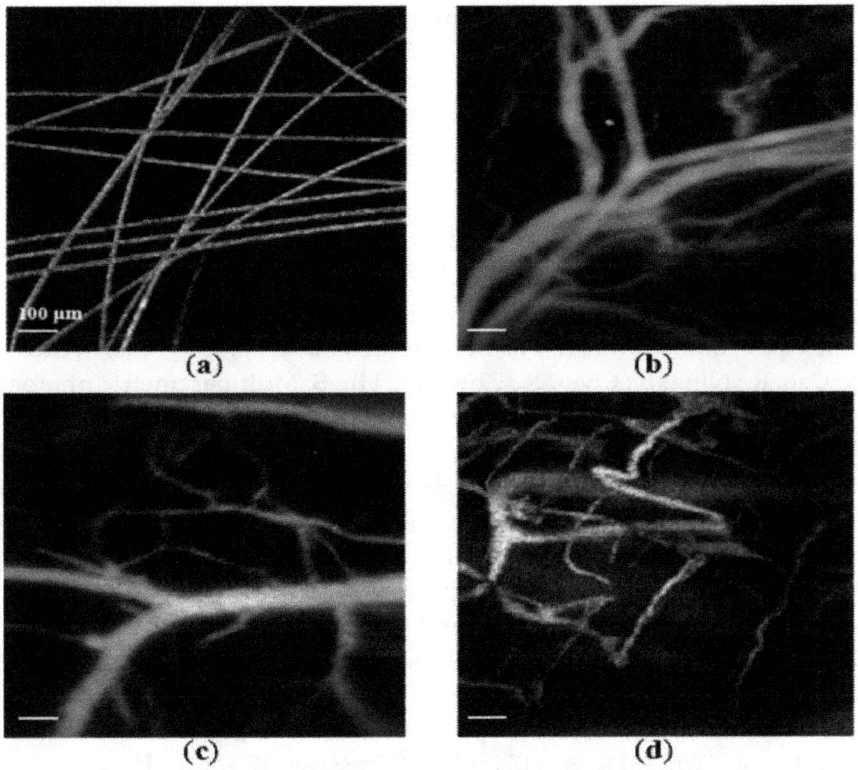

Figure 3. The MAP images of (**a**) carbon fibers, (**b**) blood vessels in a mouse ear and (**c**) brain, and (**d**) vasculature in a human lower lip. The frame size of images in (**a**–**c**) is 500 × 500 pixels, and the image in (**d**) is 250 × 250 pixels. Scale bar: 100 μm.

4. Discussion and Conclusions

In this work, we reported a miniature ORPAM imaging probe using a 2D MEMS mirror and a small flat ultrasound transducer. The performance of the system was evaluated with phantom, animal, and human experiments. The MEMS mirror, being small, light, fast, and inexpensive, considerably reduces the probe size. The imaging results suggest that this technique holds potential for both fundamental and clinical applications. For example, in brain surgery, using this probe is feasible to evaluate bypass-grafted blood vessels based on morphological and functional information, such as vessel diameter, blood flow, and oxygen saturation (sO_2). The other potential application is to detect early-stage oral cancer. By imaging the lips, small blood vessels, and especially capillary loops, can be clearly observed. The morphological changes in these capillary loops are tightly related to the occurrence of oral cancer. However, this probe has some limitations. Firstly, the imaging area is relatively small, which is mainly caused by the limited scanning angle of the MEMS mirror and the probe size. To increase the domain, either the design of MEMS mirror can be optimized to increase the scanning angle, or a new design can be proposed for the optical path. Secondly, the spatial resolution was insufficient to visualize cellar level targets. In theory, the lateral resolution is mainly determined by the numerical aperture (NA) of the focusing lens and the axial resolution depends on the center frequency and bandwidth of the ultrasonic transducer. Hence, we could achieve higher spatial resolution by using a high-NA focusing lens and a high frequency transducer with a broader bandwidth. Thirdly, the imaging speed of the system was limited by the repetition rate of the laser. If a 300 kHz repetition rate laser is applied, we could acquire a large volume data within 1 s, which would mostly eliminate the motion artifacts of in vivo experiments and extend the applications of this probe.

Author Contributions: W.Q. established the system and conducted the experiments; Q.C. analyzed the data; H.G. conducted the experiments; H.X. designed and fabricated the MEMS mirrors; L.X. conceived the concept and supervised the entire project.

Acknowledgments: This work was sponsored by National Natural Science Foundation of China (61775028, 81571722 and 61528401), Startup grant from Southern University of Science and Technology, State International Collaboration Program from Sichuan province (2016HH0019). We thank Yabing Liu for assembling the MEMS mirror.

References

1. Kim, C.; Song, K.H.; Gao, F.; Wang, L.V. Sentinel Lymph Nodes in the Rat: Noninvasive Photoacoustic and US Imaging with a Clinical US System. *Radiology* **2010**, *25*, 102–110. [CrossRef]
2. Chen, Q.; Jin, T.; Qi, W.; Mo, X.; Xi, L. Label-free photoacoustic imaging of the carido-cerebrovascular development in the embryonic zebrafish. *Biomed. Opt. Exp.* **2017**, *8*, 2359–2367. [CrossRef] [PubMed]
3. Wang, T.; Sun, N.; Cao, R.; Ning, B.; Chen, R.; Zhou, Q.; Hu, S. Multiparametric photoacoustic microscopy of the mouse brain with 300-kHz A-line rate. *Neurophotonics* **2016**, *3*, 045006. [CrossRef] [PubMed]
4. Wong, T.T.W.; Zhang, R.; Zhang, C.; Hsu, H.; Maslov, K.I.; Wang, L.; Shi, J.; Chen, R.; Shung, K.K.; Zhou, Q.; et al. Label-free automated three-dimensional imaging of whole organs by microtomy-assisted photoacoustic microscopy. *Nat. Commun.* **2017**, *8*, 1386. [CrossRef] [PubMed]
5. Maslov, K.; Zhang, H.F.; Hu, S.; Wang, L.V. Optical-resolution photoacoustic microscopy for in vivo imaging of single capillaries. *Opt. Lett.* **2008**, *33*, 929–931. [CrossRef] [PubMed]
6. Wang, L.V. Multiscale photoacoustic microscopy and computed tomography. *Nat. Photonics* **2009**, *3*, 503–509. [CrossRef] [PubMed]
7. Beard, P. Biomedical photoacoustic imaging. *Interface Focus* **2011**, *1*, 602–631. [CrossRef] [PubMed]
8. Hu, S.; Maslov, K.; Wang, L.V. Second-generation optical-resolution photoacoustic microscopy with improved sensitivity and speed. *Opt. Lett.* **2011**, *36*, 1134–1136. [CrossRef] [PubMed]
9. Zhu, L.; Li, L.; Gao, L.; Wang, L.V. Multiview optical resolution photoacoustic microscopy. *Optica* **2014**, *1*, 217–222. [CrossRef] [PubMed]
10. Wang, L.; Maslov, K.; Yao, J.; Rao, B.; Wang, L.V. Fast voice-coil scanning optical-resolution photoacoustic microscopy. *Opt. Lett.* **2011**, *36*, 139–141. [CrossRef] [PubMed]
11. Xi, L.; Sun, J.; Zhu, Y.; Wu, L.; Xie, H.; Jiang, H. Photoacoustic imaging based on MEMS mirror scanning. *Biomed. Opt. Exp.* **2010**, *1*, 1278–1283. [CrossRef] [PubMed]
12. Qi, W.; Jin, T.; Rong, J.; Jiang, H.; Xi, L. Inverted multiscale optical resolution photoacoustic microscopy. *J. Biophotonics* **2017**, *10*, 1580–1585. [CrossRef] [PubMed]
13. Jin, T.; Guo, H.; Jiang, H.; Ke, B.; Xi, L. Portable optical resolution photoacoustic microscopy (pORPAM) for human oral imaging. *Opt. Lett.* **2017**, *42*, 4434–4437. [CrossRef] [PubMed]
14. Yao, J.; Wang, L.; Yang, J.; Maslov, K.I.; Wong, T.T.W.; Li, L.; Huang, C.; Zou, J.; Wang, L.V. High-speed label-free functional photoacoustic microscopy of mouse brain in action. *Nat. Methods* **2015**, *12*, 407–410. [CrossRef] [PubMed]
15. He, Y.; Wang, L.; Shi, J.; Yao, J.; Li, L.; Zhang, R.; Huang, C.H.; Zou, J.; Wang, L.V. In vivo label-free photoacoustic flow cytography and on-the-spot laser killing of single circulating melanoma cells. *Sci. Rep.* **2016**, *6*, 39616. [CrossRef] [PubMed]
16. Yao, J.; Wang, L.; Yang, J.M.; Gao, L.S.; Maslov, K.I.; Wang, L.V.; Huang, C.H.; Zou, J. Wide-field fast-scanning photoacoustic microscopy based on a water-immersible MEMS scanning mirror. *J. Biomed. Opt.* **2012**, *17*, 080505. [CrossRef] [PubMed]
17. Lin, L.; Zhang, P.; Xu, S.; Shi, J.; Li, L.; Yao, J.; Wang, L.; Zou, J.; Wang, L.V. Handheld optical-resolution photoacoustic microscopy. *J. Biomed. Opt.* **2016**, *22*, 041002. [CrossRef] [PubMed]
18. Chen, S.L.; Xie, Z.; Ling, T.; Guo, L.J.; Wei, X.; Wang, X. Miniaturized all-optical photoacoustic microscopy based on microelectromechanical systems mirror scanning. *Opt. Lett.* **2012**, *37*, 4263–4265. [CrossRef] [PubMed]
19. Kim, J.Y.; Lee, C.; Park, K.; Lim, G.; Kim, C. Fast optical-resolution photoacoustic microscopy using a 2-axis water-proofing MEMS scanner. *Sci. Rep.* **2015**, *5*, 7932. [CrossRef] [PubMed]
20. Kim, J.Y.; Lee, C.; Park, K.; Lim, G.; Kim, C. A PDMS-Based 2-Axis Waterproof Scanner for Photoacoustic Microscopy. *Sensors* **2015**, *15*, 9815–9826. [CrossRef] [PubMed]
21. Kim, J.Y.; Lee, C.; Park, K.; Han, S.; Kim, C. High-speed and high-SNR photoacoustic microscopy based on a galvanometer mirror in nonconducting liquid. *Sci. Rep.* **2016**, *6*, 34803. [CrossRef] [PubMed]

22. Park, K.; Kim, J.Y.; Lee, C.; Jeon, S.; Lim, G.; Kim, C. Handheld Photoacoustic Microscopy Probe. *Sci. Rep.* **2017**, *7*, 13359. [CrossRef] [PubMed]
23. Hajireza, P.; Shi, W.; Zemp, R.J. Real-time handheld optical-resolution photoacoustic microscopy. *Opt. Exp.* **2011**, *19*, 20097–20102. [CrossRef] [PubMed]
24. Guo, H.; Song, C.; Xie, H.; Xi, L. Photoacoustic endomicroscopy (PAEM) based on a MEMS scanning mirror. *Opt. Lett.* **2017**, *42*, 4615–4618. [CrossRef] [PubMed]

10

Fabrication of Electromagnetically-Driven Tilted Microcoil on Polyimide Capillary Surface for Potential Single-Fiber Endoscope Scanner Application

Zhuoqing Yang [1], Jianhao Shi [1], Bin Sun [2,*], Jinyuan Yao [1], Guifu Ding [1] and Renshi Sawada [3]

1 National Key Laboratory of Science and Technology on Micro/Nano Fabrication, School of Electronics Information and Electrical Engineering, Shanghai Jiao Tong University, Shanghai 200240, China; yzhuoqing@sjtu.edu.cn (Z.Y.); sjh_timehao@163.com (J.S.); jyyao@sjtu.edu.cn (J.Y.); gfding@sjtu.edu.cn (G.D.)

2 Institute of Biomedical and Health Engineering, Shenzhen Institute of Advanced Technology, Chinese Academy of Science, Shenzhen 518055, China

3 Graduate School of Systems Life Science, Kyushu University, Fukuoka 819-0395, Japan; sawada@mech.kyushu-u.ac.jp

* Correspondence: bin.sun@siat.ac.cn

Abstract: The design and fabrication of a Micro-electromechanical Systems (MEMS)-based tilted microcoil on a polyimide capillary are reported in this paper, proposed for an electromagnetically-driven single-fiber endoscope scanner application. The parameters of the tilted microcoil were optimized by simulation. It is proved that the largest driving force could be achieved when the tilt-angle, the pitch and the coil turns of the designed microcoil were 60°, 80 μm and 20, respectively. The modal simulation of the designed fiber scanner was carried out. The prototypes of the tilted microcoils were fabricated on the surface of polyimide capillary with 1 mm-diameter using our developed cylindrical projection lithography system. The dimensions of the two tilted microcoils were as follows: one was tilt-angle 45°, line width 10 ± 0.2 μm, coil pitch 78.5 ± 0.5 μm, and the other was tilt-angle 60°, line width 10 ± 0.2 μm, coil pitch 81.5 ± 0.5 μm. Finally, a direct mask-less electroplating process was employed to fabricate the copper microcoil with 15 μm thickness on the gold (Au) seed-layer, and the corresponding line width was expanded to 40 μm.

Keywords: tilted microcoil; electromagnetically-driven; surface micromachining; polyimide capillary; MEMS

---

1. Introduction

Miniature devices have been developed extensively for medical and biological applications. Recently, to inspect the imaging within blood vessel and lactiferous ducts inside animal and human body, ultra-thin medical endoscopes have been developed by shrinking the overall diameter of the devices [1,2]. Conventional endoscopes mostly employ Charge Coupled Device (CCD) and Complementary Metal Oxide Semiconductor (CMOS) imaging sensors for image capture [3,4]. However, the main limitation of video-endoscopes is their diameters. Video-endoscopes <3 mm in diameter suffer from a reduced imaging quality when using conventional imaging technology. Consequently, a kind of flexible endoscope was ushered in by fiber-optic bundles [5,6]. It is also difficult to obtain high-resolution imaging within a thin fiber scope, due to the fact that the number of optical fibers is restricted. In order to improve the imaging quality, a smaller diameter, rapid-scanning and high-resolution optical scanner with a single fiber has recently been developed.

Weber et al. [7] developed a single-fiber scanner, which employed a micro-mirror and a micro-motor to realize linear and rotated scanning, and the outer diameter of the assembled system was 2.75 mm. Hu et al. [8] proposed a single fiber coated with nickel magnetic gel, which was actuated by an external electromagnet. Weber et al. [9] also presented an endoscopic probe with a forward-looking piezoelectric fiber scanner with an outer diameter of 2.5 mm. Assadsangabi et al. [10] reported an optical fiber scanner using a micro rotary motor, which consisted of ferrofluid, permanent magnet and activation coil. Its final packaged outer diameter was 3 mm. Obviously, the packaged dimensions in the aforementioned designs were too large for some intra-corporeal applications in which the fiber scanner needs to fit in small diameter (<2 mm) organ ducts. In addition, Tadao et al. [2] reported an electromagnetically-driven ultra-miniature single-fiber scanner that was actuated by tilted microcoils fabricated on cylindrical substrates using a laser point exposure system. A microcoil with a tilt-angle of 45° and a coil pitch of 200 μm was successfully obtained, but scanning amplitude was limited because of the small driving force generated by a large pitch microcoil.

In this work, we present an ultra-thin electromagnetically-driven scanner fabricated by a novel Micro-electromechanical Systems (MEMS)-based fabrication method called cylindrical projection lithography, which is a new fabrication technology for manufacturing functional microstructures or transducers on the surface of cylindrical substrates as micro components in some biomedical tools. The developed cylindrical projection lithography method can be used for directly patterning tilted microcoil on the surface of a polyimide capillary as an electromagnetically-driven actuator. The microcoil patterns of photoresist film can be fabricated with different tilt-angles. More importantly, a smaller line width and coil pitch can be also realized. Thus, the fabricated microcoil would efficiently enhance the electromagnetically driven force, despite its miniature size. The corresponding fabrication process also includes spray-coating technology and a direct mask-less electroplating process on a microcoil pattern with a seed layer.

We begin in the next section by describing the configuration and principle of the designed single-fiber scanner, followed by optimizing the related structural parameters. Subsequently, the cylindrical projection lithography technique and fabrication process are presented. Finally, the fabrication and characterization of the tilted microcoils are presented.

2. Design and Simulation

2.1. Single-Fiber Scanner

To realize a large scanning amplitude in the narrow space of the human body, a novel electromagnetically driven MEMS-based single-fiber scanner has been designed, as illustrated in Figure 1. This fiber scanner is composed of a single-mode optical fiber, a collimator lens, a cylindrical magnet, a jig, and two tilted microcoils (X-axis driving coil and Y-axis driving coil). A 125 μm diameter optical fiber is positioned in the middle of the polyimide capillary using a jig with a small hole in it, which is manufactured by a 3D printer. A micro collimator lens is fused at the tip of the optical fiber, and a cylindrical magnet (Cobalt Nickel) is fixed on the fiber. Finally, two tilted microcoils are fabricated on the surface of the 1 mm diameter polyimide capillary with a wall thickness of 0.1 mm (SCHOTT MORITEX Corporation, Cambridge, UK). Its melting point and dielectric constant are 400 °C and 3.4 respectively. When AC power is supplied to the tilted microcoil, the fiber will vibrate continuously in period under the effect of magnetic force torque. By supplying AC power to both of the driving coils with a 90° phase shift, the fiber can scan in two dimensions. When the frequency of the applied AC is the same as that of the fiber with magnet, the whole structure will continuously scan with the largest amplitude scanning angle.

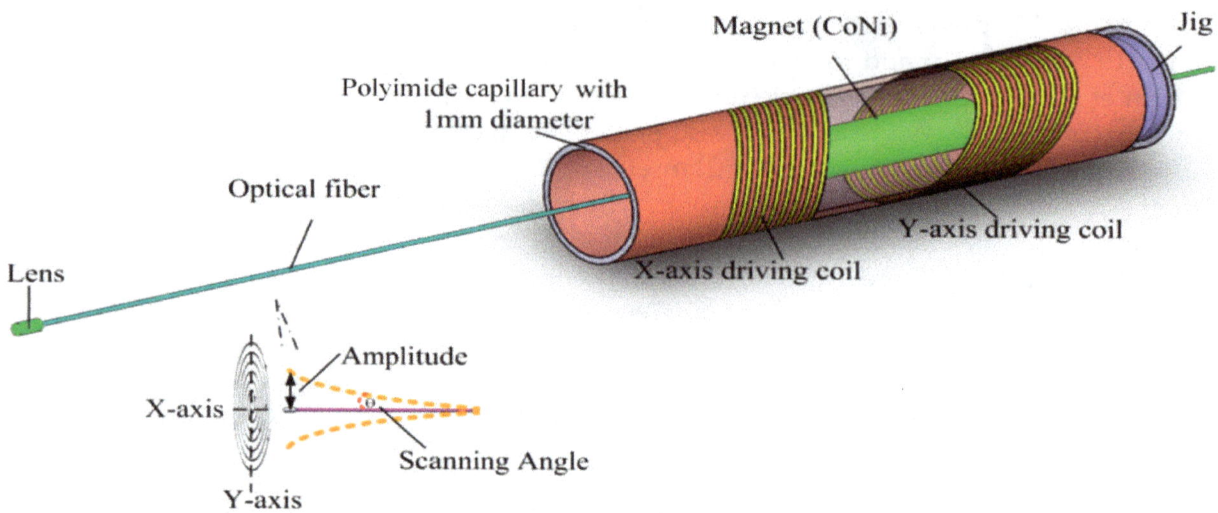

Figure 1. Sketch of proposed single-fiber scanner by electromagnetically driven tilted microcoil to which AC power is supplied.

2.2. Design of Tilted Microcoil

Theoretically, when a soft magnetic magnet is placed inside a tilted microcoil as shown in Figure 2, a magnetic force torque will be generated on the magnet and a torque T proportional to magnetic force F is exerted on the magnet given by [11].

$$T = V \times |M \times H| = VMH \sin \alpha \propto F \quad (1)$$

where, the volume of the magnet is V, M is the magnetization intensity. α is the angle between magnetization direction and external magnetic field. Here, it is equal to the value of the tilt-angle. H is the magnetic field intensity generated by tilted microcoil. Generally, the smaller the coil pitch, the greater the magnetic field intensity.

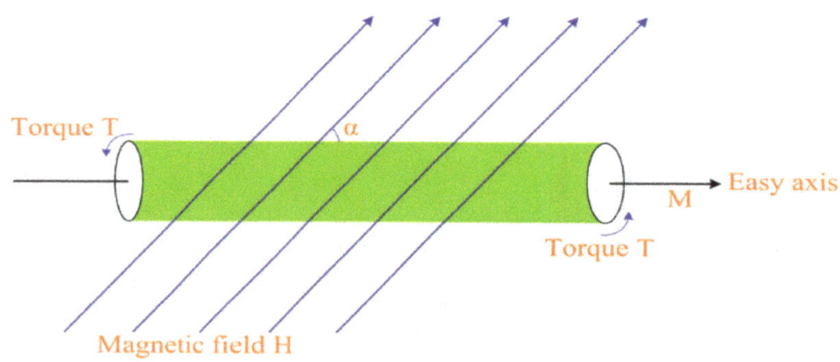

Figure 2. Schematic of torque calculation under tilt magnetic field.

The key parameters of designed tilted microcoil are shown in Figure 3a, including coil pitch, tilt-angle and turns. ANSYS MAXWELL software (V16.0, Ansys Inc., Canonsburg, PA, USA) was used for simulating the magnetic force, as well as providing us a convenient method and relative precise result. Coil pitch is a decisive factor for magnetic field intensity. Here, the coil pitch of 80 μm is designed in order to provide our fabrication with a greater ability to achieve greater magnetic field intensity. The simulation model consists of two parts: tilted microcoil model and magnet model. The tilted microcoil model was built with different parameters, such as tilt-angle, coil pitch and turns. The material property of the microcoil model is copper, which is applied with 50 mA AC power. On the other hand, a 3 mm length and 600 μm diameter magnet is established, which is made of Cobalt Nickle, whose test coercive field strength is shown in Figure 3b.

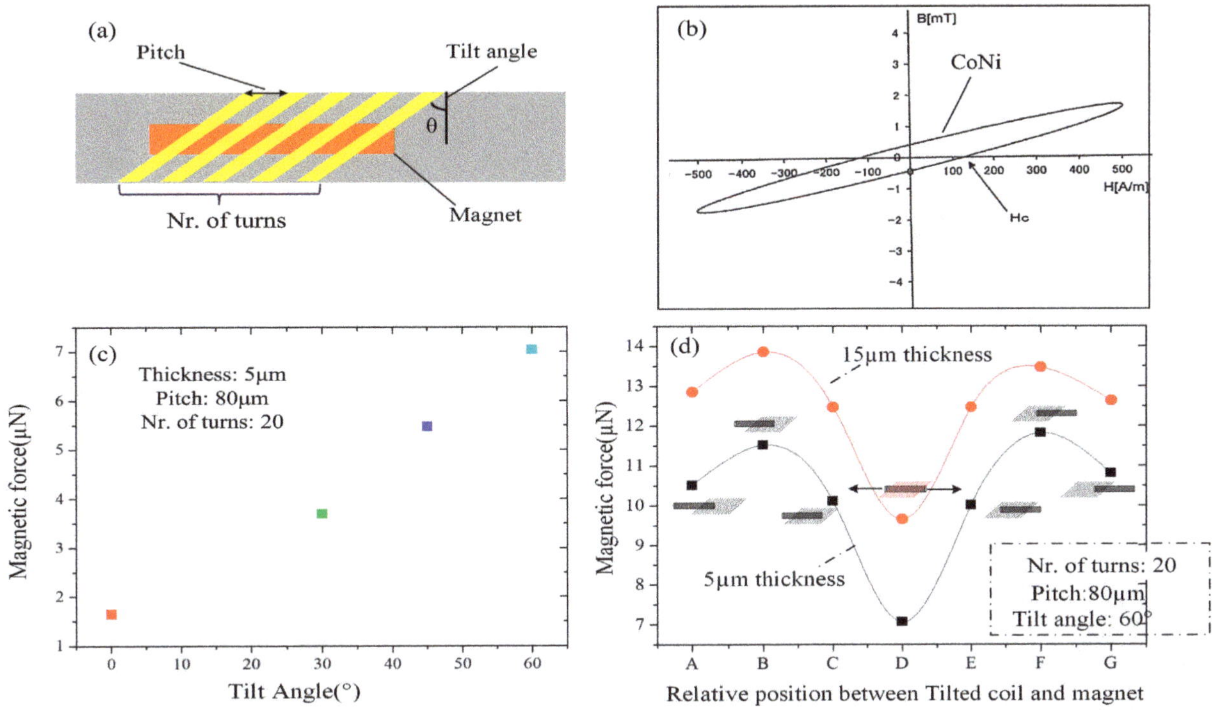

Figure 3. Parameters of designed microcoil and simulated results of magnetic force. (**a**) Key parameters of tilted microcoil and magnet; (**b**) B-H curve of CoNi magnet used; (**c**) Simulated magnetic force with different tilt-angles; (**d**) Simulated magnetic forces with relative positions between coil and magnet. (Nr. means number in the figure).

Figure 3c shows that the magnetic force gradually rises as the tilt-angle increases. This is consistent with theoretical torque calculation, where the torque also increases with the angle α. However, the tilt-angle is limited in our present fabrication process, and a larger tilt-angle (more than 60°) is difficult to realize due to the insufficient running accuracy of the stage and underexposure. In the present work, a microcoil with a 60° tilt-angle is fabricated in order to obtain, to the best of our ability, a large magnetic force.

Subsequently, the effect of the location of the magnet on the output magnetic driving force has been taken into consideration in detail. As is indicated in Figure 3d, the magnetic force was simulated at different locations between the tilted microcoil and the magnet (from position A to position E). In the simulation result, the maximum force was obtained at location B or F, where half of the magnet is placed outside the tilted microcoil. It was also simulated in two coils with different thicknesses of 5 μm and 15 μm, respectively. The results show a similar changing trend.

Next, the magnetic force with an increasing number of turns (ranging from 10 to 40) and tilt-angles of 30°, 40° and 60° was also simulated, as shown in Figure 4. The magnetic force induced by 10 turns is very small, because the magnet is inadequately magnetized. A large magnetic force was obtained in the 60° tilt-angle microcoil with 20 turns. The magnetic force generally remains constant when the turns are equal to or more than 20. This indicates that the magnet will be magnetized to saturation in the tilted magnetic field when half of its volume is placed in a sufficiently long tilted microcoil, such as 20 turns. In addition, an almost identical magnetic force is produced by the tilted coils with 20, 30, and 40 turns, which is independent of turns. These results indicate that the microcoil with 60° tilt-angle exerts a larger magnetic force on the magnet when the other parameters remain constant. The magnetic force continuously changes with the different relative position between the tilted microcoil and the magnet, with the largest one being at the B or F position. The largest magnetic force existed for the microcoil with 20 turns with different tilt-angles when the magnet is placed at the B position. Based on the simulation results and our fabrication capacity, the microcoil with a 60° tilt-angle, 20 turns, and 80 μm coil pitch is ultimately fabricated.

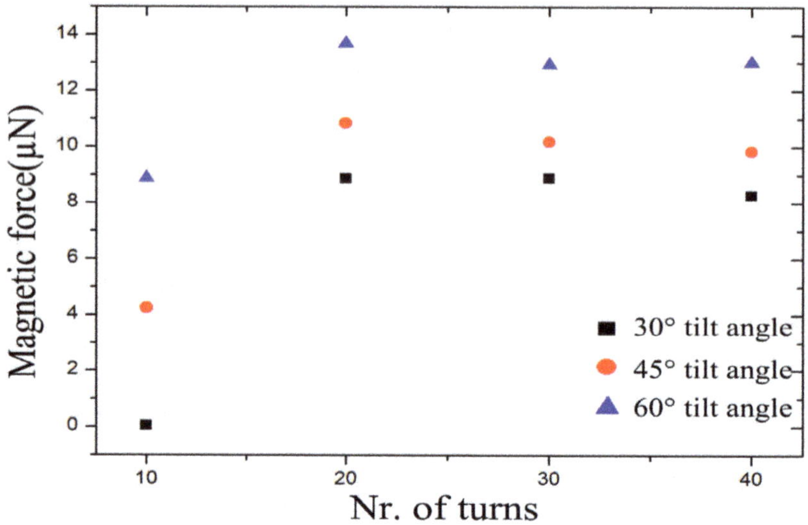

Figure 4. Simulated magnetic force with increasing turns (from 10 to 40) with tilt-angle of 30°, 45° and 60°, respectively.

2.3. *The Modal and Dynamic Analysis*

Like all mechanical structures, this fiber scanner has its own resonant frequency, and it achieves the largest amplitude under its resonant frequency. To obtain the resonant frequency of the fiber scanner, modal analysis was conducted by employing commercial ANSYS finite element analysis (FEA) software (V16.0, Ansys Inc., Canonsburg, PA, USA). The geometrical parameters and specifications of the fiber scanner model are given in Table 1. The SOLID 45 element type was chosen, and the SWEEP method was used to mesh the model, as shown in Figure 5a. The first three order modes and corresponding resonant frequencies of the fiber scanner were simulated, as shown in Figure 5b–d, respectively.

Table 1. Geometric parameters and material properties for the fiber scanner model.

Components	Geometric Parameters and Material Property	Values
Optical fiber	Elastic Modulus E_f	1.72 GPa
	Poisson ratio R_f	0.17
	Density ρ_f	2200 Kg/m^2
	Length F_1, F_2, F_3	4 mm, 3 mm, 6 mm
	Diameter D_f	125 μm
Magnet	Elastic Modulus E_m	210 GPa
	Poisson ratio R_m	0.31
	Density ρ_m	8500 Kg/m^2
	Length M_1	3 mm
	Diameter D_m	600 μm
Lens	Elastic Modulus E_l	1.72 GPa
	Poisson ratio R_l	0.17
	Density ρ_l	2200 Kg/m^2
	Length L_1	2 mm
	Diameter D_l	1 mm

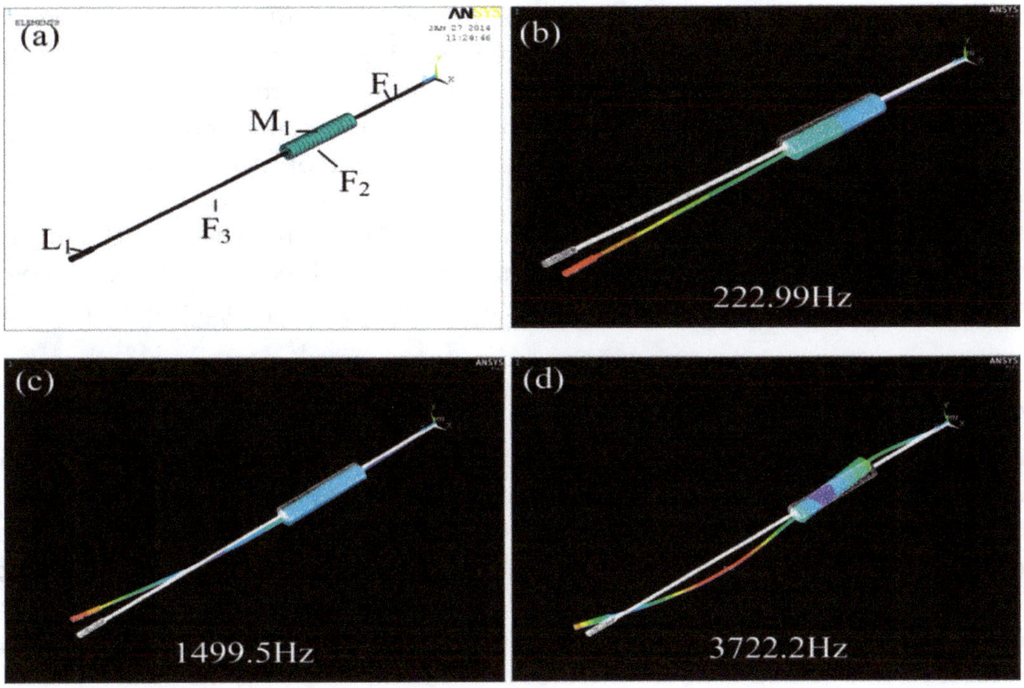

Figure 5. FEA models for modal analysis. (**a**) Whole model for fiber scanner; (**b–d**) presented structure deformation and frequency of the first three order resonant modes.

3. Fabrication of Tilted Microcoil

3.1. Exposure System

The cylindrical projection lithography system was described in detail in our previous work [12], and its basic setup is shown in Figure 6. The only difference is that the effective exposure area is improved from the previous <20 mm diameter to the present >30 mm diameter circular area, which allows the fabrication of a sufficiently long tilted microcoil with turns of up to 50 in a short time. This exposure equipment mainly consists of three parts: (a) a programmable lithography system with x, y, z, θ-stage controller, (b) a programmed control stage with alignment system, and (c) a uniform illumination system.

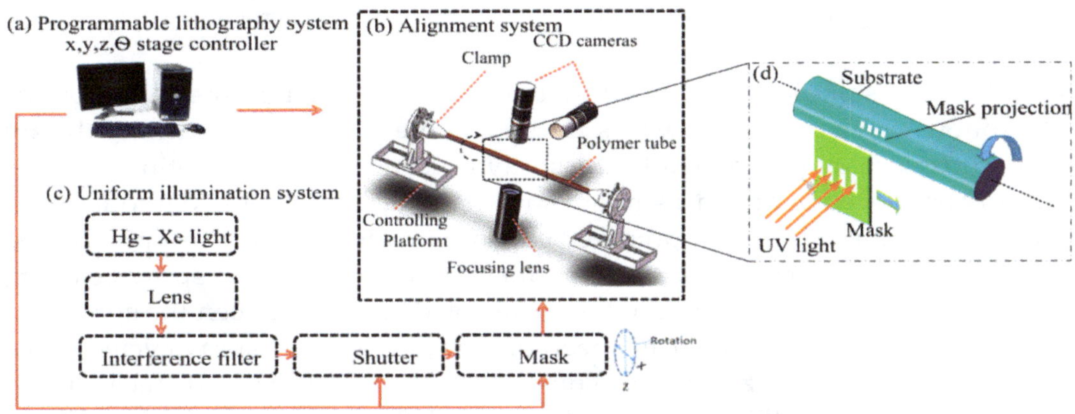

Figure 6. Programmable UV lithography system with alignment for cylindrical substrate: (**a**) programmable lithography system x, y, z, θ-stage controller; (**b**) Charge Coupled Device (CCD) camera alignment system; (**c**) Uniform illumination system; (**d**) Close-up schematic diagram of fabricated sample.

First of all, all the optical elements of the exposure equipment were aligned by a He-Ne laser, after that, the UV light from the illumination source passed through all the aligned optical elements, and the projection of the mask was focused on the surface of the photoresist-coated capillary substrate. Additionally, there are two CCD cameras; one is utilized for observing and adjusting the substrate in order to achieve a stable rotation, the other is used for observation of the alignment state. The substrate and mask were able rotate and move during the whole exposure process. The projection of the mask was able to scan along and around the substrate. Finally, the microcoil pattern was successfully transferred onto the surface of capillary substrate. As a result, the tilted microcoil could be fabricated by rotating the photoresist-coated polyimide capillary, and moving the projection of the mask, as shown in Figure 6d.

3.2. Fabrication Process

The main fabrication process for the tilted microcoil is shown in Figure 7. At the beginning, a polyimide capillary was sputtered with a 120 nm Cr coating and a 30 nm Au coating. In addition, the polyimide capillary was rotating during the sputtering process to obtain a uniform thin film. This process not only saves time, but also achieves a uniform thickness for the sputtering coating film. This is beneficial to controlling etching time. Next, in order to increase the adhesive force between the Cr and Au layers, a thermal treatment process was employed at 200 °C for 20 min after sputtering. After that, photoresist was coated onto the surface of the samples using the spray-coating system that was developed for preparing thin uniform resist coating on cylindrical substrates [13]. The surface treatment process using a UV ozone treatment unit was carried out before the spray coating.

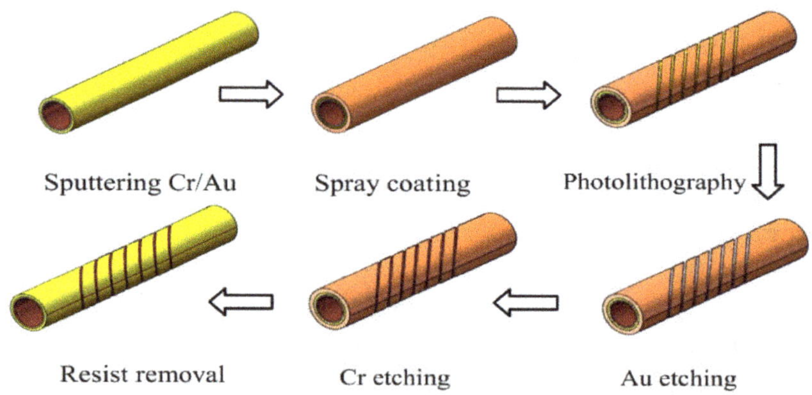

Figure 7. Main fabrication process of the tilted microcoil.

The two ends of the sample can be fixed by two clips mounted on the two motors, which can be driven synchronously at a certain rotation speed using the control panel during the spray-coating process. A heater nozzle is mounted next to the spray nozzle to realize real-time heating treatment, which is necessarily employed to obtain a smooth surface without pinholes. Without real-time heating treatment, there are some pinholes on the prepared coating, wavelike surface morphology is also visible, as was verified in our previous research [13]. Some major parameters of the spray-coating process can be independently controlled and programmed, such as the distance between the spray nozzle and the substrate, rotation speed of the sample, scan speed of the spray nozzle, spray cycles, and so on. Here, the distance between the spray nozzle and the substrate is 56 mm. A better surface with few pinholes and particles can be obtained at this distance. Shipley S1830 positive photoresist (Shipley Co. LLC, Marlborough, MA, USA) was employed as the spray-coating photoresist. The solvent was AZ5200 thinner (AZ electronic materials, Luxembourg), which consists of propylene glycol monomethyl ether acetate (PGMEA), i.e., a common solvent for the direct spraying-coating process. Finally, a 4 μm thickness of the photoresist coating was sprayed onto the circumferential surface of the sample.

For the lithography process, firstly, the sample was loaded on the cylindrical projection exposure equipment, and then it was fixed tightly by two clamps mounted on the two synchronously driven rotation stages. Next, the sample was adjusted so as to remain level and the control program, compiled in advance, was loaded into a personal computer. Finally, the sample was exposed by UV light with the shutter open. A tilted microcoil pattern of the photoresist was realized by controlling the rotation speed of the substrate and the linear movement speed of the mask. After exposure and development of the photoresist, the Cr and Au coatings were etched by wet etching. On the basis of the thickness of the coating and the etch rates, the sample was immersed in the Au etching liquid for 25 s, and then put into the Cr etching liquid for 1 min. Next, the photoresist was removed in acetone. Finally, the copper was electroplated on the Au seed-layer of the coil pattern by mask-less electroplating process. The electroplating resolution developed by our lab and Meltex Inc., Japan was employed, in which a kind of novel additive was used to obtain a high quality of electroplated film [14].

4. Characterization

4.1. Characteristics of Tilted Microcoil Patterns

The main parameter dimensions of the designed tilted microcoil pattern are decided by the lithography process. Two kinds of masks were used for patterning the tilted microcoil in the exposure process. These are one-line pattern mask and multi-line pattern mask. To save exposure time, multi-line pattern mask is the best selection, where there are 20 lines in the mask, each of which is $40 \times 170\ \mu m^2$, and the spacing between lines is 180 μm and 310 μm for 45° and 60° tilt-angles, respectively, as shown in Figure 8a.

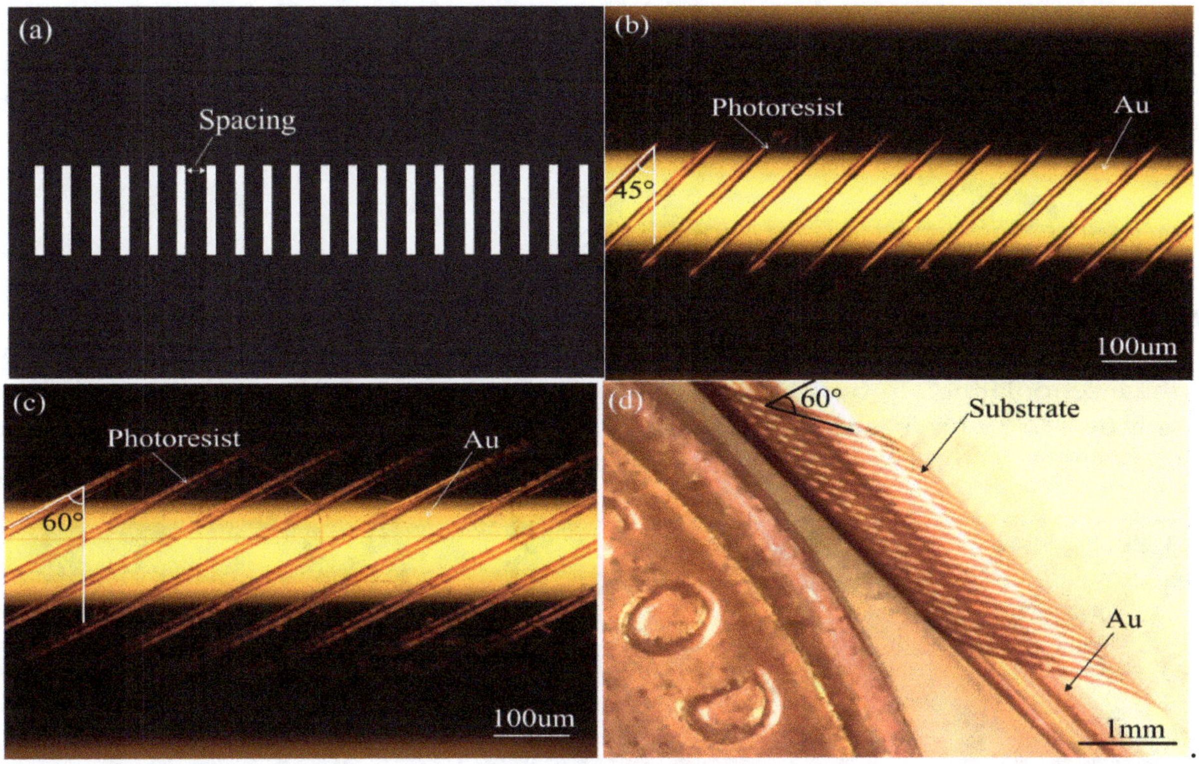

Figure 8. Mask pattern and tilt microcoil pattern. (**a**) Mask pattern with multi-lines; (**b**) Optical image of fabricated microcoil with 45° tilt-angle; (**c**) Optical image of the fabricated microcoil with 60° tilt-angle; (**d**) Photography of 20 turn microcoil with 60° tilt-angle fabricated on the 1 mm diameter ployimide capillary substrate.

According to our design and calculations, the spacings 180 μm and 310 μm are the critical distances for using 40 × 170 μm^2 lines to fabricate 45° tilt-angle and 60° tilt-angle microcoils, respectively, while avoiding overlap exposure. The tilted microcoil pattern can be realized by controlling the rotation speed of the substrate and the linear movement speed of the mask synchronously, as mentioned above. The distances of linear movement can be decided according to the tilt-angle, are are 3180 μm and 5444 μm for 45° tilt-angle and 60° tilt-angle microcoils, respectively. The exposure time is selected based on the size of the line pattern. In our experiment, 10 min, 20 min, 30 min, 40 min and 50 min were attempted successively. For the mask with a 40 × 170 μm^2 line pattern, 40 min exposure time was sufficient for our designed microcoils. The rotation speed of the substrate and the movement speed of the mask are also closely related to the exposure time, and can be calculated and evaluated based on the exposure time. Mask movement is separated into two parts: forward movement, for 0°–180° rotation of the substrate; and backward movement, for 180°–360° rotation. The distance of forward movement is 3180 μm for 45° tilt-angle microcoils and 5444 μm for 60° tilt-angle microcoils. However, to obtain a continuous coil line, the distance for backward movement is 3000 μm for 45° tilt-angle microcoils and 5134 μm for 60° tilt-angle microcoils, when considering the subtraction between movement distance and line spacing on the mask. The rotation speed and movement speed are decided as follows: forward movement speed, backward movement speed and rotation speed for the 45° tilt-angle microcoil are approximately 2.65 μm/s, 2.50 μm/s and 0.15 deg/s, respectively. Forward movement speed, backward movement speed and rotation speed for the 60° tilt-angle microcoil are approximately 4.54 μm/s, 4.28 μm/s and 0.15 deg/s, respectively.

A representative optical image of the photoresist pattern of the microcoil with 45° tilt-angle fabricated on the polyimide capillary by the cylindrical projection lithography technique is shown in Figure 8b. The photoresist pattern of microcoil with a tilt-angle of 45° was patterned with 10 ± 0.2 μm coil width, 78.5 ± 0.5 μm coil pitch and 20 turns. In addition, the photoresist pattern microcoil with tilt-angle 60° was also successfully patterned with 10 ± 0.2 μm coil width, 81.5 ± 0.5 μm coil pitch and 20 turns, as shown in Figure 8c. A photograph of the 20 turn microcoil with 60° tilt-angle on the 1 mm diameter polyimide capillary after Au etching, Cr etching and photoresist removal is presented in Figure 8d.

4.2. Characteristics of Electroplated Tilted Microcoil

The SEMs of the electroplated copper microcoil are shown in Figure 9a. Copper electroplating would be produced directly on the Au coil line used as the seed layer without photoresist mold. In addition, the Cu coil line grows along the Au coil line vertically, and slightly expands both sides during the electroplating. In our case, the Cu coil line width finally increases to 40 μm, and the thickness grows to 15 μm based on a 10 μm Au coil line. The microcoil with a tilt-angle of 60°, line width of 40 μm, and thickness of 15 μm was successfully obtained, as shown in Figure 9b,c.

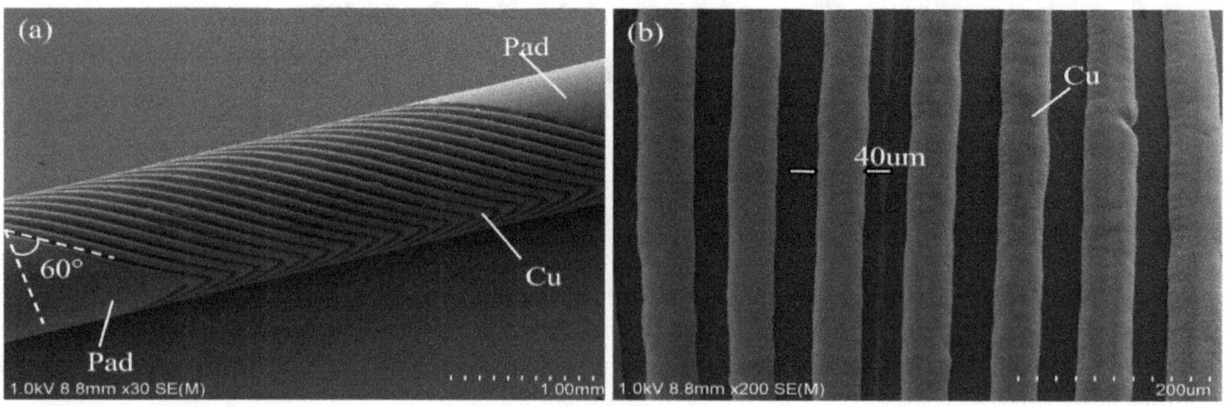

Figure 9. *Cont.*

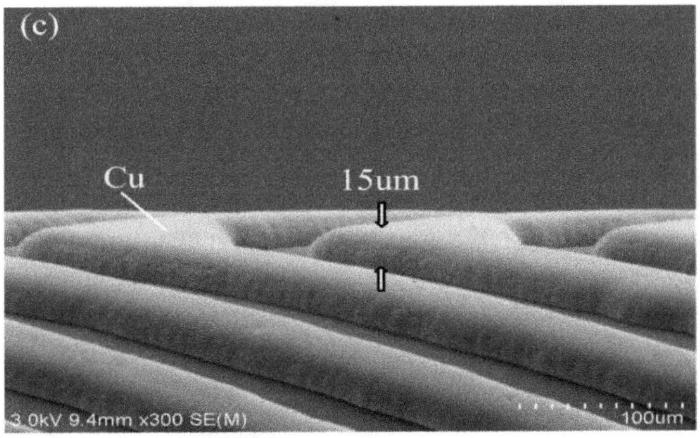

Figure 9. SEMs of the electroplated tilted microcoil. (**a**) Intact coil; (**b**) line width and spacing; (**c**) thickness of Cu microcoil.

5. Conclusions

We proposed an ultra-thin single-fiber scanner that is electromagnetically driven by tilted microcoils. It can be fabricated by a specific MEMS process. The parameters of the tilted microcoil were designated as 60° tilt-angle, 80 μm coil pitch, and 20 turns based on the simulation and optimization results for magnetic force. The modal response of the designed scanner was simulated. The tilted microcoils were fabricated on a polyimide capillary surface by the developed MEMS-based fabrication process. The process includes spray coating, cylindrical projection lithography, and mask-less electroplating micromachining. In particular, the photoresist pattern of the microcoil has been obtained successfully and with high resolution using this lithography method. The dimensions of the two fabricated tilted microcoils were as follows: 45° tilt-angle, 10 μm ± 0.2 μm line width, 78.5 ± 0.5 μm coil pitch and 20 turns; and 65° tilt-angle, 10 μm ± 0.2 line width, 81.5 ± 0.5 μm coil pitch and 20 turns. Finally, a direct mask-less electroplating process was used to obtain a 15 μm thick copper microcoil.

Acknowledgments: The authors would like to express their gratitude for the support from the National Natural Science Foundation of China (No. 61571287) and Shanghai Pujiang Program (14PJ1405800). The authors would also like to thank A. Toda at Meltex Inc., Japan for his help on electroplating coil experiment work.

Author Contributions: Z.Y. and B.S. conceived and designed the experiments; J.S. performed the experiments; J.Y. and G.D. analyzed the data; R.S. contributed reagents/materials/analysis tools; Z.Y. wrote the paper.

References

1. Seibel, E.J. 1-mm catheterscope. In Proceedings of the SPIE 2008 Optical Fibers and Sensors for Medical Diagnostics and Treatment Applications VIII, San Jose, CA, USA, 19–21 January 2008; pp. 685207–685208.
2. Matsunaga, T.; Hino, R.; Makishi, W.; Esashi, M.; Haga, Y. Electromagnetically driven ulutra-miniature single fiber scanner for high-resolution endoscopy fabricated on cylindrical substrates using MEMS process. In Proceedings of the 23rd IEEE International Conference on Micro Electro Mechanical Systems, Hong Kong, China, 24–28 January 2010; p. 999.
3. Kamiuchi, H.; Kuwana, K.; Fukuyo, T.; Yamashita, H.; Chiba, T.; Dohi, T.; Masamune, K. 3-D endoscope using a single CCD camera and pneumatic vibration mechanism. *Surg. Endosc.* **2013**, *27*, 1642–1647. [CrossRef] [PubMed]
4. Catanzaro, A.; Faulx, A.; Isenberg, G.A.; Wong, R.C.; Cooper, G.; Sivak, M.V.; Chak, A. Prospective Evaluation of 4-mm Diameter Endoscopes for Esophagoscopy in Sedated and Unsedated Patients. *Gastrointest. Endoscopy* **2003**, *57*, 300–304.
5. Liu, X.; Huang, Y.; Kang, J.U. Dark-field illuminated reflectance fiber bundle endoscopic microscope. *J. Biomed. Opt.* **2011**, *16*, 046003. [CrossRef] [PubMed]

6. Kester, R.T.; Bedard, N.; Gao, L.; Tkaczyk, T.S. Real-time snapshot hyperspectral imaging endoscope. *J. Biomed. Opt.* **2011**, *16*, 056005. [CrossRef] [PubMed]
7. Niklas, W.; Hans, Z.; Andreas, S. Endoscopic optical probes for linear rotational scanning. In Proceedings of the 2013 IEEE 26th International Conference on Micro Electro Mechanical Systems, Taipei, Taiwan, 20–24 January 2013; p. 1065.
8. Hu, H.P.; Chiao, J.C. A compact fiber optical scanner using electromagnetic actuation. In Proceedings of the International Society for Optics and Photonics Photonics: Design, Technology, and Packaging II, Brisbane, Australia, 12–14 December 2005; Vol. 6038.
9. Niklas, W.; Tobias, M.; Hans, Z.; Andreas, S. Tunable MEMS fiber scanner for confocal microscopy. In Proceedings of the 2014 IEEE 27th International Conference on Micro Electro Mechanical Systems (MEMS), San Francisco, CA, USA, 26–30 January 2014; p. 881.
10. Babak, A.; Min, H.T.; Simon, W.; Kenichi, T. Ferrofluid-assisted micro rotary motor for minially invasive endoscopy application. In Proceedings of the 2014 IEEE 27th International Conference on Micro Electro Mechanical Systems (MEMS), San Francisco, CA, USA, 26–30 January 2014; p. 200.
11. Niklas, W.; Daniel, H.; Hans, Z.; Andreas, S. Polymer/Silicon Hard Magnetic Micromirrors. *J. Microelectr. Syst.* **2012**, *21*, 1098–1106.
12. Lee, K.D.; Hiroshima, H.; Zhang, Y.; Itoh, T.; Maeda, R. Cylindrical projection lithography for microcoil structure. *Microelectr. Eng.* **2011**, *88*. [CrossRef]
13. Uchiyama, S.; Hayase, M.; Takagi, H.; Itoh, T.; Zhang, Y. Spray Coating Deposition of Thin Resist Film on Fiber Substrates. *Jpn. J. Appl. Phys.* **2012**, *51*, 116502. [CrossRef]
14. Toda, A. *Electroplating of Copper Film on Capillary*; Meltex Report No.53; Meltex Inc.: Tokyo, Japan, 2012. (In Japanese)

11

MEMS Actuators for Optical Microendoscopy

Zhen Qiu [1] and Wibool Piyawattanametha [1,2,*]

1 Department of Biomedical Engineering, Institute for Quantitative Health Science and Engineering, Michigan State University, East Lansing, MI 48824, USA; qiuzhen@egr.msu.edu

2 Departments of Biomedical Engineering, Faculty of Engineering King Mongkut's Institute of Technology Ladkrabang (KMITL), Bangkok 10520, Thailand

* Correspondence: piyawatt@msu.edu or wibool@gmail.com

Abstract: Growing demands for affordable, portable, and reliable optical microendoscopic imaging devices are attracting research institutes and industries to find new manufacturing methods. However, the integration of microscopic components into these subsystems is one of today's challenges in manufacturing and packaging. Together with this kind of miniaturization more and more functional parts have to be accommodated in ever smaller spaces. Therefore, solving this challenge with the use of microelectromechanical systems (MEMS) fabrication technology has opened the promising opportunities in enabling a wide variety of novel optical microendoscopy to be miniaturized. MEMS fabrication technology enables abilities to apply batch fabrication methods with high-precision and to include a wide variety of optical functionalities to the optical components. As a result, MEMS technology has enabled greater accessibility to advance optical microendoscopy technology to provide high-resolution and high-performance imaging matching with traditional table-top microscopy. In this review the latest advancements of MEMS actuators for optical microendoscopy will be discussed in detail.

Keywords: MEMS actuators; microendoscopy; confocal; two-photon; wide-filed imaging; photoacoustic; fluorescence; scanner

---

1. Introduction

Actuation and scanning mechanisms have played important roles in novel microendoscopic imaging systems. Common challenges in the development of these miniature instruments are in both design freedom and the integration of miniaturized opto-mechanical components. Microelectromechanical systems (MEMS) fabrication technologies play a valuable and instrumental role in solving the aforementioned issues in order to achieve similar performance as traditional microscopy counterparts. In optical microendoscopy, actuation and scanning mechanisms enable three-dimensional (3D) image formation in the tiny devices with ultra-compact form factors. The technical challenges in designing such kinds of components include the generation of a distortion-free scanning pattern with sufficient speed to mitigate in vivo motion artifacts with millimeter package dimensions. To realize in vivo tissue imaging on living subjects, 5 Hz or faster frame rates are usually required to accommodate movements induced by several factors, such as respiratory displacement, heart beating, and organ peristalsis.

The size of the MEMS actuators determines their mounted locations at either the proximal or distal end of the instrument. A much greater control of the focal volume, including axial scanning for imaging into the tissue, can be achieved with the MEMS actuators positioned distally. However, their typical sizes mounted at the distal end of the instrument should be less than 5.5 mm (for example, fitting the Olympus therapeutic endoscope) in order to be compatible with the tool channel of a standard medical endoscope [1].

A spiral scanner consists of a tubular piezoelectric actuator (small diameter <1 mm) that drives the distal tip of a single-mode (SM) optical fiber using modulated sinusoidal waveforms around the resonant frequency [2]. This approach has been successfully implemented in the scanning fiber endoscope (SFE) with wide-field fluorescence imaging and in representative multi-photon microendoscopes. Compared to the raster scanning, the spiral scan pattern can achieve higher frame rates with large amplitude. Micro-motor-based rotational scanning mechanisms steer the laser beam circumferentially around the longitudinal axis of the endoscope after a 45° deflection off a reflective mirror or prism. Similar methods have been widely used in optical coherence tomography (OCT) and photoacoustic (PA) endoscopes. The galvo-scanner, reliable but aging technology, is a meso-scale electromechanical mechanism that performs beam scanning by deflecting a mounted mirror coated with aluminum or gold depending on the effective wavelength range. The relatively large size limits its use to steering a focused beam into the proximal end of a coherent bundle of optical fibers. This technique has been used in fiber bundle-based confocal microendoscopy (Cellvizio, Mauna Kea Technologies, Paris, France) [3]. The bulky galvo scanner at the proximal end provides deflections in the slow axis and is used with a resonant mirror that performs fast-axis scanning.

Micromirrors have been developed with microelectromechanical systems (MEMS) technologies that use either electrothermal or electrostatic actuators to achieve large deflection angles and high dynamic bandwidths with excellent linearity. These scanners can be batch fabricated on silicon wafers to achieve devices with relatively high yield. MEMS actuators and scanners usually require sophisticated micro-fabrication processes but have great flexibility in scanning speed and device dimensions/geometries. Based on different working principles, there are some typical types of actuation mechanisms for MEMS actuators in microendoscopes [4–7], including bulky piezoelectric tubing, electrostatic comb-drive or plates, electro-thermal, electro-magnetic, and thin-film piezoelectric materials. Thus far, electrostatic devices are most commonly applied in microendoscope development because of their relative fast scan speeds with ultra-low power consumption (from very low current consumption). However, one of the disadvantages of the electrostatic MEMS devices, relative high driving voltage (>100 V), might become a major concern for clinically translational use in the event of electrical short circuit from the MEMS devices. Recently, some novel electrostatic resonant 2D scanners operating at low driving voltage can potentially resolve this issue. On the other hand, the novel thin-film piezoelectric materials actuated MEMS devices have excellent performance with relatively low driving voltage (<20 V) and ultra-low power consumption and may be the future for scanners and actuators in endomicroscopy [8–10]. The low fill-in factor (<50%) of existing micromirrors is a common problem that may be solved by micro-assembly or advanced manufacturing processes [7].

This review is intended to present some representative examples of many exciting optical microendoscopy being pursued around the world based on MEMS actuators.

2. Overview of Optical Imaging Modalities

Various optical imaging modalities implemented so far with MEMS actuation technologies will be given as a preview here, including OCT, PA, confocal microscopy (CM), and multiphoton microscope.

By using the short coherence length of a broadband light source, the resolution of OCT can achieve around 1 μm to 15 μm, which usually depends on the light source employed, including supercontinuum white light lasers. OCT imaging system usually has deep tissue penetration up to 3 mm, which is sufficient for imaging of the whole epithelial layer. Furthermore, to realize 3D imaging, 2D lateral scans need to be realized by a moving stage or a scanning mirror (SM). Two-dimensional (2D) MEMS actuators are often used for 3D imaging, although there are some alternative approaches with conventional cable-based actuation and scanning mechanisms driven by rotation motors and pulling stations. The OCT imaging system has been successfully applied to ophthalmology and widely used in clinics since its first seminal report [11]. In addition, researchers have made tremendous efforts on the miniaturization and clinical translation of the OCT system for many kinds of applications on hollow organs [12], including colon, esophagus, bladders, and lung.

Recently, photoacoustic (PA) microscopy has become an emerging and promising imaging technology with several advantages [13], in terms of the tissue penetration, high spatial resolution, and contrast. Based on the light-tissue-sound interaction, the novel imaging modality acquires 3D images through detecting an acoustic wave generated by rapid thermoelastic expansion induced by pulsed laser beam absorption in the tissue specimens. In summary, two representative photoacoustic microscopic imaging systems have been demonstrated, including optical resolution photoacoustic microscopy (so called OR-PAM) and acoustic resolution photoacoustic microscopy (so called AR-PAM). MEMS actuation technologies enable compact photoacoustic microendoscopes and have been developed by several research groups, which will be introduced in detail later.

Based on the continuous-wave (CW) laser, confocal microscopy provides imaging contrast with subcellular resolution optical sectioning capability via a pinhole [14]. The confocal microscope acquires 3D images by stacking two-dimensional lateral (x-y) images (plane by plane) along the z-axis, by utilizing a two-dimensional galvo-scanner and piezo-actuated objective lens. Due to the conventional pre-objective scanning configuration, only a limited field-of-view (FOV) can be realized with a high numerical aperture (NA). Reflective and fluorescence imaging modes are often used for confocal microscopy. While operating in the reflective mode, the confocal microscopy relies on the backscattered light from the tissue and provide morphological information of tissues. On the other hand, fluorescence imaging in conjunction of fluorophore labeling will provide a signal from microstructures with relatively high specificity, high sensitivity, and bright contrast. Bench-top commercial confocal microscopic imaging system with bulky objective lenses have been widely used for ex vivo or intra-vital imaging in biomedical research laboratories. By taking advantage of the MEMS-based actuation technologies, confocal microendoscopes have been developed based on different architectures, including conventional single-axis with pre-objective scanning and new dual-axis with post-objective scanning [1], which will be introduced later in the section on MEMS-based confocal microendoscopy. The traditional single-axis architecture uses high-NA objective lenses that provide high resolution, but limit the working distance significantly. In the novel dual-axis confocal architecture, relatively larger FOV and longer working distance can be realized by the system design consisting of a low numerical aperture lens and scanning elements located right at the post-objective position.

Different from the working principle of confocal microscopy, the two-photon microscopic imaging system is mainly based in nonlinear light-tissue interactions [15,16]. The fluorescence emission signal can be generated while two lower-energy (longer wavelength) photons in the near-infrared (NIR, more than 800 nm) regime arrive at tissue biomolecules simultaneously. To collect the weak fluorescence emission signal, sensitive detectors, such as avalanche photodiodes (APDs) and photomultiplier tubes (PMTs), are usually employed. High peak intensity femtosecond (fs) pulse lasers (~10–200 fs) are required for the two-photon microscopic imaging because the probability of the simultaneous two photon absorption by a single fluorophore is relatively low. With a high numerical aperture objective lens, the fluorescence emission signal will be acquired only from the focus plane. In addition, with the longer wavelength used in two-photon microscopic imaging, it enables deep tissue penetration and stronger imaging contrast with relatively lower photo-bleaching and photo-damage to the tissue specimens. Thanks to the rapid development of advanced fiber optics and fiber laser technologies, ultra-compact MEMS-actuated two photon microendoscopes have been successfully demonstrated for basic biological studies (like neural circuit imaging) and clinically translational applications [17]. For delivering a high-intensity, ultrafast pulse laser with minimal distortion, photonic crystal fibers (PCFs) have been developed and widely used in microendoscopic imaging systems [17].

3. MEMS-Based Optical Coherence Tomography (OCT) Microendoscopy

Since the first electro-thermal MEMS 2D scanner-based OCT endoscopic prototype [18] was demonstrated, researchers have developed several types of MEMS-based OCT microendoscopes [19,20]. Although traditional electromagnetic micro-motor based OCT catheters have already been widely used for in vivo imaging on small animal models or human patients [21–23], mass-producible MEMS actuator-enabled OCT microendoscopes will very likely become the future trend because MEMS-based micro-devices have many advantages, especially in terms of the miniaturization potential and repeatability. MEMS-based micro-devices may be based on various working principles and actuation mechanisms, such as electrostatic [24–29], electrothermal [18,30–33], bulky PZT-based fiber scan tube [34–39], and electromagnetics [40].

Among the variety of micro-devices, the electrostatic comb-drive-actuated MEMS scanner is a popular one [24–29]. For example, one of the representative MEMS-based OCT microendoscopes, as shown in Figure 1 [28], has utilized an electrostatic MEMS scanner [25] driven by angled vertical comb (AVC) actuators for a large tilting angle. The effective mirror aperture's diameter is as large as 1 mm, which is sufficient to reflect the light beam for side-view high-resolution imaging with the MEMS-based endoscopic catheter. The single-mode fiber (SMF), fiber collimator, and the MEMS scanner are fully integrated in an aluminum-based packaging. The detailed fiber-based optical system design of the time-domain OCT imaging system and the real-time data acquisition system with high sampling speed are illustrated in Figure 2a. Three-dimensional OCT image volumes acquired in vitro from a hamster cheek pouch are shown in Figure 2b. Both horizontal (also called *en-face*) and vertical cross-sectional plane images extracted from the 3D OCT volume, in Figure 2c, have demonstrated high-resolution morphological changes inside the tissue specimen.

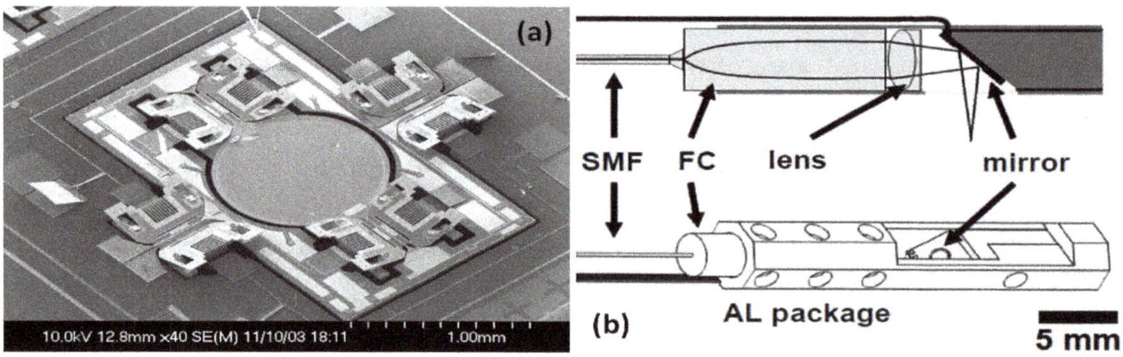

Figure 1. (**a**) Scanning electron micrograph of the MEMS two-axis optical scanner. The scanner has a large 1 mm diameter mirror and uses angled vertical comb (AVC) actuators to produce a large angle scan for high-resolution imaging. (**b**) Optical schematic and mechanical drawing of the optical coherence tomography (OCT) catheter endoscope. SMF: single mode fiber, FC: fiber collimator, AL: aluminum.

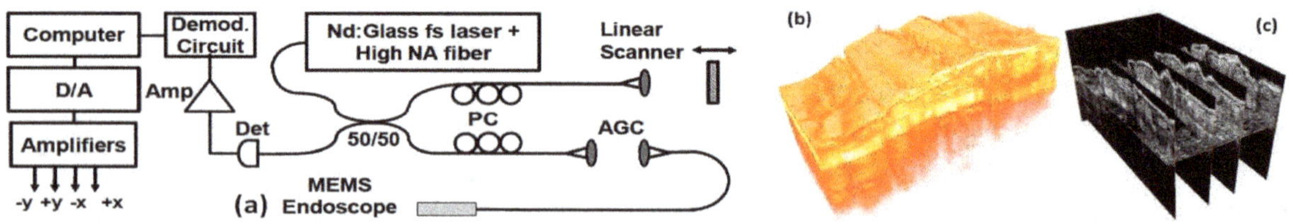

Figure 2. (**a**) OCT system schematic for imaging with the MEMS endoscope. PC: polarization control, AGC: air-gap coupling, Det: detector, Amp: amplifier, D/A: digital to analog Converter; OCT images acquired with the MEMS scanning catheter. (**b**) Three-dimensional rendering of the OCT volume dataset from a hamster cheek pouch; and (**c**) the serial cross-sections and *en-face* plane extracted from a 3D OCT volume of a hamster cheek pouch acquired in vitro.

Most recently, a novel MEMS-based OCT microendoscope with circumferential-scanning has been developed by the engineering team led by Xie from the University of Florida [41] through a unique optical design utilizing multiple electrothermal MEMS scanners. An array of ultra-compact electro-thermally actuated MEMS scanners (Figure 3a) are integrated at the distal end of the catheter to reflect collimated beams, as shown in Figure 3b,c. Flexible printed circuit boards (FPCB) provide driving current for electrothermal scanners. All of the micro-optical components and MEMS-based circumferential scanning systems have been fully integrated and assembled in a compact form factor (Figure 3e) for potential in vivo imaging application in the human gastrointestinal (GI) tract. The fiber-based collimating system is used for laser excitation, as shown in Figure 3f.

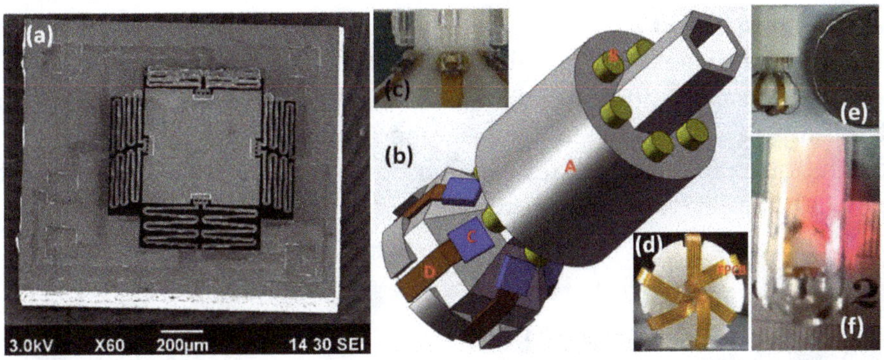

Figure 3. Electrothermal MEMS scanner-based OCT catheter. (**a**) A SEM image of the MEMS scanner. (**b**) The schematic 3D drawing of the probe design. A: 3D-printed probe head; B: C-lens collimators; C: the MEMS chips; D: FPCB. (**c**) A zoom-in picture showing the C-lens collimators and MEMS chips. (**d**) A back-view picture showing the flexible printed circuit boards (FPCBs) folded into the hollow hole. (**e**) A photo of the assembled probe (pictured with a Chinese Yuan coin). (**f**) Photograph of the OCT probe with laser beam scanning. Reproduced with permission from [41]; published by OSA, 2018.

4. MEMS-Based Photoacoustic Microendoscopy

A MEMS scanner-based photoacoustic microscope (PAM) system's conceptual design has been demonstrated by Chen [42] by taking advantages of both an optical micro-ring resonator and electrostatic comb-drive-actuated MEMS scanner. The ultrasensitive micro-ring resonator with broad bandwidth, developed by Ling [43], is one type of micro-/nano-photonic device which sense an ultrasonic signal using optical approaches. As shown in Figure 4a, a fiber-based optical system setup with pulse laser excitation (wavelength 532 nm), MEMS mirror driving system, real-time data acquisition system has been described in the schematic drawing. The electrostatic MEMS scanner within the package, in Figure 4b, provides the lateral laser beam point-scanning in raster scanning mode at a slow rate. This new PAM imaging system can provide ex vivo optical resolution photoacoustic images of the tissue. To detect the weak photoacoustic signal, the micro-ring resonator is located right under the tissue specimen with acoustic signal coupling media, such as water or ultrasonic gel.

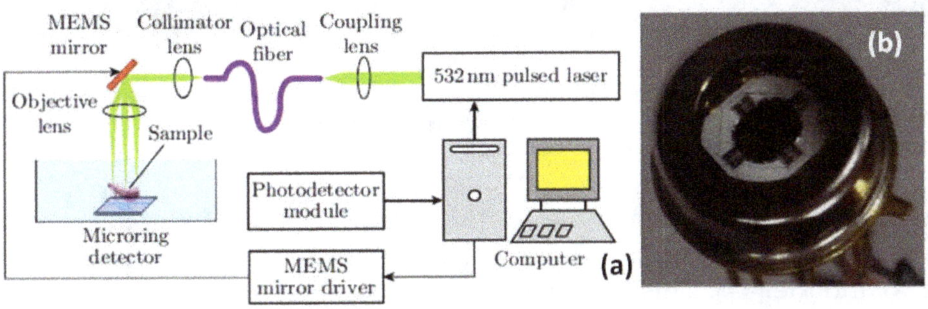

Figure 4. MEMS-based optical resolution photoacoustic microscope. (**a**) Schematic of the MEMS-based optical resolution photoacoustic microscopy (OR-PAM) system and (**b**) photography of the MEMS mirror.

To realize the photoacoustic microscopic system in more portable or endoscope-friendly form factor, researchers have been making tremendous efforts on the miniaturization of the imaging system design and the distal scanhead with MEMS technologies. A new handheld photoacoustic microscope (PAM) probe [40], as shown in Figure 5, has been developed recently for potential clinical application. The distal scanhead of the handheld PAM system, 17 mm in diameter and a weight of 162 g, mainly consists of the fiber-based collimator, ultrasound detector, acoustic and photonic beam coupler, and beam scanning system. The handheld PAM system has integrated a newly custom-developed electromagnetic MEMS 2D scanner, shown in Figure 5a. The schematic drawing of the full imaging system is illustrated in Figure 5b, including the high-speed data acquisition system, ultrasonic transducer, and fiber based optics. High-resolution imaging quality with a large FOV using this handheld PAM system has been demonstrated by imaging the blood vessel of a mouse ear, shown in Figure 6. The PAM imaging system has also been used to delineate a human mole to demonstrate its clinical application in delineating melanoma which has the highest death rate among skin cancers and may cause about 9730 deaths the United States.

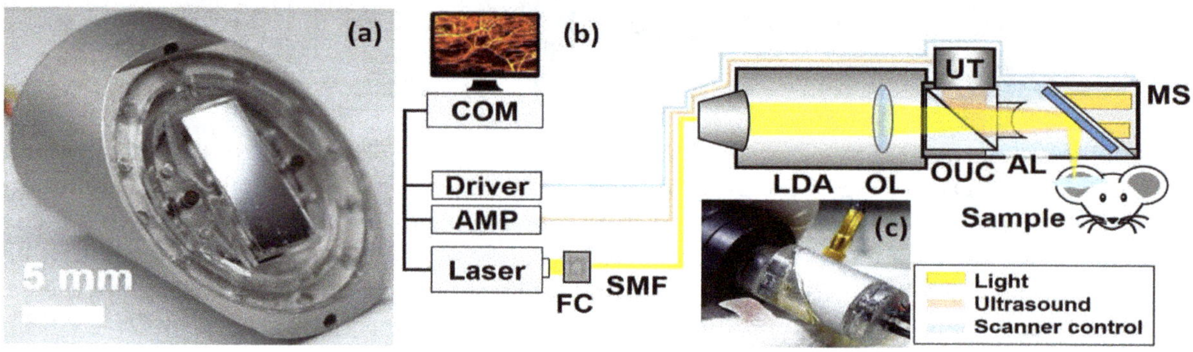

Figure 5. Handheld photoacoustic microscopy (PAM) probe. (**a**) Electromagnetic scanner. (**b**) Schematic of the handheld system. AL: acoustic lens; AMP: amplifier; COM: computer; EM: electromagnets; FC: fiber collimator; LDA: light delivery assembly; MS: MEMS scanner; OL: objective lens; OUC: opto-ultrasound combiner; SMF: single mode fiber; UT: ultrasonic transducer. (**c**) Photograph of the handheld PAM probe.

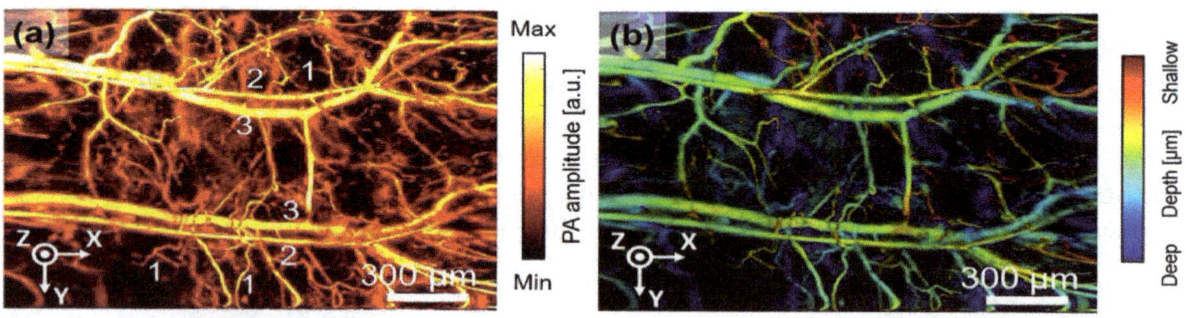

Figure 6. Extension of field-of-view (FOV). (**a**) Single PA MAP image of a mouse ear with an extended FOV (2.8 × 2 mm). (**b**) Depth map image corresponding to PA MAP image (**a**).

Based on an advanced ultra-compact electrothermal MEMS 2D scanner, a novel miniaturized MEMS-based photoacoustic (PA) microendoscope has been recently developed through collaborative team work led by Xi and Xie [44]. This work has been the most advanced PA microendoscopic imaging system and is close to clinical application. The cross-sectional view photograph of the endoscopic packaging is shown in Figure 7a, including a GRIN lens-based fiber-based collimator, electrothermal MEMS scanner, and optical and acoustic coupler. The new MEMS-based PA microendoscope can acquire high-resolution photoacoustic images of tissue specimens. The image performance of this new photoacoustic microendoscope has been demonstrated on a mouse ear, as shown in Figure 8c.

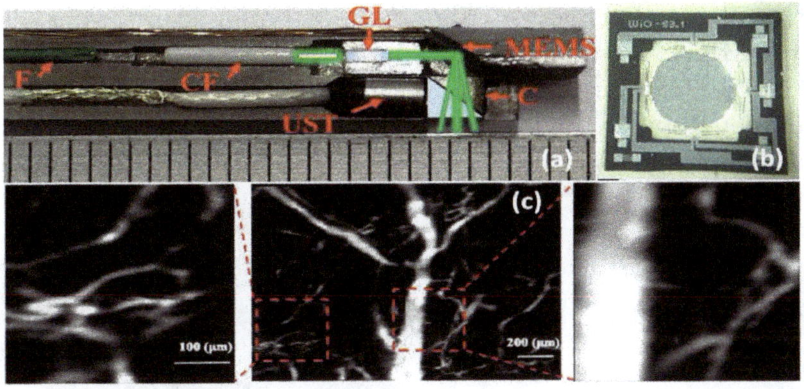

Figure 7. MEMS-based photoacoustic (PA) microendoscope. (**a**) Photograph of the assembled imaging probe. (**b**) Photograph of the electrothermal MEMS mirror. F: fiber; CF: ceramic ferrule; GL: GRIN lens; MEMS mirror; UST, ultrasound transducer; C, cube. (**c**) High-resolution photoacoustic imaging of a mouse ear, the MAP image (left) was acquired with 20 sub images and two typical subimage (right) indicated by the dashed rectangle. Reproduced with permission from [44]; published by OSA, 2017.

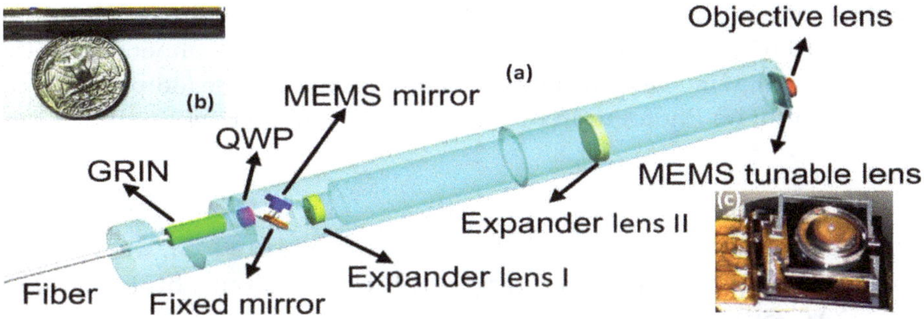

Figure 8. Electrothermal MEMS scanner-based confocal microendoscope. (**a**) Schematic 3D drawing of the microendoscope design. (**b**) Photograph of the assembled microendoscopic probe with US coin as a reference. (**c**) Photograph of an assembled tunable lens on the electrothermal MEMS scanner.

Thus far, several miniaturized photoacoustic microendoscopes have been developed using electromagnetic [46–48] or electrothermal scanners [44]. To co-axially steer both laser and ultrasonic beams, a water-immersible electromagnetic MEMS scanner [48] has been custom-made to operate in the ultrasound coupling media. Due to the high detection sensitivity and broader bandwidth with very compact form factor, a micro-ring resonator [43,49–52] has attracted more attention and been fully explored, such as the transparent micro-ring for microendoscope applications [51,52].

5. MEMS-Based Confocal Microendoscopy

Compared to other relatively new imaging modalities, confocal microscopy has been studied for decades. MEMS-based confocal microendoscopes were invented a long time ago since the first seminal work demonstrated by Kino and Dickensheets [53]. Later, researchers have focused on improving the lateral or axial resolution and depth imaging while miniaturizing the confocal microendoscopes using MEMS technologies. For instance, the new MEMS-based 3D confocal microendoscope with a tunable Z-focus has been developed by Xie's team [45] using an advanced electrothermal MEMS scanner with tunable objective lens mounted in the center of the moving Z-axis stage with large translational movement (>300 μm) at low voltage. As shown in Figure 8, the MEMS-actuated tunable objective lens is located at the distal end, which is very close to the tissue specimen. By being fully packaged in stainless steel tubing, the fiber-based microendoscope could potentially be applied for clinical applications on humans (Figure 8b).

Another interesting electrothermally-actuated MEMS fiber scanner has also been invented and fully integrated into the MEMS-based confocal microendoscope [54]. A SEM image of the compact electrothermal MEMS fiber scanner is shown in Figure 9b. As shown in Figure 9, the team from KAIST [54] has recently developed a novel scanning fiber-enabled ultra-thin confocal microendoscope which can be easily inserted into the miniature tool channel of the medical laparoscope, shown in Figure 9c.

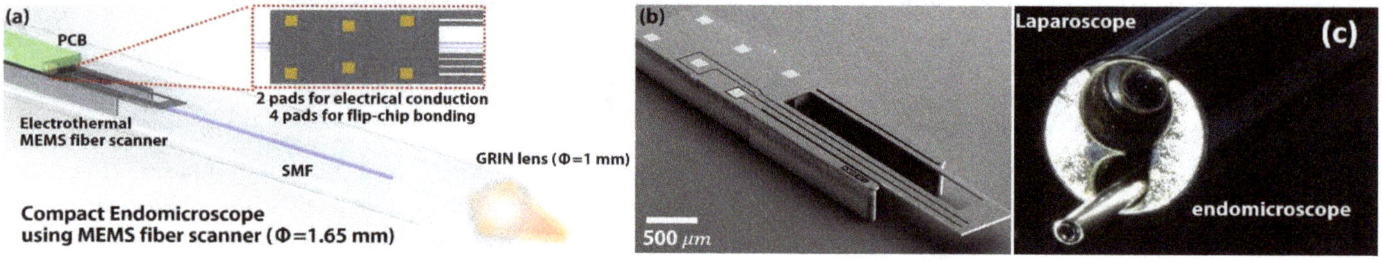

Figure 9. Electrothermal MEMS fiber scanner-based confocal microendoscope. (**a**) Schematic drawing of the catheter with a Lissajous scanner. The MEMS fiber scanner is fabricated for flip-chip bonding, which minimized the electrical packaging dimensions, resulting in the scanner package being 1.65 mm in diameter. (**b**) Top-view SEM image of the fabricated microactuator. The footprint dimension indicates 1 mm × 5 mm × 0.43 mm; (**c**) Photograph of the packaged catheter assembled to the laparoscopic functional channel.

Compared to the conventional single-axis confocal architecture [45], the novel dual-axis confocal (DAC) configuration offers superior dynamic range in the Z-axis with higher axial resolution. Based on the fully-scalable DAC optics architecture, miniaturization using 2D/3D MEMS scanners and micro-optics have been performed during the past ten years. Both electrostatic MEMS scanners and thin-film piezo-electrical (PZT: lead zirconate titanate)-based MEMS scanners have been developed for MEMS-based DAC microendoscopy.

A monolithic thin-film piezo-electrical MEMS scanner [55] (footprint in less than 3.2 mm by 3.0 mm), with both vertical (Z-axis) and lateral (X-axis or Y-axis) scanning capabilities, has been demonstrated for the first time to perform horizontal and vertical cross-sectional imaging. The schematic drawing (Figure 10a) illustrates the integration of the thin-film PZT-based MEMS scanner with multidimensional freedom inside the optical design of the DAC microendoscope. A photograph of the thin-film PZT based MEMS device, which provides large translational motion for Z-axis focus change (>200 μm) and wide tilting angle (>± 5° mechanically) for lateral scanning, is shown in Figure 10b.

Although new thin-film PZT-based MEMS scanners show promising technical advantages over conventional MEMS devices, their micro-machining processes are still challenging due to the complexity of preparation and patterning of thin-film piezo-electrical materials. On the other hand, the traditional electrostatic MEMS scanner [56–60] has recently been fully explored with unique mechanical flexure designs to meet the requirements from 3D confocal microendoscopic imaging systems [61–65]. As shown in Figure 11, a novel monolithic electrostatic MEMS scanner with switchable lateral and vertical scanning capabilities have been successfully demonstrated with a compact footprint (<3.2 mm × 3.0 mm) for DAC microendoscopes. The new electrostatic scanner is based on the parametric resonance working principle with an in-plane comb-drive configuration. Through design optimization, the driving voltage can be close to 40 V, which is safe for human patients. With cross-sectional depth imaging, MEMS-based DAC microendoscopes may potentially be used for molecular contrast agent-based multi-color fluorescence imaging [66–69] for colorectal cancer early detection in the human gastrointestinal tract.

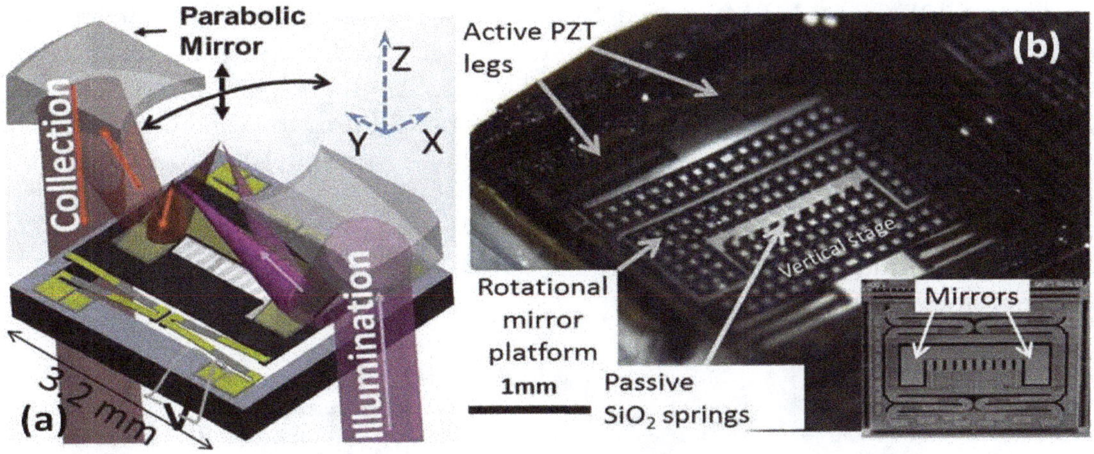

Figure 10. MEMS-based dual-axis confocal (DAC) microendoscope. (**a**) Schematic drawing of the MEMS vertical-rotational stage scanning for cross-sectional imaging with the DAC microendoscope. (**b**) Photograph of the vertical-rotational MEMS scanning stage based on an active outer vertical displacement and a passive inner resonant scanning. Inset: Variant with solid dog-bone mirror surface for the DAC microscope.

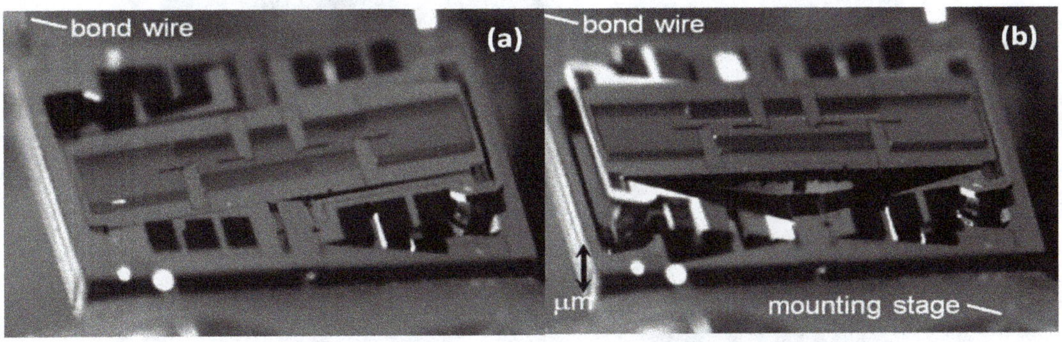

Figure 11. Electrostatic MEMS scanner with switchable lateral and vertical scanning capability. (**a**) Demonstration of the lateral X-axis and Y-axis scanning for horizontal cross-sectional imaging. (**b**) Demonstration of the translational Z-axis scanning for vertical cross-sectional imaging.

By combining two separate electrostatic MEMS scanners, lateral (XY) and vertical (Z-axis) scanners [70], respectively, a new 3D MEMS scan engine-based DAC microendoscope with multi-color achromatic optics design could perform real-time 3D volumetric imaging in the tissue specimen for both clinical applications and system biology studies on live rodents. Furthermore, monolithic multiple degree-of-freedom or a 3D thin-film PZT-actuated micro-stage [8–10] will also potentially provide the 3D imaging without increasing the optical design complexity. As alternative approaches for miniature confocal system design, tunable optics-based [71] and micro-grating-based spectral encoded confocal microendoscopes [72] can realize depth imaging and *en-face* imaging with fewer scanning components.

6. MEMS-Based Multiphoton Microendoscopy

Not only being used in OCT and confocal system, electrostatic MEMS scanners have already demonstrated their critical roles for miniaturized multiphoton microendoscopic imaging system development since the first prototype was demonstrated by Piyawattanametha in 2006 for mice brain in vivo imaging [73,74]. Extended applications [75–77] have also been studied using the electrostatic MEMS 2D scanner-enabled multiphoton microendoscope, including femtosecond laser-based microsurgery [77].

Recently, handheld and endoscopic multiphoton microscopes have been developed with custom-made electrostatic MEMS 2D scanners [78] and Er-doped fiber laser [79,80]. For example, as shown in Figure 12, a new MEMS based two-photon fluorescent microendoscope [78] with a compact distal end is packaged in the stainless steel tube. The 2D MEMS resonant gimbal-based scanner can perform a lateral scan around the X- and Y-axes. With administration of Hoechst (nucleic acid stain), in vivo fluorescence imaging has been demonstrated in the distal colon of CDX2P-NLS Cre;adenomatosis polyposis coli (CPC;Apc) mouse model, which mimics human colorectal cancer diseases, as shown in Figure 13. A single-frame from a video sequence is shown in Figure 13a while the post-processed image after averaging (5 frames) is shown in Figure 13b. Compared to the images of H and E slides, the sub-cellular high-resolution microscopic imaging system could potentially provide histology-like imaging.

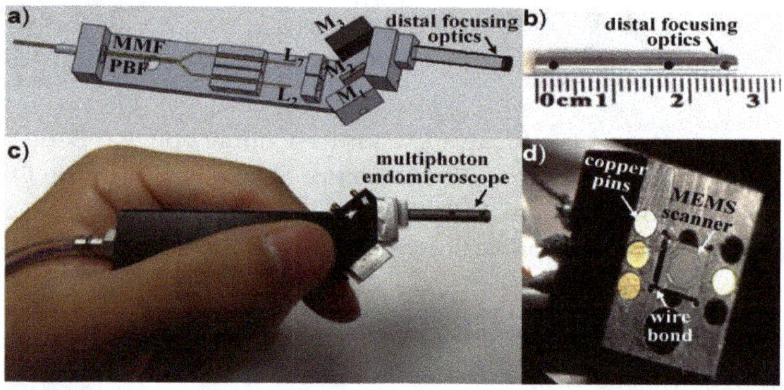

Figure 12. MEMS-based two-photon microendoscope. (**a**) Schematic CAD drawing of the optical circuit. (**b**) Distal end of focusing optics. (**c**) Handheld instrument which is used to perform repetitive imaging in small animal models of human disease. (**d**) Photograph of the MEMS scanner wire bonded on the substrate.

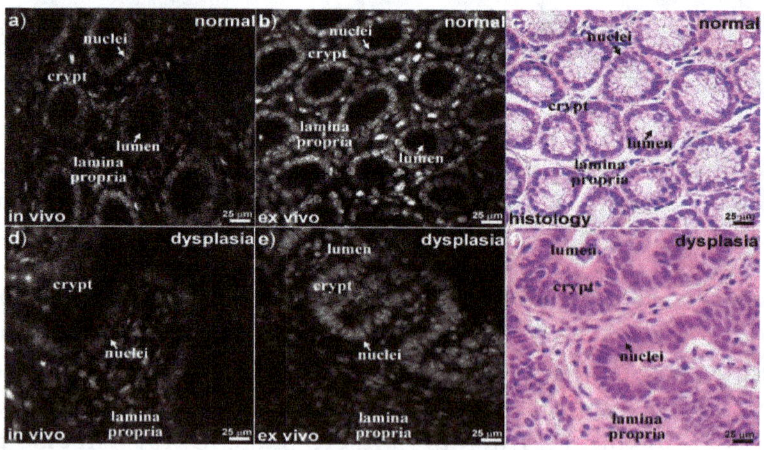

Figure 13. Fluorescent imaging results using the MEMS-based two-photon microendoscope. (**a**) Two-photon excited fluorescence image of normal colonic mucosa. (**b**) In-vivo image from normal averaged over five frames. (**c**) Corresponding histology of normal colon. Single frame from video of dysplastic crypts from colon of CPC; adenomatosis polyposis coli (Apc) mouse (**d**) In vivo at 5 frames/s and (**e**) In vivo image (averaged over five frames). (**f**) Corresponding histology of dysplasia.

Due to the footprint size of the electrostatic MEMS scanner, the distal end of the microendoscopic scanhead could not be easily miniaturized to less than 2.0 mm. However, the bulk PZT tube-based fiber scanner could potentially be fabricated with an ultra-thin wall and an outer diameter less than 1.5 mm so that the piezo tube fiber scanner enabled multiphoton microscope's distal end could be very small. Fiber scanner-based miniaturized multiphoton microscope was first demonstrated by Helmchen and Denk in 2001 for in vivo imaging on rodents' brains [81]. In addition, similar to the very small piezo tube-based fiber scanner [82,83], a bulk piezo sheet-based 2D raster-mode fiber scanner has also been investigated for multiphoton microendoscopic label-free imaging on unstained tissue specimens [84].

Based on the extensive experience on the multiphoton imaging system development, the team led by Li at Johns Hopkins University has recently developed a novel piezo tube-based fiber scanner-enabled miniaturized two-photon and second harmonic imaging system [85]. Aimed for label-free functional histology in vivo, the new fiber-optic scanning two-photon endomicroscope mainly consists of several key components, including a flexible double cladding fiber (DCF) for laser excitation and harvesting emission light, GRIN lens, and the very small piezo tube-based fiber scanner. A miniaturized custom-made objective with longitudinal focal shift has been developed by collaborating with GRINTECH (GmbH, Jena, Germany). A phase diffractive grating is sandwiched between two GRIN elements, as shown in Figure 14b.

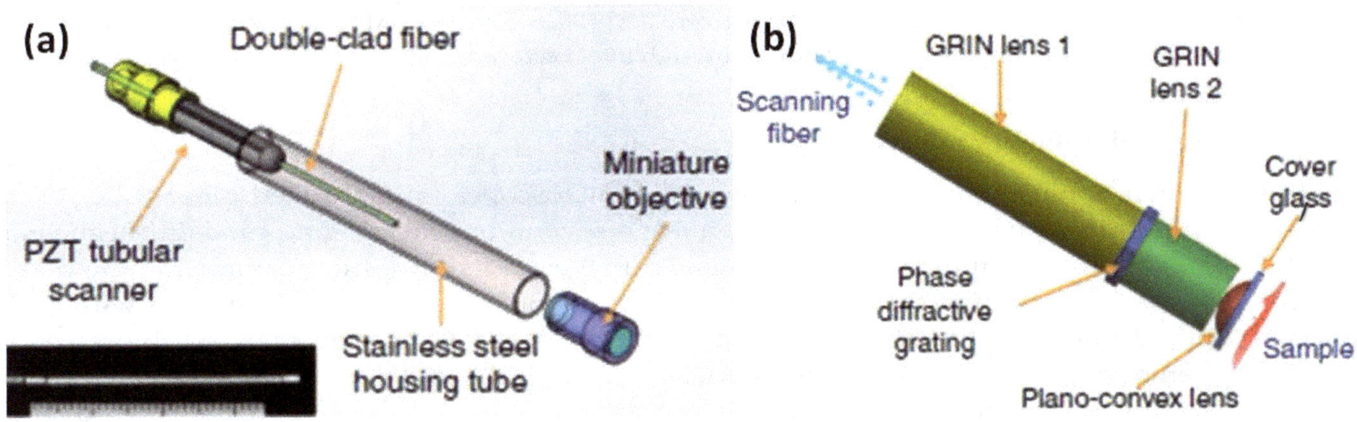

Figure 14. Fiber optic scanning two-photon endomicroscope. (**a**) Schematic drawing of the mechanical assembly based on double cladding fiber (DCF), the bottom inset is the photograph of the endomicroscope with an outer diameter of about 2.1 mm and a rigid length of about 35 mm. (**b**) Miniature custom-made objective and longitudinal focal shift. A phase diffractive grating is sandwiched between two GRIN elements. The fiber- and sample-side WDs are designed to be 200 μm in air and water.

The novel fiber optic multiphoton microendoscope developed by Liang [85] performs both two-photon fluorescence (2PF) and second harmonic generation (SHG) label-free structural imaging in vivo on small animal and human patients. As shown in Figure 15a,b, the overlay of intrinsic 2PF and SHG images have been acquired ex vivo from mouse liver. The emission signal was detected through two spectral channels: 496–665 nm (green, 2PF signal) and 435–455 nm (red, SHG signal). Figure 15c,d show the in vivo two-photon auto-fluorescence images of the mucosa of mouse small intestine, while the two detection channels are 417–477 nm for NADH (green) and 496–665 nm for FAD (red). Time-lapse SHG images of a cervical collagen fiber network have been acquired through intact ectocervical epithelium of cervices dissected from preterm-birth mouse models Figure 15e and normal pregnant mice (Figure 15f) at gestation day 15.

Electrostatic comb-drive actuated MEMS scanner and piezo fiber scanners have demonstrated their great potential in the development of multiphoton microendoscopes. In addition to those two actuation mechanisms, electrothermal MEMS scanners [86,87] have also been proposed for fiber scanning in the multiphoton imaging system although it may not be quite ready for clinical applications yet.

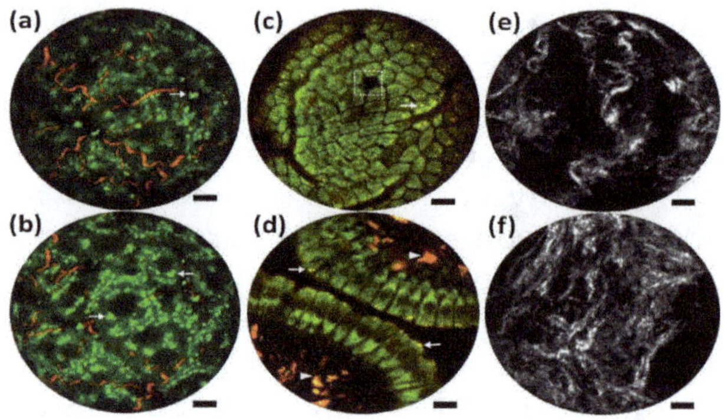

Figure 15. Endomicroscopy two-photon fluorescence (2PF) and second harmonic generation (SHG) label-free structural imaging. (**a**,**b**) Overlay of intrinsic 2PF and SHG ex vivo images of mouse liver. (**c**,**d**) Two-photon autofluorescence in vivo images of the mucosa of mouse small intestine. The two detection channels are 417–477 nm for NADH (green) and 496–665 nm for FAD (red). (**e**,**f**) SHG images of the cervical collagen fiber network acquired through intact ectocervical epithelium of cervices. Scale bars are 10 µm.

7. Fluorescence Wide-Field Endoscopy

Since its first application in the scanning-probe microscopes, miniaturized piezo tube based fiber scanner have demonstrated its great potential in several optical imaging modalities, such as OCT [34,36], or multiphoton [82,88]. By taking advantages of its ultra-thin form factor, the piezo tube has also been used in the scanning fiber endoscope (SFE) for wide-field imaging with both reflective [2] and fluorescent modes [89]. Compared to other MEMS scanner-based fluorescence imaging systems [90], the SFE-based endoscopic imaging system could have a much smaller outer diameter. Recently, Savastano and Zhou have demonstrated multimodal laser-based angioscopy [91] for structural, chemical, and biological imaging of atherosclerosis using the miniature catheter imaging system. As shown in Figure 16a, the scanning fiber endoscope excites tissues by scanning blue (424 nm), green (488 nm), and red lasers (642 nm) in a spiral pattern. Backscattered (reflectance) light and the fluorescent signal is collected by a ring of multimode fibers located in the periphery of the scanner housing and shaft and conducted to a data acquisition computer for image reconstruction. The optical system can be packaged with an outer diameter of 2.1 mm (left) or 1.2 mm (right) endoscopes, as shown in Figure 16b.

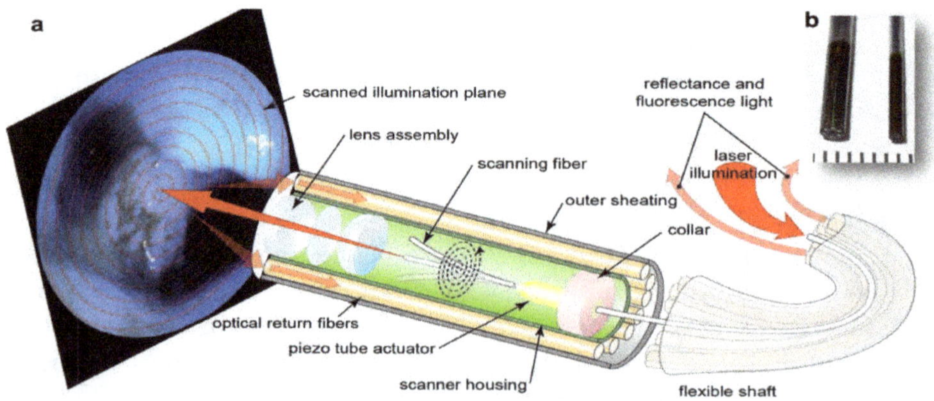

Figure 16. Scanning fiber endoscope optics and fluorescence spectrometry of major structural constituents of atherosclerotic plaques. (**a**) The scanning fiber endoscope excites tissues by scanning blue (424 nm), green (488 nm), and red lasers (642 nm) in a spiral pattern. Backscattered (reflectance) light and fluorescent signal is collected by a ring of optical fibers located in the periphery of the scanner housing and shaft, and conducted to a computer for image generation. (**b**) The optical system can be mounted in 2.1 mm (left) or 1.2 mm (right) endoscopes.

A description and summary of performance for several different MEMS scanning mechanisms that are currently being developed for in vivo endomicroscopy are summarized in Table 1.

Table 1. MEMS scanning mechanisms developed for in vivo optical endomicroscopy.

Imaging Modality	Scan	Res (μm)	FOV	Frame Rate (Hz)	Applications	Advantages	Disadvantages
Fluorescent Wide-Field	Piezo	100–300	~70–90°	~30	GI, respiratory, ear, urinary, reproductive tracts,	High imaging speed, inexpensive laser source, minimal moving parts, commercial devices exist	Relatively low resolution and contrast, no depth sectioning
Single-axis Confocal	Piezo, PZT, Electrostatic, Electrothermal, Magnetic	0.5–5	0–150°	>2	GI, respiratory, ear, urinary, reproductive tracts	High sensitivity provide functional information miniaturization through proximal or distal ends commercial devices exist	Limited contrast and wavelength, limited tissue penetration (<100 μm), limited working distance, increased aberration due to high NA optics
Dual-axis Confocal	Electrostatic	3–6	250–1000 μm	>15	Skin, GI tract, liver, head and neck, pancreas,	Effective out-of-focus rejection of scattered light for high contrast, deep tissue penetration (~400 μm), relatively isotropic resolution	Low NA optics limits sensitivity, challenging alignment of a dual-beam configuration
OCT	Piezo, PZT, Electrostatic, Electrothermal, Magnetic	1–15	2000–5000 μm	>60	GI, respiratory, ear, urinary, reproductive tracts	Impressive miniaturization, high sensitivity, dynamic range, high imaging speed, deep tissue penetration (a few mm)	Label-free imaging, expensive detector array, Short dynamic range along depth
Two-photon	Piezo, PZT, Electrostatic, Electrothermal, Magnetic	0.5–2	200–500 μm	>5	GI, respiratory, tracts	High resolution and contrast, deep tissue penetration (~500 μm ~1 mm) less photobleaching and phototoxicity, Commercial devices exist	Relatively expensive laser source and optics, need dispersion compensation or special fibers to maintain pulse shape
Optical resolution photoacoustic microscope (OR-PAM)	Electrostatic and Electrothermal	~5	1000 μm	10	Breast, brain	High spatial resolution and contrast high imaging speed, deep tissue penetration (a few mm)	Relatively expensive laser source progress on miniaturization is still ongoing

8. Conclusions

In this review, we present a review of the latest advancements of MEMS actuator-based optical microendoscopy. High precision in manufacturing coupled with various optical/mechanical functionalities derived from MEMS fabrication techniques make these components well suited to integrate into many optical based microendoscopy. Nonetheless, it is crucial to gain understandings of other underlying principles, such as life-cycle, sizes, speed, material properties, force, operating ranges, and power consumptions to achieve optimum performance before uniting all components altogether. In addition, clinical considerations, such as usage simplicity and ergonomics, cannot be overlooked as those parameters are used to dictate the overall designs and selections of MEMS actuators for optical microendoscopy. Overall, electrostatic-based actuation is one of the most popular actuators employed in endoscopic-based imaging despite the fact that it provides both relatively moderate actuation force and limited scanning ranges. However, the advantages are their ease of fabrication, lower complexity of integration to endoscope packages, and relative fast scanning speed to help reduce motion artifacts. All in all, MEMS actuator-based optical microendoscopy has been showing great promise to deliver high-performance imaging on par with traditional microscopy in aiding medical diagnosis procedures.

Abbreviations

The following abbreviations are used in this manuscript:

PCF	Photonics band gap fiber
PZT	Lead zirconate titanate
OCT	Optical coherent tomography
DAC	Dual-axis confocal
FOV	Field-of-view
PMT	Photomultiplier tubes
APD	Avalanche photodiode
NA	Numerical aperture
DCF	Double clad fiber
PAM	Photoacoustic microscope
PA	Photoacoustic
UST	Ultrasound transducer
3D	Three-dimensional
MEMS	Microelectromechanical Systems
GRIN	Graded index
CPC;Apc	CDX2P-NLS Cre;adenomatosis polyposis coli
GI	Gastrointestinal
WD	Working distance

References

1. Piyawattanametha, W.; Wang, T.D. MEMS-Based Dual Axes Confocal Microendoscopy. *IEEE J. Sel. Top. Quantum Electron. (JSTQE)* **2010**, *16*, 804–814. [CrossRef] [PubMed]
2. Lee, C.M.; Engelbrecht, C.J.; Soper, T.D.; Helmchen, F.; Seibel, E.J. Scanning fiber endoscopy with highly flexible, 1-mm catheterscopes for wide-field, full-color imaging. *J. Biophotonics* **2010**, *3*, 385–407. [CrossRef] [PubMed]
3. Mauna Kea Technologies, Paris, France. Available online: http://www.maunakeatech.com (accessed on 28 November 2018).
4. Elahi, S.F.; Wang, T.D. Future and advances in endoscopy. *J. Biophotonics* **2011**, *4*, 471–481. [CrossRef] [PubMed]
5. Flusberg, B.A.; Cocker, E.D.; Piyawattanametha, W.; Jung, J.C.; Cheung, E.L.; Schnitzer, M.J. Fiber-optic fluorescence imaging. *Nat. Methods* **2005**, *2*, 941. [CrossRef] [PubMed]
6. Khemthongcharoen, N.; Jolivot, R.; Rattanavarin, S.; Piyawattanametha, W. Advances in imaging probes and optical microendoscopic imaging techniques for early in vivo cancer assessment. *Adv. Drug Deliv. Rev.* **2014**, *74*, 53–74. [CrossRef] [PubMed]
7. Solgaard, O.; Godil, A.A.; Howe, R.T.; Lee, L.P.; Peter, Y.A.; Zappe, H. Optical MEMS: From micromirrors to complex systems. *J. Microelectromechan. Syst.* **2014**, *23*, 517–538. [CrossRef]
8. Liu, L.; Xie, H. 3-D confocal laser scanning microscopy based on a full-MEMS scanning system. *IEEE Photonics Technol. Lett.* **2013**, *25*, 1478–1480. [CrossRef]
9. Qiu, Z.; Pulskamp, J.S.; Lin, X.; Rhee, C.H.; Wang, T.; Polcawich, R.G.; Oldham, K. Large displacement vertical translational actuator based on piezoelectric thin films. *J. Micromech. Microeng.* **2010**, *20*, 075016. [CrossRef] [PubMed]
10. Choi, J.; Qiu, Z.; Rhee, C.H.; Wang, T.; Oldham, K. A three-degree-of-freedom thin-film PZT-actuated microactuator with large out-of-plane displacement. *J. Micromech. Microeng.* **2014**, *24*, 075017. [CrossRef]
11. Huang, D.; Swanson, E.A.; Lin, C.P.; Schuman, J.S.; Stinson, W.G.; Chang, W.; Hee, M.R.; Flotte, T.; Gregory, K.; Puliafito, C.A. Optical coherence tomography. *Science* **1991**, *254*, 1178–1181. [CrossRef]
12. Fujimoto, J.G.; Pitris, C.; Boppart, S.A.; Brezinski, M.E. Optical coherence tomography: An emerging technology for biomedical imaging and optical biopsy. *Neoplasia* **2000**, *2*, 9–25. [CrossRef]
13. Wang, L.V.; Gao, L. Photoacoustic microscopy and computed tomography: From bench to bedside. *Annu. Rev. Biomed. Eng.* **2014**, *16*, 155–185. [CrossRef]

14. Paddock, S.W.; Eliceiri, K.W. Laser scanning confocal microscopy: History, applications, and related optical sectioning techniques. In *Confocal Microscopy*; Humana Press: New York, NY, USA, 2014; pp. 9–47.
15. Denk, W.; Strickler, J.H.; Webb, W.W. Two-photon laser scanning fluorescence microscopy. *Science* **1990**, *248*, 73–76. [CrossRef]
16. Helmchen, F.; Denk, W. Deep tissue two-photon microscopy. *Nat. Methods* **2005**, *2*, 932. [CrossRef]
17. Fu, L.; Gu, M. Fibre-optic nonlinear optical microscopy and endoscopy. *J. Microsc.* **2007**, *226*, 195–206. [CrossRef]
18. Pan, Y.; Xie, H.; Fedder, G.K. Endoscopic optical coherence tomography based on a microelectromechanical mirror. *Opt. Lett.* **2001**, *26*, 1966–1968. [CrossRef]
19. Sun, J.; Xie, H. MEMS-based endoscopic optical coherence tomography. *Int. J. Opt.* **2011**, *2011*. [CrossRef]
20. Gora, M.J.; Suter, M.J.; Tearney, G.J.; Li, X. Endoscopic optical coherence tomography: Technologies and clinical applications [Invited]. *Biomed. Opt. Express* **2017**, *8*, 2405–2444. [CrossRef]
21. Tran, P.H.; Mukai, D.S.; Brenner, M.; Chen, Z. In vivo endoscopic optical coherence tomography by use of a rotational microelectromechanical system probe. *Opt. Lett.* **2004**, *29*, 1236–1238. [CrossRef]
22. Gora, M.J.; Sauk, J.S.; Carruth, R.W.; Gallagher, K.A.; Suter, M.J.; Nishioka, N.S.; Kava, L.E.; Rosenberg, M.; Bouma, B.E.; Tearney, G.J. Tethered capsule endomicroscopy enables less invasive imaging of gastrointestinal tract microstructure. *Nat. Med.* **2013**, *19*, 238. [CrossRef]
23. Yuan, W.; Brown, R.; Mitzner, W.; Yarmus, L.; Li, X. Super-achromatic monolithic microprobe for ultrahigh-resolution endoscopic optical coherence tomography at 800 nm. *Nat. Commun.* **2017**, *8*, 1531. [CrossRef] [PubMed]
24. Zara, J.M.; Yazdanfar, S.; Rao, K.D.; Izatt, J.A.; Smith, S.W. Electrostatic micromachine scanning mirror for optical coherence tomography. *Opt. Lett.* **2003**, *28*, 628–630. [CrossRef] [PubMed]
25. Piyawattanametha, W.; Patterson, P.R.; Hah, D.; Toshiyoshi, H.; Wu, M.C. Surface-and bulk-micromachined two-dimensional scanner driven by angular vertical comb actuators. *J. Microelectromechan. Syst.* **2005**, *14*, 1329–1338. [CrossRef]
26. Milanovic, V.; Matus, G.A.; McCormick, D.T. Gimbal-less monolithic silicon actuators for tip-tilt-piston micromirror applications. *IEEE J. Sel. Top. Quantum Electron.* **2004**, *10*, 462–471. [CrossRef]
27. Jung, W.; McCormick, D.T.; Zhang, J.; Wang, L.; Tien, N.C.; Chen, Z. Three-dimensional endoscopic optical coherence tomography by use of a two-axis microelectromechanical scanning mirror. *Appl. Phys. Lett.* **2006**, *88*, 163901. [CrossRef]
28. Aguirre, A.D.; Herz, P.R.; Chen, Y.; Fujimoto, J.G.; Piyawattanametha, W.; Fan, L.; Wu, M.C. Two-axis MEMS scanning catheter for ultrahigh resolution three-dimensional and *en-face* imaging. *Opt. Express* **2007**, *15*, 2445–2453. [CrossRef] [PubMed]
29. Lu, C.D.; Kraus, M.F.; Potsaid, B.; Liu, J.J.; Choi, W.; Jayaraman, V.; Cable, A.E.; Hornegger, J.; Duker, J.S.; Fujimoto, J.G. Handheld ultrahigh speed swept source optical coherence tomography instrument using a MEMS scanning mirror. *Biomed. Opt. Express* **2014**, *5*, 293–311. [CrossRef]
30. Jain, A.; Kopa, A.; Pan, Y.; Fedder, G.K.; Xie, H. A two-axis electrothermal micromirror for endoscopic optical coherence tomography. *IEEE J. Sel. Top. Quantum Electron.* **2004**, *10*, 636–642. [CrossRef]
31. Sun, J.; Guo, S.; Wu, L.; Liu, L.; Choe, S.W.; Sorg, B.S.; Xie, H. 3D in vivo optical coherence tomography based on a low-voltage, large-scan-range 2D MEMS mirror. *Opt. Express* **2010**, *18*, 12065–12075. [CrossRef]
32. Samuelson, S.R.; Wu, L.; Sun, J.; Choe, S.W.; Sorg, B.S.; Xie, H. A 2.8-mm imaging probe based on a high-fill-factor MEMS mirror and wire-bonding-free packaging for endoscopic optical coherence tomography. *J. Microelectromech. Syst.* **2012**, *21*, 1291–1302. [CrossRef]
33. Wang, D.; Fu, L.; Wang, X.; Gong, Z.; Samuelson, S.R.; Duan, C.; Jia, H.; Ma, J.S.; Xie, H. Endoscopic swept-source optical coherence tomography based on a two-axis microelectromechanical system mirror. *J. Biomed. Opt.* **2013**, *18*, 086005. [CrossRef]
34. Liu, X.; Cobb, M.J.; Chen, Y.; Kimmey, M.B.; Li, X. Rapid-scanning forward-imaging miniature endoscope for real-time optical coherence tomography. *Opt. Lett.* **2004**, *29*, 1763–1765. [CrossRef]
35. Chen, T.; Zhang, N.; Huo, T.; Wang, C.; Zheng, J.G.; Zhou, T.; Xue, P. Tiny endoscopic optical coherence tomography probe driven by a miniaturized hollow ultrasonic motor. *J. Biomed. Opt.* **2013**, *18*, 086011. [CrossRef]
36. Zhang, N.; Tsai, T.H.; Ahsen, O.O.; Liang, K.; Lee, H.C.; Xue, P.; Li, X.; Fujimoto, J.G. Compact piezoelectric transducer fiber scanning probe for optical coherence tomography. *Opt. Lett.* **2014**, *39*, 186–188. [CrossRef]

37. Park, H.C.; Song, C.; Kang, M.; Jeong, Y.; Jeong, K.H. Forward imaging OCT endoscopic catheter based on MEMS lens scanning. *Opt. Lett.* **2012**, *37*, 2673–2675. [CrossRef]
38. Park, H.C.; Seo, Y.H.; Jeong, K.H. Lissajous fiber scanning for forward viewing optical endomicroscopy using asymmetric stiffness modulation. *Opt. Express* **2014**, *22*, 5818–5825. [CrossRef]
39. Park, H.C.; Seo, Y.H.; Hwang, K.; Lim, J.K.; Yoon, S.Z.; Jeong, K.H. Micromachined tethered silicon oscillator for an endomicroscopic Lissajous fiber scanner. *Opt. Lett.* **2014**, *39*, 6675–6678. [CrossRef]
40. Kim, K.H.; Park, B.H.; Maguluri, G.N.; Lee, T.W.; Rogomentich, F.J.; Bancu, M.G.; Bouma, B.E.; de Boer, J.F.; Bernstein, J.J. Two-axis magnetically-driven MEMS scanning catheter for endoscopic high-speed optical coherence tomography. *Opt. Express* **2007**, *15*, 18130–18140. [CrossRef]
41. Luo, S.; Wang, D.; Tang, J.; Zhou, L.; Duan, C.; Wang, D.; Liu, H.; Zhu, Y.; Li, G.; Zhao, H.; et al. Circumferential-scanning endoscopic optical coherence tomography probe based on a circular array of six 2-axis MEMS mirrors. *Biomed. Opt. Express* **2018**, *9*, 2104–2114. [CrossRef]
42. Chen, S.L.; Xie, Z.; Ling, T.; Guo, L.J.; Wei, X.; Wang, X. Miniaturized all-optical photoacoustic microscopy based on microelectromechanical systems mirror scanning. *Opt. Lett.* **2012**, *37*, 4263–4265. [CrossRef]
43. Ling, T.; Chen, S.L.; Guo, L.J. Fabrication and characterization of high Q polymer micro-ring resonator and its application as a sensitive ultrasonic detector. *Opt. Express* **2011**, *19*, 861–869. [CrossRef] [PubMed]
44. Guo, H.; Song, C.; Xie, H.; Xi, L. Photoacoustic endomicroscopy based on a MEMS scanning mirror. *Opt. Lett.* **2017**, *42*, 4615–4618. [CrossRef] [PubMed]
45. Liu, L.; Wang, E.; Zhang, X.; Liang, W.; Li, X.; Xie, H. MEMS-based 3D confocal scanning microendoscope using MEMS scanners for both lateral and axial scan. *Sens. Actuators A Phys.* **2014**, *215*, 89–95. [CrossRef] [PubMed]
46. Park, K.; Kim, J.Y.; Lee, C.; Jeon, S.; Lim, G.; Kim, C. Handheld Photoacoustic Microscopy Probe. *Sci. Rep.* **2017**, *7*, 13359. [CrossRef] [PubMed]
47. Zaman, R.T.; Yousefi, S.; Long, S.R.; Saito, T.; Mandella, M.; Qiu, Z.; Chen, R.; Contag, C.H.; Gambhir, S.S.; Chin, F.T.; et al. A Dual-Modality Hybrid Imaging System Harnesses Radioluminescence and Sound to Reveal Molecular Pathology of Atherosclerotic Plaques. *Sci. Rep.* **2018**, *8*, 1–13. [CrossRef] [PubMed]
48. Yao, J.; Wang, L.; Yang, J.M.; Maslov, K.I.; Wong, T.T.; Li, L.; Huang, C.H.; Zou, J.; Wang, L.V. High-speed label-free functional photoacoustic microscopy of mouse brain in action. *Nat. Methods* **2015**, *12*, 407. [CrossRef] [PubMed]
49. Hsieh, B.Y.; Chen, S.L.; Ling, T.; Guo, L.J.; Li, P.C. All-optical scanhead for ultrasound and photoacoustic dual-modality imaging. *Opt. Express* **2012**, *20*, 1588–1596. [CrossRef]
50. Zhang, C.; Ling, T.; Chen, S.L.; Guo, L.J. Ultrabroad bandwidth and highly sensitive optical ultrasonic detector for photoacoustic imaging. *ACS Photonics* **2014**, *1*, 1093–1098. [CrossRef]
51. Dong, B.; Chen, S.; Zhang, Z.; Sun, C.; Zhang, H.F. Photoacoustic probe using a microring resonator ultrasonic sensor for endoscopic applications. *Opt. Lett.* **2014**, *39*, 4372–4375. [CrossRef]
52. Li, H.; Dong, B.; Zhang, Z.; Zhang, H.F.; Sun, C. A transparent broadband ultrasonic detector based on an optical micro-ring resonator for photoacoustic microscopy. *Sci. Rep.* **2014**, *4*, 4496. [CrossRef]
53. Dickensheets, D.L.; Kino, G.S. Micromachined scanning confocal optical microscope. *Opt. Lett.* **1996**, *21*, 764–766. [CrossRef] [PubMed]
54. Seo, Y.H.; Hwang, K.; Jeong, K.H. 1.65 mm diameter forward-viewing confocal endomicroscopic catheter using a flip-chip bonded electrothermal MEMS fiber scanner. *Opt. Express* **2018**, *26*, 4780–4785. [CrossRef] [PubMed]
55. Qiu, Z.; Rhee, C.H.; Choi, J.; Wang, T.D.; Oldham, K.R. Large stroke vertical PZT microactuator with high-speed rotational scanning. *J. Microelectromechan. Syst.* **2014**, *23*, 256–258. [CrossRef] [PubMed]
56. Maitland, K.C.; Shin, H.J.; Ra, H.; Lee, D.; Solgaard, O.; Richards-Kortum, R. Single fiber confocal microscope with a two-axis gimbaled MEMS scanner for cellular imaging. *Opt. Express* **2006**, *14*, 8604–8612. [CrossRef] [PubMed]
57. Shin, H.J.; Pierce, M.C.; Lee, D.; Ra, H.; Solgaard, O.; Richards-Kortum, R. Fiber-optic confocal microscope using a MEMS scanner and miniature objective lens. *Opt. Express* **2007**, *15*, 9113–9122. [CrossRef] [PubMed]
58. Liu, J.T.; Mandella, M.J.; Ra, H.; Wong, L.K.; Solgaard, O.; Kino, G.S.; Piyawattanametha, W.; Contag, C.H.; Wang, T.D. Miniature near-infrared dual-axes confocal microscope utilizing a two-dimensional microelectromechanical systems scanner. *Opt. Lett.* **2007**, *32*, 256–258. [CrossRef]

59. Piyawattanametha, W.; Ra, H.; Qiu, Z.; Loewke, K.E.; Mandella, M.J.; Contag, C.H.; Wang, T.D.; Friedland, S.; Liu, J.T.; Kino, G.S.; et al. In vivo near-infrared dual-axis confocal microendoscopy in the human lower gastrointestinal tract. *J. Biomed. Opt.* **2012**, *17*, 021102. [CrossRef]
60. Jung, I.W.; López, D.; Qiu, Z.; Piyawattanametha, P. 2-D MEMS Scanner for Handheld Multispectral Dual-Axis Confocal Microscopes. *J. Microelectromechan. Syst.* **2018**, *27*. [CrossRef]
61. Li, H.; Duan, X.; Qiu, Z.; Zhou, Q.; Kurabayashi, K.; Oldham, K.R.; Wang, T.D. Integrated monolithic 3D MEMS scanner for switchable real time vertical/horizontal cross-sectional imaging. *Opt. Express* **2016**, *24*, 2145–2155. [CrossRef]
62. Qiu, Z.; Liu, Z.; Duan, X.; Khondee, S.; Joshi, B.; Mandella, M.J.; Oldham, K.; Kurabayashi, K.; Wang, T.D. Targeted vertical cross-sectional imaging with handheld near-infrared dual axes confocal fluorescence endomicroscope. *Biomed. Opt. Express* **2013**, *4*, 322–330. [CrossRef]
63. Qiu, Z.; Khondee, S.; Duan, X.; Li, H.; Mandella, M.J.; Joshi, B.P.; Zhou, Q.; Owens, S.R.; Kurabayashi, K.; Oldham, K.R.; et al. Vertical cross-sectional imaging of colonic dysplasia in vivo with multi-spectral dual axes confocal endomicroscopy. *Gastroenterology* **2014**, *146*, 615–617. [CrossRef] [PubMed]
64. Li, H.; Qiu, Z.; Duan, X.; Oldham, K.R.; Kurabayashi, K.; Wang, T.D. 2D resonant microscanner for dual axes confocal fluorescence endomicroscope. In Proceedings of the 2014 IEEE 27th International Conference on Micro Electro Mechanical Systems (MEMS), San Francisco, CA, USA, 26–30 January 2014; pp. 805–808. [CrossRef]
65. Shahid, W.; Qiu, Z.; Duan, X.; Li, H.; Wang, T.D.; Oldham, K.R. Modeling and simulation of a parametrically resonant micromirror with duty-cycled excitation. *J. Microelectromechan. Syst.* **2014**, *23*, 1440–1453. [CrossRef] [PubMed]
66. Zhou, J.; Joshi, B.P.; Duan, X.; Pant, A.; Qiu, Z.; Kuick, R.; Owens, S.R.; Wang, T.D. EGFR overexpressed in colonic neoplasia can be detected on wide-field endoscopic imaging. *Clin. Transl. Gastroenterol.* **2015**, *6*, e101. [CrossRef]
67. Khondee, S.; Rabinsky, E.F.; Owens, S.R.; Joshi, B.P.; Qiu, Z.; Duan, X.; Zhao, L.; Wang, T.D. Targeted therapy of colorectal neoplasia with rapamycin in peptide-labeled pegylated octadecyl lithocholate micelles. *J. Control. Release* **2015**, *199*, 114–121. [CrossRef] [PubMed]
68. Campbell, J.L.; SoRelle, E.D.; Ilovich, O.; Liba, O.; James, M.L.; Qiu, Z.; Perez, V.; Chan, C.T.; de la Zerda, A.; Zavaleta, C. Multimodal assessment of SERS nanoparticle biodistribution post ingestion reveals new potential for clinical translation of Raman imaging. *Biomaterials* **2017**, *135*, 42–52. [CrossRef] [PubMed]
69. Davis, R.; Campbell, J.; Burkitt, S.; Qiu, Z.; Kang, S.; Mehraein, M.; Miyasato, D.; Salinas, H.; Liu, J.; Zavaleta, C. A Raman Imaging Approach Using CD47 Antibody-Labeled SERS Nanoparticles for Identifying Breast Cancer and Its Potential to Guide Surgical Resection. *Nanomaterials* **2018**, *8*, 953. [CrossRef]
70. Jeong, J.W.; Kim, S.; Solgaard, O. Split-frame gimbaled two-dimensional MEMS scanner for miniature dual-axis confocal microendoscopes fabricated by front-side processing. *J. Microelectromechan. Syst.* **2012**, *21*, 308–315. [CrossRef]
71. Cu-Nguyen, P.H.; Grewe, A.; Hillenbrand, M.; Sinzinger, S.; Seifert, A.; Zappe, H. Tunable hyperchromatic lens system for confocal hyperspectral sensing. *Opt. Express* **2013**, *21*, 27611–27621. [CrossRef]
72. Kang, D.; Martinez, R.V.; Whitesides, G.M.; Tearney, G.J. Miniature grating for spectrally-encoded endoscopy. *Lab Chip* **2013**, *13*, 1810–1816. [CrossRef]
73. Piyawattanametha, W.; Barretto, R.P.; Ko, T.H.; Flusberg, B.A.; Cocker, E.D.; Ra, H.; Lee, D.; Solgaard, O.; Schnitzer, M.J. Fast-scanning two-photon fluorescence imaging based on a microelectromechanical systems two-dimensional scanning mirror. *Opt. Lett.* **2006**, *31*, 2018–2020. [CrossRef]
74. Piyawattanametha, W.; Cocker, E.D.; Burns, L.D.; Barretto, R.P.; Jung, J.C.; Ra, H.; Solgaard, O.; Schnitzer, M.J. In vivo brain imaging using a porTable 2.9 g two-photon microscope based on a microelectromechanical systems scanning mirror. *Opt. Lett.* **2009**, *34*, 2309–2311. [CrossRef] [PubMed]
75. Hoy, C.L.; Durr, N.J.; Chen, P.; Piyawattanametha, W.; Ra, H.; Solgaard, O.; Ben-Yakar, A. Miniaturized probe for femtosecond laser microsurgery and two-photon imaging. *Opt. Express* **2008**, *16*, 9996–10005. [CrossRef] [PubMed]
76. Jung, W.; Tang, S.; McCormic, D.T.; Xie, T.; Ahn, Y.C.; Su, J.; Tomov, I.V.; Krasieva, T.B.; Tromberg, B.J.; Chen, Z. Miniaturized probe based on a microelectromechanical system mirror for multiphoton microscopy. *Opt. Lett.* **2008**, *33*, 1324–1326. [CrossRef] [PubMed]

77. Hoy, C.L.; Ferhanoğlu, O.; Yildirim, M.; Piyawattanametha, W.; Ra, H.; Solgaard, O.; Ben-Yakar, A. Optical design and imaging performance testing of a 9.6-mm diameter femtosecond laser microsurgery probe. *Opt. Express* **2011**, *19*, 10536–10552. [CrossRef] [PubMed]
78. Duan, X.; Li, H.; Qiu, Z.; Joshi, B.P.; Pant, A.; Smith, A.; Kurabayashi, K.; Oldham, K.R.; Wang, T.D. MEMS-based multiphoton endomicroscope for repetitive imaging of mouse colon. *Biomed. Opt. Express* **2015**, *6*, 3074–3083. [CrossRef] [PubMed]
79. Zhao, Y.; Sheng, M.; Huang, L.; Tang, S. Design of a fiber-optic multiphoton microscopy handheld probe. *Biomed. Opt. Express* **2016**, *7*, 3425–3437. [CrossRef] [PubMed]
80. Huang, L.; Mills, A.K.; Zhao, Y.; Jones, D.J.; Tang, S. Miniature fiber-optic multiphoton microscopy system using frequency-doubled femtosecond Er-doped fiber laser. *Biomed. Opt. Express* **2016**, *7*, 1948–1956. [CrossRef] [PubMed]
81. Helmchen, F.; Fee, M.S.; Tank, D.W.; Denk, W. A miniature head-mounted two-photon microscope: High-resolution brain imaging in freely moving animals. *Neuron* **2001**, *31*, 903–912. [CrossRef]
82. Engelbrecht, C.J.; Johnston, R.S.; Seibel, E.J.; Helmchen, F. Ultra-compact fiber-optic two-photon microscope for functional fluorescence imaging in vivo. *Opt. Express* **2008**, *16*, 5556–5564. [CrossRef]
83. Ducourthial, G.; Leclerc, P.; Mansuryan, T.; Fabert, M.; Brevier, J.; Habert, R.; Braud, F.; Batrin, R.; Vever-Bizet, C.; Bourg-Heckly, G.; et al. Development of a real-time flexible multiphoton microendoscope for label-free imaging in a live animal. *Sci. Rep.* **2015**, *5*, 18303. [CrossRef]
84. Rivera, D.R.; Brown, C.M.; Ouzounov, D.G.; Pavlova, I.; Kobat, D.; Webb, W.W.; Xu, C. Compact and flexible raster scanning multiphoton endoscope capable of imaging unstained tissue. *Proc. Natl. Acad. Sci. USA* **2011**, *108*, 17598–17603. [CrossRef] [PubMed]
85. Liang, W.; Hall, G.; Messerschmidt, B.; Li, M.J.; Li, X. Nonlinear optical endomicroscopy for label-free functional histology in vivo. *Light Sci. Appl.* **2017**, *6*, e17082. [CrossRef] [PubMed]
86. Chen, S.C.; Choi, H.; So, P.T.; Culpepper, M.L. Thermomechanical actuator-based three-axis optical scanner for high-speed two-photon endomicroscope imaging. *J. Microelectromechan. Syst.* **2014**, *23*, 570–578. [CrossRef] [PubMed]
87. Zhang, X.; Duan, C.; Liu, L.; Li, X.; Xie, H. A non-resonant fiber scanner based on an electrothermally-actuated MEMS stage. *Sens. Actuators A Phys.* **2015**, *233*, 239–245. [CrossRef] [PubMed]
88. Zhang, Y.; Akins, M.L.; Murari, K.; Xi, J.; Li, M.J.; Luby-Phelps, K.; Mahendroo, M.; Li, X. A compact fiber-optic SHG scanning endomicroscope and its application to visualize cervical remodeling during pregnancy. *Proc. Natl. Acad. Sci. USA* **2012**, *109*, 12878–12883. [CrossRef] [PubMed]
89. Miller, S.J.; Joshi, B.; Wang, T.D.; Lee, C.M.; Seibel, E.J.; Gaustad, A. Targeted detection of murine colonic dysplasia in vivo with flexible multispectral scanning fiber endoscopy. *J. Biomed. Opt.* **2012**, *17*, 021103. [CrossRef] [PubMed]
90. He, B.; Xi, L.; Samuelson, S.R.; Xie, H.; Yang, L.; Jiang, H. Microelectromechanical systems scanning-mirror-based handheld probe for fluorescence molecular tomography. *Appl. Opt.* **2012**, *51*, 4678–4683. [CrossRef] [PubMed]
91. Savastano, L.E.; Zhou, Q.; Smith, A.; Vega, K.; Murga-Zamalloa, C.; Gordon, D.; McHugh, J.; Zhao, L.; Wang, M.M.; Pandey, A.; et al. Multimodal laser-based angioscopy for structural, chemical and biological imaging of atherosclerosis. *Nat. Biomed. Eng.* **2017**, *1*, 0023. [CrossRef] [PubMed]

12

Advances in Capacitive Micromachined Ultrasonic Transducers

Kevin Brenner [1,†], **Arif Sanli Ergun** [1,2,†], **Kamyar Firouzi** [1,†], **Morten Fischer Rasmussen** [1,†], **Quintin Stedman** [1,†] and **Butrus (Pierre) Khuri–Yakub** [1,*,†]

1 E.L. Ginzton Lab., Stanford University, Stanford, CA 94305, USA; brennerk@stanford.edu (K.B.); sanli.ergun@gmail.com (A.S.E.); kfirouzi@stanford.edu (K.F.); mofi@stanford.edu (M.F.R.); qstedman@stanford.edu (Q.S.)

2 Department of Electrical and Electronics Engineering, TOBB University of Economics and Technology, Ankara 06560, Turkey

* Correspondence: pierreky@stanford.edu

† These authors contributed equally to this work.

Abstract: Capacitive micromachined ultrasonic transducer (CMUT) technology has enjoyed rapid development in the last decade. Advancements both in fabrication and integration, coupled with improved modelling, has enabled CMUTs to make their way into mainstream ultrasound imaging systems and find commercial success. In this review paper, we touch upon recent advancements in CMUT technology at all levels of abstraction; modeling, fabrication, integration, and applications. Regarding applications, we discuss future trends for CMUTs and their impact within the broad field of biomedical imaging.

Keywords: capacitive micromachined ultrasonic transducer (CMUT); acoustics; micromachining; capacitive; transducer; modelling; fabrication

---

1. Introduction

The capacitive micromachined ultrasonic transducer (CMUT) started with an idea to make a better airborne ultrasound transducer operating in the MHz frequency range [1]. Later, a simple underwater experiment showed the huge advantage in bandwidth over piezoelectric transducers and motivated the development of a sealed CMUT for immersion applications [2]. A CMUT consists of a flexible top plate suspended over a gap. Transduction is achieved electrostatically, in contrast with piezoelectric transducers. The merit of the CMUT derives from having a very large electric field in the cavity of the capacitor, a field of the order of 10^8 V/m or higher results in an electro-mechanical coupling coefficient that competes with the best piezoelectric materials. The availability of micro-electro-mechanical-systems (MEMS) technologies makes it possible to realize thin vacuum gaps where such high electric fields can be established with relatively low voltages. Thus, viable devices can be realized and even integrated directly on electronic circuits such as complimentary metal-oxide-semiconductor (CMOS). A further and very important development was the discovery of collapse mode operation of the CMUT. In this mode of operation, the CMUT cells are designed so that part of the top plate is in physical contact with the substrate, yet electrically isolated with a dielectric, during normal operation. The transmit and receive sensitivities of the CMUT are further enhanced thus providing a superior solution for ultrasound transducers [3]. In short, the CMUT is a high electric field device, and if one can control the high electric field from issues like charging and breakdown, then one has an ultrasound transducer with superior bandwidth and sensitivity, amenable for integration with electronics, manufactured using traditional integrated circuits fabrication technologies with all its advantages, and can be made flexible for wrapping around a cylinder or even over human tissue.

In this paper, we will review the various aspects of CMUT technology: theory of operation, fabrication with surface and bulk micromachining, electronic integration methods, characterization, and applications. Beyond this overview, further details in the above-named topics will be left to the references.

2. Theory and Modeling of Capacitive Ultrasonic Transduction

A CMUT element typically consists of several cells connected in parallel. Each cell is composed of a flexible top plate (also referred to as top electrode) anchored around its edges. A shallow gap is formed between this flexible top plate and a fixed bottom plate. These two plates are made electrically conductive (partially or completely) to form a capacitor with the gap in-between (Figure 1a), making the CMUT cell a variable capacitor. A CMUT presents a challenging modeling problem as multiple physics are involved in its operation. As with any other MEMS device, at the basic level, the mechanics of the plate needs to be modeled along with the electrodynamics. Moreover, a CMUT interacts with an acoustic medium such as air or water to radiate or sense ultrasound; so, the interaction of the acoustic medium with the CMUT plate also needs to be modeled.

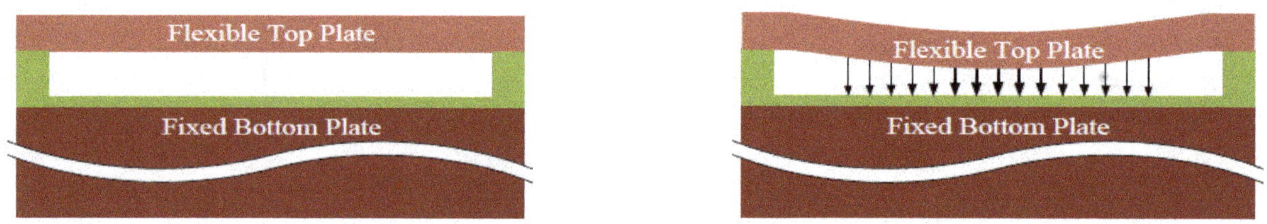

(a) (b)

Figure 1. Capacitive micromachined ultrasonic transducer (CMUT) cell illustration. (**a**) A CMUT cell is composed of a flexible top plate and a fixed bottom plate. (**b**) A direct current (DC) bias is applied during the operation that deflects the top plate.

Mechanical systems can be converted into electrical circuits by using the analogy between the mechanical and the electrical domains. One way to implement this analogy is to replace the forces in the mechanical domain by voltage sources and velocities by electrical currents. The models of this type are called equivalent circuit models. This methodology serves as a powerful tool for the analysis of electromechanical systems. Equivalent circuit models have been widely used for design and optimization of variety of transducer technologies such as piezoelectric [4] and an CMUTs [5,6].

Advancement in contemporary computing and equivalent circuits has enabled more detailed two-dimensional and three-dimensional finite element (FE) models to calculate the collapse voltage, output pressure, bandwidth, sensitivity, and crosstalk. Finite element models are designed to solve to the exact coupled-field theory of electrostatics, solid mechanics, and acoustics. A variety of finite element tools have been deployed, including but not limited to, ANSYS, COMSOL, COVENTOR, LS-DYNA, PZFlex, as well as custom-made modeling tools [7].

In the following sub-sections, we first explain the basic electromechanics of CMUTs using a simple parallel plate model. Next, we review the basics of equivalent circuit and finite element modeling.

2.1. Basic Electromechanics of CMUTs

To the first order, in one dimension, a CMUT can be modeled by a parallel plate capacitor with a moving top electrode as shown in Figure 2. The mechanics of a parallel plate can be approximated by a mass-spring-damper system model, with a spring constant k_p, mass constant m_p, and damping constant r_p. The medium acoustic impedance is simply modeled using a damper, r_m, and a mass, m_m. Under direct current (DC) bias, the top electrode is attracted towards the bottom electrode. At equilibrium, the deflection due to the electrostatic force is counter balanced by the mechanical spring force of the membrane. Assuming the top electrode is displaced by x, the capacitance of the parallel plate capacitor is given by

$$c(x) = \frac{A\epsilon_o\epsilon_r}{g_{eff} - x}. \tag{1}$$

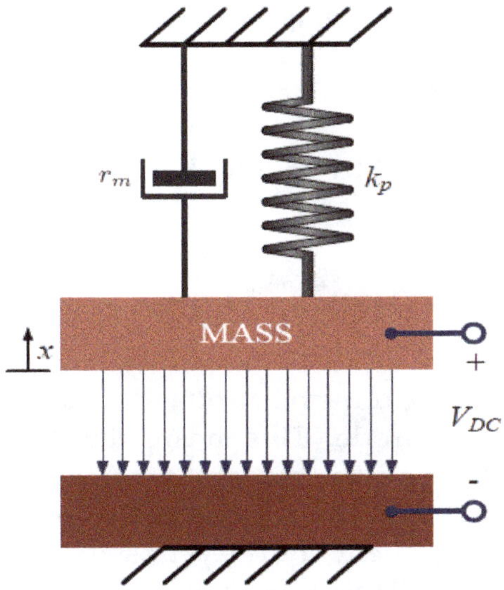

Figure 2. Simplified mass-spring-damper CMUT model.

The effective gap height g_{eff} is given as $g_{eff} = (t_i + t_m)/\epsilon_r + g_o$, where A is the area of the top electrode, ϵ_o is the permittivity of vacuum, ϵ_r is the relative permittivity of the insulator and the membrane material (assumed here to be the same), g_o is the initial gap distance under zero bias voltage, and t_i and t_m are the insulator and the membrane thickness, respectively. Note that because of the presence of the oxide layer, the effective gap is different than the physical gap, and thus, the relative permittivity is different than that of Vacuum. The dynamics of a CMUT can be studied via the Newton's second law, namely,

$$m_p\frac{d^2x}{dt^2} + r_p\frac{dx}{dt} + k_px = f_{el} + f_{ac} - p_o, \tag{2}$$

where f_{el} is the force due to electrical loading, f_{ac} is the force due to acoustic loading, and p_o is the atmospheric pressure. r_p represents the intrinsic viscoelastic damping of the top plate, which is usually negligible, and thus, we henceforth assume $r_p = 0$. Both forces can be estimated using the principle of minimum potential energy:

$$f_{el} = \frac{-\epsilon_o\epsilon_rAV(t)^2}{2(g_{eff} - x)^2}, \; f_{ac} = -p(t)A, \tag{3}$$

where $p(t)$ is the acoustic pressure. As seen, this equation is nonlinear in the displacement x. For most conventional applications, a CMUT, however, is biased by a large DC voltage (V_{dc}), and then modulated through a small AC voltage (V_{ac}) in the transmit mode or a small acoustic pressure in the receive mode (leading to induction of a small V_{ac}). This assumption serves as a basis for linearization of the electrostatic force at V_{dc} and x_{dc}. After expanding the total voltage and displacement as $V = V_{dc} + V_{ac}$ and $x = x_{dc} + x_{ac}$, and dropping the second order terms, the linearized equation of motions becomes:

$$(m_p + m_m)\frac{d^2 x_{ac}}{dt^2} + r_m \frac{dx_{ac}}{dt} + (k_p - k_s)x_{ac} = \frac{-\epsilon_o \epsilon_r A V_{dc} V_{ac}(t)}{2(g_{eff} - x_{dc})^2}, \tag{4}$$

with

$$k_s = \frac{\epsilon_o \epsilon_r A {V_{dc}}^2}{(g_{eff} - x_{dc})^3}, \tag{5}$$

where k_s is known as the spring softening effect, which is a function of the DC bias, and implies the resonance frequency of the CMUT shifts as the DC bias increases. As the top electrode moves closer to the bottom electrode due to the applied voltage, the electrical field increases, and the top electrode displaces further, acting as if the spring constant of the top electrode decreases under the influence of the applied voltage. Also, m_m and r_m are the effect of acoustic loading, which we shall discuss in-depth later in this section.

The DC components can be calculated by solving $k_p x_{dc} = f_{el} - p_o$. In absence of the atmospheric pressure, this leads to

$$V_{dc} = \sqrt{\frac{2k_p x_{dc}}{\epsilon_o \epsilon_r A}}(g_{eff} - x_{dc}), \tag{6}$$

which implies an important phenomenon; if the bias voltage is increased beyond a certain value, the top electrode collapses onto the bottom electrode. This means that the displacement of the top electrode can result in an increase in the electric field to the point where the attractive electrostatic force cannot be balanced by the spring force, resulting in the collapse of the top electrode onto the bottom electrode. Mathematically, this occurs when the gradient of the electrostatic force is larger than the gradient of the mechanical force. One can calculate the collapse voltage by equating the gradient of the electrostatic force to zero:

$$V_{coll} = \sqrt{8kg_{eff}^3 / 27\epsilon_o \epsilon_r A}, \tag{7}$$

and thus, it can be seen that displacement at V_{coll} is $g_{eff}/3$.

2.2. Small-Signal (Linear) Equivalent Circuit Model

Using the linear model presented above, a CMUT can be considered as a two-port network composed of an electrical domain and a mechanical domain (Figure 3). Such an equivalent circuit is a useful tool that captures the small-signal behavior of the CMUT in one dimension. One can perform a variety of simulations, such as calculating the electrical impedance and the small-signal transmit (TX) and receive (RX) sensitivities as a function of frequency.

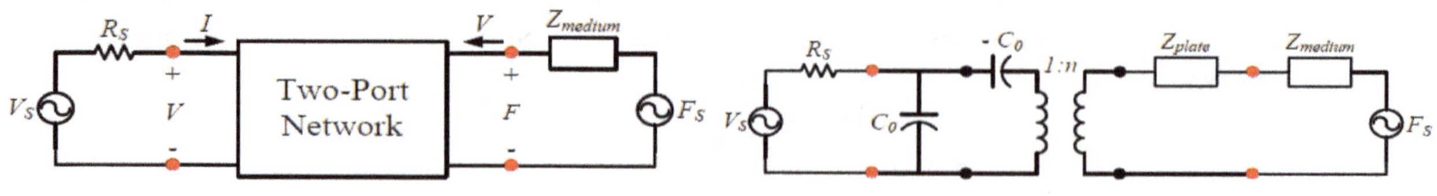

(a) (b)

Figure 3. CMUT Network model. (**a**) General two-port network representation that relates voltage and current (V and I) to force and velocity (F and V). (**b**) Small-signal equivalent circuit model (in transmit mode, $F_s = 0$, and in receive mode, $V_s = 0$). R_s represents the electric source resistance.

In the electrical part, C_o is the clamped capacitance of the device at the bias voltage and $-C_o$ represents the spring softening capacitance. V_s and R_s represent the input voltage source and its electric resistance. The mechanical membrane and medium acoustic impedances constitute the mechanical part. F_s is the force due to an acoustic pressure source, i.e., $F_s = pA$. The two parts are coupled together through an electromechanical transformer, picturing a CMUT as a device that transforms electrical energy to mechanical energy and vice versa. For a parallel plate capacitor, the electric field and transformer ratio are given by

$$E_o = \frac{V_{dc}}{g_{eff} - x_{dc}}, \; C_o = \frac{\epsilon_o \epsilon_r A}{g_{eff} - x_{dc}}, \; n = E_o C_o. \tag{8}$$

Note also that it is easy to verify $n = \sqrt{k_s C_o}$. When the transducer is operated in vacuum, the mechanical port of the circuit is short-circuited. For immersion devices, the mechanical port is simply terminated by the radiation impedance. In transmit mode, $F_s = 0$, and in receive mode, $V_s = 0$.

The maximum small signal output pressure of the transducer can be easily calculated using the equivalent circuit method. The maximum output pressure is obtained at the resonant frequency of the membrane, where all the reactive elements cancel each other out in the mechanical part of the circuit. At this frequency, the output pressure per volt is simply

$$p_{max} = \frac{n}{A} = \frac{\epsilon_o V_{dc}}{(g_{eff} - x_{dc})^2}, \tag{9}$$

and for a bias voltage close to the collapse voltage, is $p_{max} = \sqrt{3k\epsilon_o / 2A g_{eff}}$. In equivalent circuit modeling, the mechanical impedance of the plate is determined by subjecting the plate to a harmonic loading, semi-analytically using either the classical plate theory [5] or finite element method [8,9], in cases where analytical solutions are either tedious or do not exist. This can be used to derive the impedance of plates of various shapes such as circular, rectangular, or hexagonal geometries, or under different boundary (clamping) conditions.

The medium in which the transducer is operating presents an impedance (Z_{medium}) to the transducer that must be included in the small-signal equivalent circuit model (see Figure 3b) and can be considered as $Z_{medium} = Z_a A$, where Z_a is the characteristic acoustic impedance of the plate as a radiator of sound (not to be confused with mechanical impedance). However, since the transducer is in general a small resonator (compared to the wavelength) Z_a can be quite different than that of a plane wave. For a circular piston transducer of radius a, within an infinite rigid baffle, this acoustic impedance is given by [10]

$$Z_a = Z_o \Big(1 - \frac{J_1(2ka)}{ka} + j\frac{H_1(2ka)}{ka}\Big), \tag{10}$$

where J_1 is the Bessel function of the first kind and the first order and H_1 is the Struve function of the first order. Z_o is the plane wave impedance ($Z_o = \rho_o c_o$), where ρ_o and c_o are the density and speed of sound in the loading fluid. $k = \omega / c_o$ is the wave number. Note that Z_a has both real and imaginary parts. The real part contributes to the acoustic damping through r_m and is known as the radiation impedance. r_m is the mechanism by which a CMUT radiates sound. The imaginary part contributes to the mass term through m_m, and thereby results in shift in the resonance frequency. In summary, $r_m = j\omega A\mathrm{Re}\{Z_a\}$ and $m_m = j\omega A\mathrm{Im}\{Z_a\}$.

Having a complete model, one can now determine the resonance frequency as well as transmit and receive sensitivities. The resonance frequency and fractional bandwidth (FBW) are

$$\omega_o = \sqrt{\frac{k_p - k_s}{m_p + m_m}}, \; FBW = \frac{r_m}{\sqrt{(m_p + m_m)(k_p - k_s)}}. \tag{11}$$

For transmit and receive sensitivities, S_{TX} and S_{RX}, it can be shown that

$$S_{TX} = \left|\frac{P_{out}}{V_{in}}\right| = S_{TX,max}\Xi(\omega), \; S_{RX} = \left|\frac{I_{out}}{P_{in}}\right| = S_{RX,max}\Xi(\omega), \tag{12}$$

where $S_{TX,max} = n/A$, $S_{RX,max} = nA/r_m$ and

$$\Xi(\omega) = \left[1 + \left(\frac{\omega}{r_m}(m_p + m_m)\right)^2 \left(1 - \frac{\omega_o}{\omega}\right)^2\right]^{-\frac{1}{2}}. \tag{13}$$

2.3. Finite Element Modeling

An equivalent circuit model using lumped parameters serves to provide a good approximation but such an approach has many limitations and may not represent all the underlying physics. Finite element analysis is ideal for analyzing such multi-physics systems. The underlying physics for the CMUT operation can be described using partial differential equations with some boundary conditions. Depending on the shape, geometry, and mode of operation of CMUTs, a diverse array of finite element procedures have been developed over the years. In the finite element method, the simulation domain is divided into many small elements, called finite elements, over which a much simpler function is used to approximate the true solution. A set of linear equations is formulated based on minimizing the error between this approximate solution and the true solution.

Conventional CMUTs have been simulated using finite element analysis as described by [11,12]. Depending on the geometry and structure of the CMUT, Finite element models have been implemented in two-dimensions (2D), two-dimensions with axial symmetry (2D-Axisym.), and three-dimensions (3D) models. In the simplest form, the equations of linear elasticity (both static and dynamic) have been used to capture the mechanics of the vibrating plate. Finite element methods have made it possible to include various mechanical nonlinearities with ease. Perhaps the most prevalent one is geometric nonlinearity (also referred to as stress stiffening) in thin CMUT plates (where the thickness to diameter ratio is less than 5%). Stress stiffening is a nonlinear signature, where the vibrating plate stiffens as it is being deformed due to the second order effects of the strain.

The plate is usually anchored at the edges and is immersed in an acoustic medium (i.e., a domain that is governed by the acoustic wave equation). Often, the acoustic domain is terminated at the outer edges (at a certain distance from the plate) via some form of absorbing boundary conditions (ABC) or a perfectly matched layer (PML). This is usually used in the transmit mode and intended to absorb all out-going waves, and thus, model a CMUT cell pulsating in an infinite half-space. To investigate the operation of a single CMUT cell, generally a spherical absorbing boundary is used to emulate the acoustic radiation condition (Figure 4a). For investigating an array of CMUT cells, it is practically not possible to model all the cells, unless the array has a small number of cells or has a specific type of symmetry. The standard procedure to model an array of CMUT cells is known as the wave-guide model, where a single cell CMUT is modeled, however, with periodic boundary conditions (both in 2D and 3D). The wave-guide model is more subtle in axially symmetric geometries, where symmetry boundary conditions (as opposed to periodic conditions) have been widely adopted to mimic the effect the neighboring cells with a good accuracy [12–14] (see Figure 4b). The wave-guide models are also used in the receive mode, in the regimes where the incident wavelength is much larger than the dimensions of the CMUT cell.

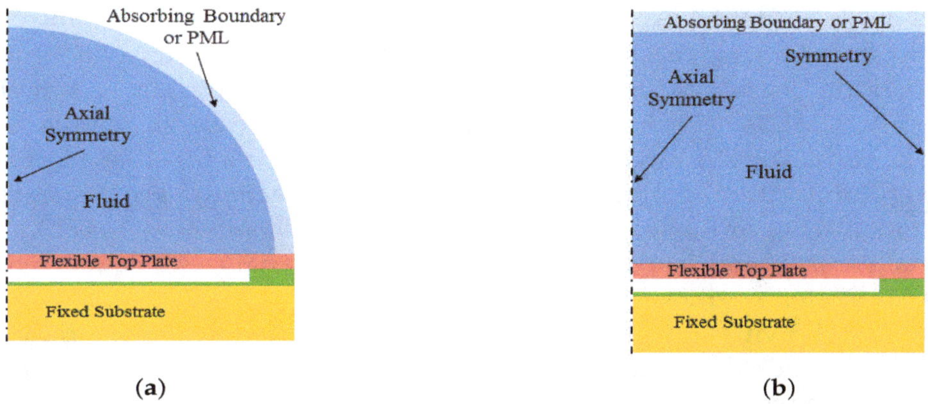

Figure 4. Geometry and boundary conditions of 2D-Axisym. CMUT finite element (FE) models. (**a**) Single cell model. (**b**) Wave-guide model.

Care should be taken, however, when using the wave-guide model. The model shown in Figure 4b generates sound waves in the fluid when the membrane is excited. The field quickly converges into plane waves as it propagates away from the membrane and the wave-fronts become parallel to the membrane plane and absorbing boundary. Below a certain cut-off frequency the fluid wave-guide only supports plane-waves, which is ideal for the purpose of modeling the CMUT cell. However if the frequency is high enough, there are also waves propagating at an oblique angle. The cut-off frequency of the wave-guide is given by $f_c = 1.22v_L/2r_{out}$, where v_L is the sound velocity in the fluid and r_{out} is the radius of the wave-guide. Above this frequency, due to the oblique incidence on the absorbing boundary, some part of the incidence wave gets reflected at the absorbing boundary. This results in standing waves in the wave-guide.

Perhaps the most challenging FE modeling of CMUTs is the electrostatic force (or variable capacitance), which is inversely proportional to the deformed gap. As such, different Element technologies have been applied, depending on the Software being used. We elaborate on two here: (1) ANSYS: the electrical ports are added to the membrane by segmenting the gap into many parallel plate capacitors as shown in Figure 5. This approach neglects the fringing fields and assumes that the electric field is always perpendicular to the electrodes. (2) COMSOL: the gap is meshed and modeled by solving the actual equation of electrostatics with a deformed mesh. The last part is necessary as the gap changes in response to the pressure or electrical fields. The coupling between the electric field and vibrating plate is through the electromechanical force that is calculated at the top electrode by the Maxwell's stress tensor [15].

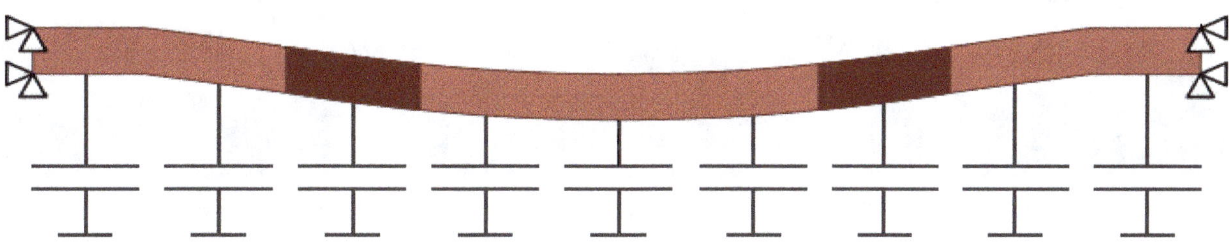

Figure 5. CMUT electrostatic gap segmentation. The electrostatic force is approximated by adding several parallel plate capacitors between the top and bottom electrodes.

Using the above model one can perform static, harmonic (small signal frequency domain), and transient (large signal time domain) analyses. For small signal analyses, static calculation is first used to pre-stress the plate prior to the harmonic analysis. The static analysis is also needed to calculate the collapse voltage. Next, a harmonic (frequency domain) analysis is performed to determine various CMUT characteristics in the linear regime.

Recent advancements in FE modeling and computer technologies have also enabled exploring a diverse array of sophisticated designs with the ultimate goal of improving performance measures such as sensitivity and bandwidth, These designs include but are not limited to collapsed mode operation and squeeze-film airborne CMUTs. Each of these developments introduces unique challenges in modeling. For example, for collapsed mode operation the mechanical as well as electrical contacts between the substrate and the vibrating plate should be taken into account. Furthermore, the whole electromechanical operation is nonlinear, leading to a need for time-domain analyses [13,14], which are generally computationally costly and less efficient than frequency analyses. Squeeze-film airborne CMUTs are devices with vented cavities and aim at increasing the bandwidth of airborne CMUTs. Modeling CMUTs with vented cavities is particularly challenging as it involves many different physical phenomena. Namely, the air inside the cavity as well as the vent holes will result in additional loading which needs to be modeled as well. The main challenge for simulating CMUTs with vented cavities lies in modeling the squeeze film, the vent channels, and the interaction of the squeeze film with the acoustic medium, for which one should consider modeling the squeeze film losses using both the Reynolds equation as well as the Navier-Stokes equations [16–18].

3. Fabrication Technologies

3.1. *Sacrificial Release Process*

The first method developed for fabricating CMUTs was the sacrificial release process [1]. This is a surface micromachining processes where the vacuum gap is created by etching a sacrificial layer between the top plate and the substrate. A vacuum-sealing step allows devices suitable for immersion applications [2].

A typical sacrificial release process is shown in Figure 6. First, a silicon nitride insulator layer is deposited on the wafer, followed by a sacrificial polysilicon layer. The sacrificial layer is patterned to define the post area between cells (a). Then, another layer of sacrificial polysilicon is deposited (b). This second sacrificial layer is used to create channels into the cell for the sacrificial polysilicon etch.

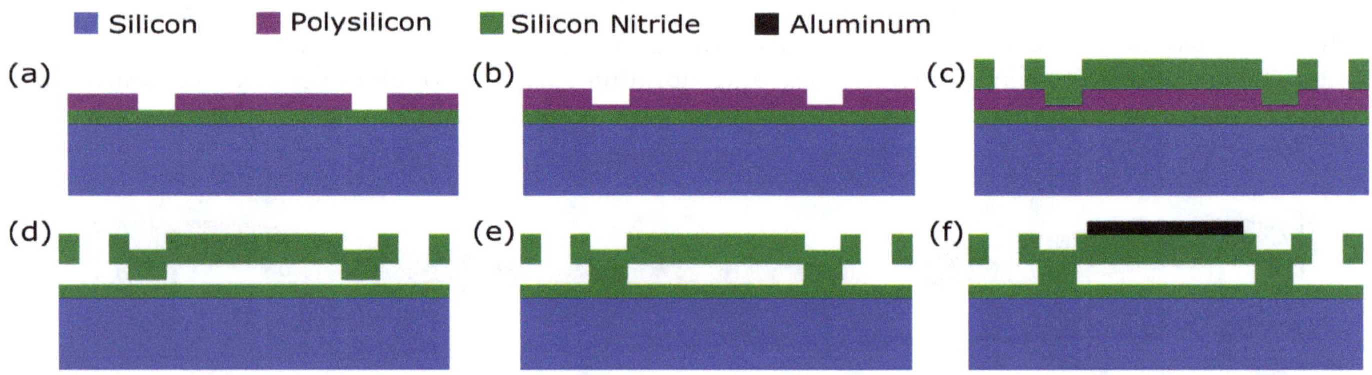

Figure 6. Sacrificial release CMUT fabrication process. (**a**) Deposit silicon nitride. Deposit and pattern the sacrificial polysilicon layer. (**b**) Deposit the polysilicon sacrificial layer for the etch channels into the cells. (**c**) Deposit and pattern the silicon nitride top plate layer. (**d**) Etch the sacrificial polysilicon layer. (**e**) Deposit silicon nitride using low-pressure chemical vapor deposition (LPCVD) to seal the cells. (**f**) Deposit and pattern the aluminum electrodes and interconnects.

Next, silicon nitride is deposited to form the top plate. Holes are made in the top silicon nitride layer to allow access to the sacrificial etch channels (c). A potassium hydroxide (KOH) wet etch is then used to remove the sacrificial polysilicon layer (d). The KOH enters through the openings in the top silicon nitride layer, then proceeds through the etch channels formed by the second sacrificial polysilicon deposition and into the cells. KOH has high selectivity to polysilicon over silicon nitride, so the silicon nitride structure remains undamaged.

The sacrificial release step leaves a gap, which is vented to the atmosphere. The gap is sealed by performing low-pressure chemical vapor deposition (LPCVD) of silicon nitride. This seals off the narrow etch channels (e). The LPCVD is performed at very low pressure, so the gap is effectively vacuum-filled when it is sealed.

Finally, aluminum is deposited to form the top electrode, electrical contacts, and interconnects (f). Sputtering is usually used in order to get conformal coverage. The substrate wafer is highly doped so that it can be used as the back electrode.

In the sacrificial release process, the gap height is set by the combined thicknesses of the two polysilicon depositions (a) and (b), and the top plate thickness is set by a silicon nitride deposition (c). This can make achieving good uniformity challenging compared to a wafer-bonding process. In addition, roughness in the silicon nitride layer can decrease the effective gap height, causing deviations in device performance from the design values [19]. Also, the plate material can have substantial intrinsic stress, which alters the device properties.

On the other hand, sacrificial release processes have several advantages. They are relatively simple and reliable. They avoid the yield challenges of a wafer bonding step. Additionally, it is possible to design sacrificial release processes with a low maximum processing temperature (250 °C) [20], allowing postprocess CMOS integration [21].

Vias and 2D Arrays

Additional steps can be added to the sacrificial release process to allow electrical connectivity from the backside using through-wafer via [22,23]. An example of such a device based on the work of Moini et al. [24] is shown in Figure 7a. Holes for the vias are made through the wafer using deep reactive ion etching (DRIE). The holes are lined with conductive silicon and then filled with undoped polysilicon. Conductive polysilicon is also used to make the bottom electrodes for the CMUTs. Processes like this allow the fabrication of 2D arrays with backside electrical contacts, such as the ring array shown in Figure 7b.

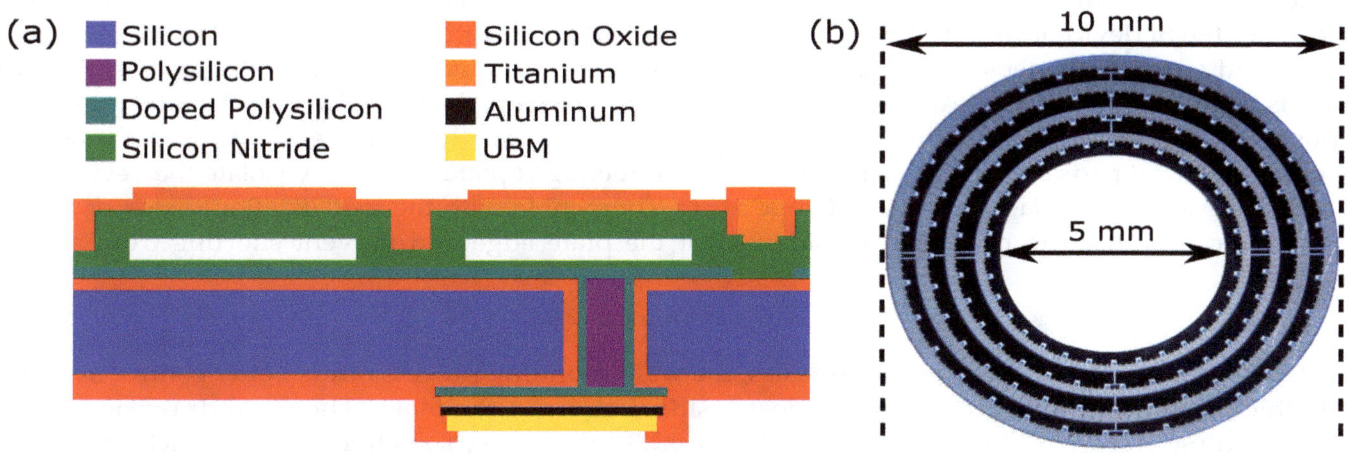

Figure 7. (**a**) Structure of a sacrificial release CMUT with vias for backside electrical contacts. (**b**) A four-ring 2D CMUT array fabricated using a sacrificial release process and through-wafer vias, as decribed in [25]. Reproduced with permission from Moini, A., Capacitive Micromachined Ultrasonic Transducer (CMUT) Arrays for Endoscopic Ultrasound.

With backside electrical contacts, it is feasible to construct 2D arrays with individually-addressable elements. Rectangular 2D arrays have been fabricated for volumetric imaging [23], and ring arrays have been fabricated for forward-looking imaging on the ends of catheters [24].

3.2. Wafer Bonding—Basic Process

In this technique, a combination of surface micromachining and silicon on insulator (SOI) technologies are used to fabricate the CMUT [26]. This wafer bonding process greatly simplifies the fabrication and brings new levels of uniformity and control, especially regarding the plate thickness, which is now defined by the device layer of the SOI wafer.

The wafer bonding fabrication process is illustrated below in Figure 8. The starting point of this process is a prime-grade heavily-doped Si wafer. Care should be taken to ensure the carrier density is high enough in both the prime and SOI wafer to limit depletion during operation. The CMUT gap height is then defined by a thermal oxidation of the prime wafer. The gap dimensions and geometry are then defined, lithographically, and transferred into the oxide with a wet or dry etch down to the Si. Next, a second thermal oxidation is used to passivate the exposed Si and prevent shorting between the bottom of the gap and the conducting plate that will ultimately be formed from the SOI wafer. It should be noted that this oxidation should be as high of quality as possible to avoid hysteresis in the device operation from trap charging or ion drift. At this point, a second lithography step can be used to flatten any bumps that may have formed along the upper edge of the cavity due to increase Si flux [27], which can drop the yield of the SOI bonding. Commonly, a ring pattern (around the gap) and etch can simply remove these bumps. At this point, a critical RCA clean is performed followed by immediate direct bonding of the SOI wafer.

During bonding, the oxidized Si wafer is brought in contact with the SOI wafer, at which point a weak van der Waals attraction holds the two wafers together, coupled with weak hydrogen bonding. Another thermal oxidation ($\approx$1100 °C) is then used to covalently bond the two wafers. The next steps involve releasing of the handle and buried oxide (BOX) from the SOI wafer to form the CMUT plates. First, the bulk of the SOI handle is removed using mechanical grinding, typically leaving $\approx$100 μm depending on the grinding uniformity and control. A wet etch in KOH or tetramethylammonium hydroxide (TMAH) is then used to strip the remaining handle, using the BOX as an etch stop. Finally, the BOX layer is removed by another wet etch in hydrofluoric (HF) acid or its derivative, such as buffered oxide etchant (BOE), this time using the Si device layer (i.e., CMUT plate) as the etch stop. At this point, the CMUTs are physically formed and subsequent steps are related to device isolation and contacts. In this basic process, top-side contacts to the bottom electrode are formed by etching via down to the Si wafer. Metal contacts are then deposited by sputtering both within the via and atop the plate. Finally, a device isolation etch is used to separate the metal pads and etch down through the conducting Si plate electrically isolate the device and/or define the array. As a last step, a low-temperature (compatible with the metallization) oxide or nitride deposition can be used to passivate the sidewall of the plate edge and prevent shorting from surface conduction.

Compared to the sacrificial release process, the wafer bonding process offers better control over the plate thickness and gap height, and much less residual stress in the plate. The main drawback of the wafer bonding process is that the wafer-bonding step, itself, is very sensitive to issues such as surface roughness [28] and cleanliness, and as such, can have a low yield. An additional drawback to thw wafer bonding process is the cost and logistical complexity of procuring suitable SOI wafers. To avoid this, silicon nitride can be deposited on a standard wafer and bonded to the substrate wafer form the top plate [29].

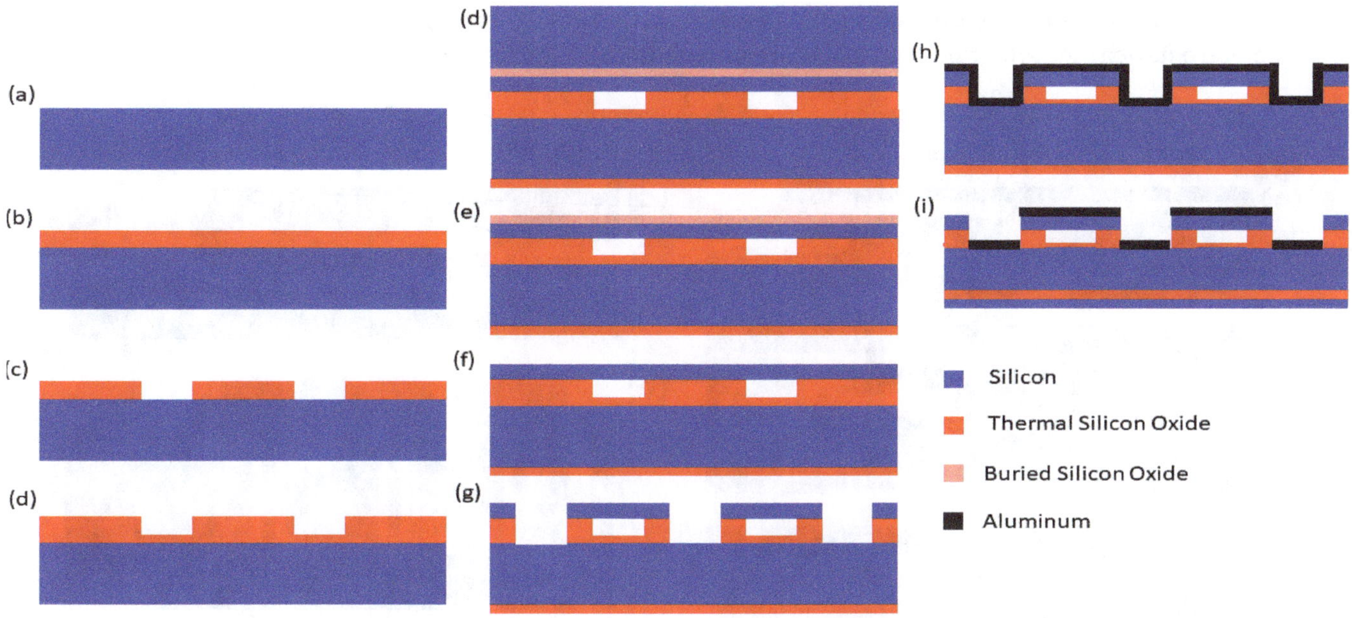

Figure 8. Process flow for a wafer-bonded CMUT. (**a**) Starting prime wafer. (**b**) Thermal oxidation. (**c**) Etch to form cavity. (**d**) Thermal oxidation. (**e**) Silicon on insulator (SOI) wafer bonding. (**f**) SOI handle. (**g**) Removing burried oxide. (**h**) Sputtering metallization. (**i**) Metal pattern and device isolation.

3.2.1. Wafer Bonding—LOCOS Process

The LOCOS (local oxidation of silicon) process is a variant of the wafer-bonding process that allows excellent gap height control and reduced parasitic capacitance when compared to the basic wafer bonding process [30]. The process uses local oxidation, a method used to isolate neighboring MOS transistors in which a silicon nitride mask is used to prevent the diffusion of oxidants to the silicon surface in particular locations so that oxide only grows in specific areas.

A typical LOCOS CMUT structure is shown in Figure 9a. The elevated silicon area in the center of the cells is created using a local oxidation step. This step may be masked with silicon oxide [30] or silicon nitride [31]. A second LOCOS step produces the silicon oxide posts which support the top plate. In this way, the gap height can be made small while keeping the post area thick, unlike the simple wafer bonding process where the gap height and post height are coupled. Gap heights as small as 40 nm have been achieved using this process [30]. In the device shown in Figure 9a, there is no metal layer on the top plate. Instead, highly-doped silicon is used to provide conductivity.

3.2.2. Wafer Bonding—Thick BOX, Pre-Charged

A variety of modifications to the basic process flow for wafer-bonded CMUTs exist, each addressing a specific aspect of performance. Charging is one aspect of CMUT performance that has received considerable attention due to its impact on the device reliability. Specifically, charge trapping and ion drift in the insulating layer within the gap can be responsible for hysteresis in the electrostatic deflection of the plate. In response to such charging, the use of an SOI wafer with a thick BOX layer to form the bottom electrodes has been proposed as one solution [32]. The structure is shown in Figure 9b. The purpose of this is to localize the electrical field, which is the underlying cause of charging, to within the gap by patterning vias through the thick BOX layer. In addition, these backside contacts allow a flat and continuous front face on the transducer array, which improves imaging and simplifies packaging. On the flip side of charging, this can be advantageously exploited with pre-charged CMUTs. Here, charging in the gap insulator is used to electrostatically deflect the CMUT plate and reduce or entirely remove the DC pull in voltage [33].

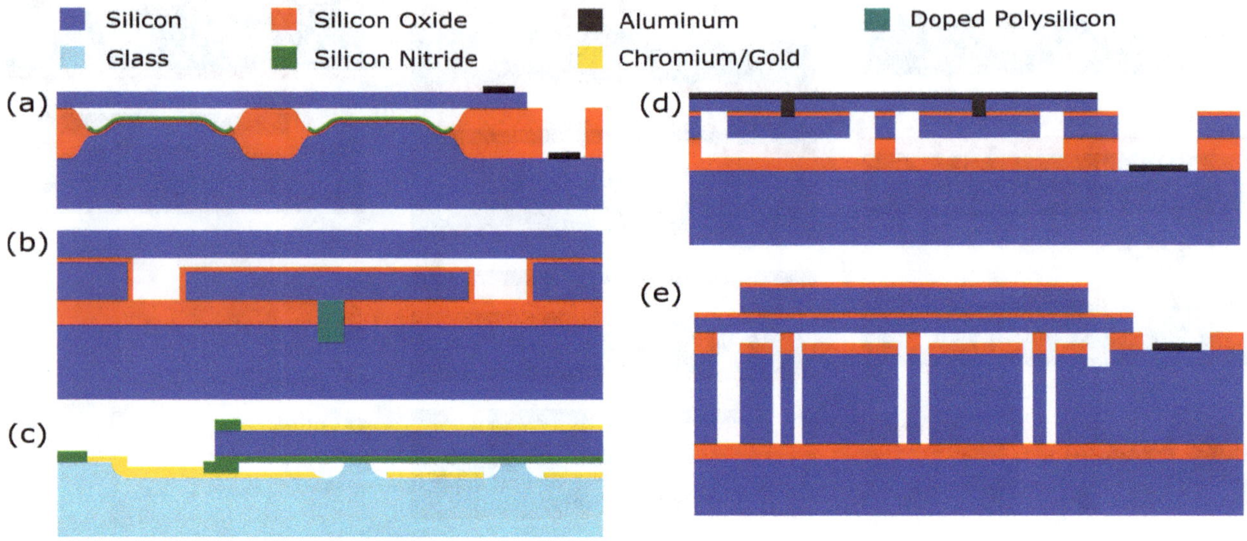

Figure 9. (**a–c**) Wafer-bonded CMUT structures. (**a**) Local oxidation of silicon (LOCOS) wafer-bonded CMUT. (**b**) Thick buried oxide (BOX) CMUT. (**c**) Anodic-bonded CMUT. (**d–e**) Structures to improve average displacement shown for comparison. (**d**) Piston CMUT fabricated with a double wafer-bonding process. (**e**) Post CMUT.

3.2.3. Wafer Bonding—High-K Insulator

Another approach to suppressing charging involves tailoring the dielectric constant of the insulating layer. Like the introduction of high-K gates in the CMOS industry, high-K insulators can play a role in suppressing charging within the CMUT gap. Specifically, high-K insulators have been shown to suppress the field-emission that occurs between the plate and bottom electrode under high-fields [34]. In parallel to modifications to the dielectric constant, the use of improved deposition techniques, such as atomic layer deposition (ALD) can further suppress charging by reducing the trap density in the insulating layer.

3.2.4. Wafer Bonding—Anodic Bonding and Transparent

A valuable departure from the standard (direct) wafer bonding process is the use of anodic bonding, which can enable CMUTs with low thermal budgets and/or transparency. Anodic bonding is typically used to bond glass to a substrate and is facilitated by ion drift within the glass to form an interfacial bond. The structure is shown in Figure 9c. CMUTs with plates formed through such anodic bonding have been demonstrated with simplified processing, greater tolerance to surface roughness, and high reliability [35]. Moreover, anodic bonding has been employed to improve the transparency of CMUTs to enable coupling with optical measurement techniques [36].

3.2.5. Wafer Bonding—Flexible

In general, electronics are beginning to tap into a new frontier of applications enabled by mechanical flexibility. CMUTs also follow this trend and have experienced interesting developments in flexible devices and arrays, enabling a variety of high-impact applications ranging from conformal patches to swallow-able pills. In general, the approach to flexible CMUT arrays can take two paths; creating the array from entirely flexible components or embedding rigid isolated CMUTs within a flexible medium. These two types of flexible CMUTs are illustrated in Figure 10. Regarding entirely flexible CMUTs, the fabrication typically involves forming the device through micromachining of polymer layers. These polymer layers are supported by a rigid substrate and later released through a chemical etch. One recent demonstration used a combination the polymer SU-8 (as a bulk material) and Parylene-C (to seal the cavity) to fabricate CMUTs on a Si wafer [37]. A thin liftoff layer was then used to release the polymer CMUT array from the Si after fabrication. Another recent approach leveraged a rolling lamination process to form an entirely flexible CMUT array [38].

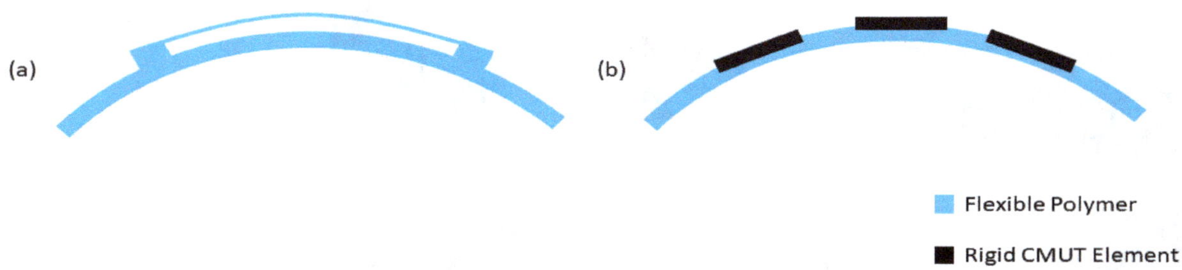

Figure 10. Approaches to fabricating flexible CMUTs. (**a**) CMUT fabricated from entirely flexible polymers. (**b**) Isolated rigid CMUTs embedded within a flexible substrate.

3.2.6. Wafer Bonding—Bendable Arrays

Regarding the second path towards flexible arrays, rigid CMUTs can be embedded within a flexible medium [39], a variety of recent works have shown progress in forming such arrays by back-filling of mechanically-isolated devices with a polymer layer. For example, recent work on a circular pill-shaped imaging platform has demonstrated a process flow whereby a bonded CMUT array is first fashioned on a Si wafer, then isolated with a through-Si etch, followed by trench filling with polydimethylsiloxane (PDMS) [40]. This process flow for fabricating a pill-shaped device is shown below in Figure 11. Similar to the wafer-bonded process flow, the starting point is a CMUT with the SOI BOX layer removed. Next, a top-side metalization is sputtered. The top-side oxide is then etched to begin the device isolation. A second top-side etch into Si is performed, followed by a nitride passivation. Next, under bump metalization (UBM) is applied to the back-side of the wafer. The device isolation is completed with a backside etch and trench filling with a polymer to form the flexible substrate.

3.3. Device Structures to Improve Average Displacement

In a conventional CMUT structure, the edges of the cells are clamped and the spring force arises from the bending of a plate of uniform thickness. This results in an average displacement which is much less than the peak displacement (1/3 in the case of circular cells [41]). A number of device structures have been developed to improve the average displacement by creating plates that move more like pistons.

One approach is to make the plate thicker in the center. A thick center area can be fabricated on the bottom of the top plate using a double wafer bonding process, producing the structure in Figure 9d [42]. Here, two SOIs are bonded together and the device layer of one is used to form the piston while the device layer of the other is used to form the plate. More simply, a mass of a material such as gold can be deposited and patterned on the top of the plate [43].

Another structure called a post CMUT uses compliant posts to provide the spring force rather than the flexural movement of the plate [44]. The structure is shown in Figure 9e. The springs are defined using DRIE and the plate is created by wafer bonding [45].

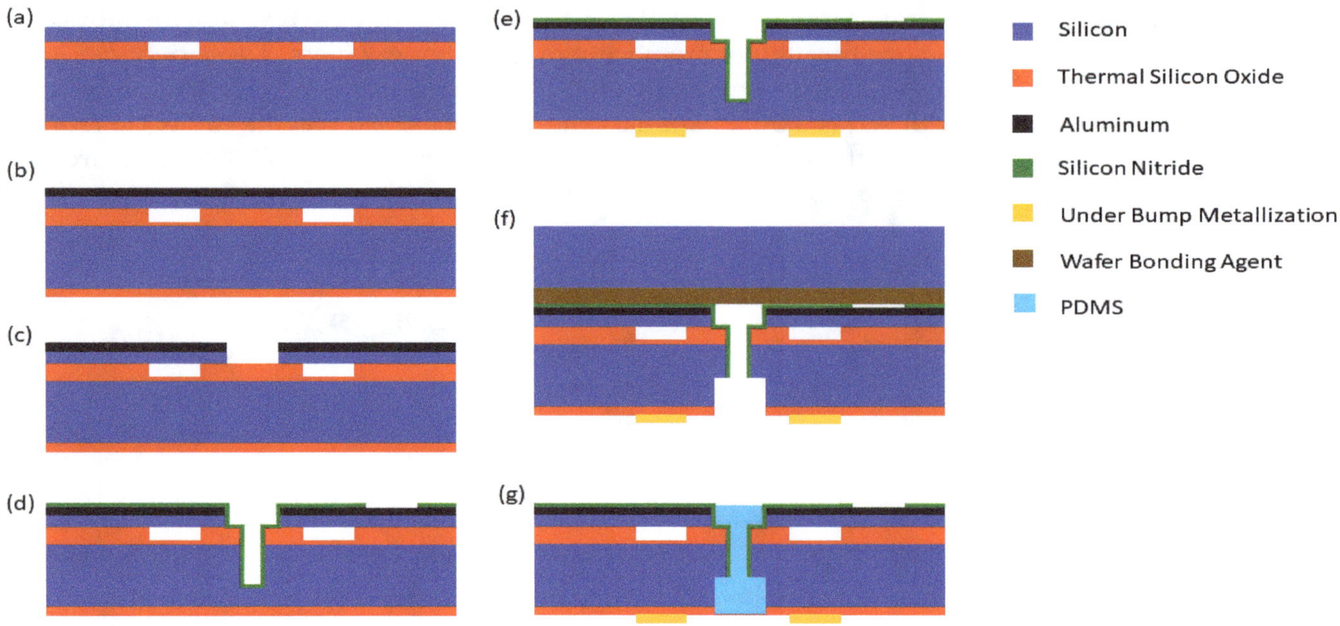

Figure 11. Process flow for fabricating a bendable CMUT array. (**a**) A wafer-bonded CMUT after stripping the SOI BOX. (**b**) Sputtering top-side metallization. (**c**) Top-side isolation etch. (**d**) Second top-side isolation with nitride passivation. (**e**) Deposit of under bump metalization (UBM). (**f**) Secure to supporting wafer. (**g**) Back-side isolation and polydimethylsiloxane (PDMS) filling.

In addition to improving average displacement, the piston and post CMUTs decouple the compliance of the plate from the mass, which allows greater design flexibility. However, they both present fabrication challenges. In the piston structure, any misalignment of the piston mass can change the dynamic behavior of the cell. Fabrication of post CMUTs with high yield has proved complex and challenging [45].

4. Integration of Ultrasonic Transducer Arrays with Electronic Circuits

In ultrasound imaging systems, ultrasound probes typically do not contain any active electronics when the element count is low (<256), and all the front-end electronics is in the imaging system. For CMUT arrays this poses a slight problem in the receive chain because of the typically high electrical input impedance of CMUT array elements. High input impedance combined with long cables result in loss of valuable signal-to-noise ratio (SNR) for the CMUTs.

This problem is mitigated by including low noise amplifiers and/or buffers inside the probe, which amplify the signal before driving the cables. Even probes with piezoelectric transducers can benefit from using active electronics.

When the element count is high such that the number of channels in the imaging system cannot match the number of elements in the array, the ultrasound probe will definitely contain a certain amount of electronics that would take care of some of the front-end processing and reduce the number of transducer channels to match the number of channels in the imaging system. In this respect, CMUT technology has a distinctive advantage over piezoelectric transducer technology because of the variety of electronic integration possibilities it provides. Figure 12 shows three common approaches to electronic integration applied to CMUT arrays.

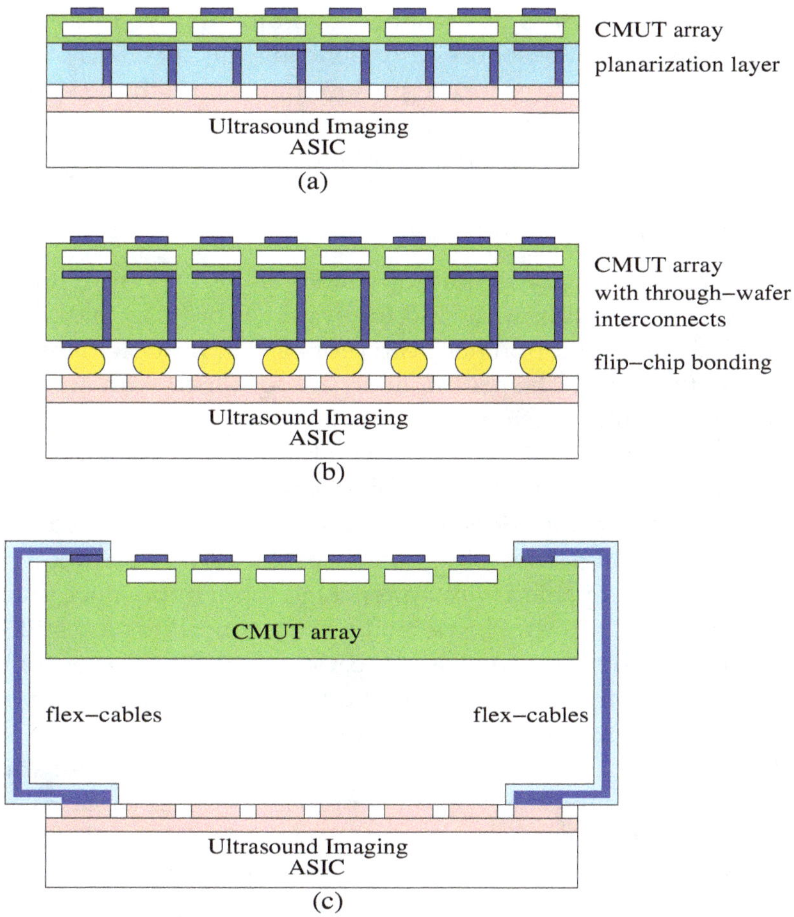

Figure 12. Schemes for electronic integration: (**a**) monolithic integration, (**b**) multi-chip integration, (**c**) hybrid integration.

A unique integration option for CMUTs had been the monolithic integration of the CMUT array with the electronics in which the CMUT array is built on top of the electronic circuitry directly [46–48]. Recently, monolithic integration of piezoelectric micromachined ultrasonic transducers (PMUT) with CMOS electronics have also been achieved by virtue of the same advantage, the compatibility of micromachining processes with CMOS processes [49,50]. Monolithic integration has always been considered the gold standard because of the compactness of the result and the elimination of extra integration steps associated with multi-chip approaches. However, this approach requires high volume production to be economically feasible, which is probably the reason why it did not find commercial traction until low cost, portable high volume ultrasound scanners became possible. (e.g., Butterfly Network Inc., Guilford, CT, USA). Whether a one-dimensional array or a two-dimensional array, monolithic integration provides the best interface (in terms of parasitics) between the CMUT array and the electronics. In monolithic integration, first the electronic circuitry (ASIC) is fabricated using a CMOS technology or similar, then the ASIC wafer is planarized using low temperature deposition and chemical-mechanical polishing (CMP) steps, which is followed by the CMUT fabrication using the sacrificial release process. There has been some success reported on using a low-temperature bonding process for CMUT fabrication as well [51].

Multi-chip integration [23,52] has been used to connect 2D CMUT arrays to the electronics for some time now. In this approach the electronics and the CMUT array are built separately and brought together using a variety of integration options: flip-chip bonding with solder reflow, with gold stud bumps and anisotropic conductive films (ACF) or with thermo-compression bonding. These integration methods, though more practical to apply, are not unique to CMUTs and have been applied to piezoelectric matrix arrays with great success as well [53,54]. For full 2D arrays where the number of individual connections is very high, fanning out interconnects to the sides where conventional interconnect schemes (wire bonding) can be used become impractical. In that case, flip-chip bonding the 2D CMUT array onto the electronics becomes a necessity. The amount of electronic integration that can be incorporated into a CMUT probe varies depending on many parameters, ranging from size to power consumption to the type of application. We will now look into some of these varieties and their associated electronics.

4.1. Analog Front End Integration for SNR Improvement

CMUTs typically have higher electrical input impedance and suffer from the parasitic capacitance of the interconnection between the transducer array and the system more than piezoelectric transducer arrays do. To alleviate this problem, a simple solution has been proposed and implemented. An array of low noise preamplifiers is integrated into the probe. The preamplifiers are equipped with active or passive switches that isolate them from the transmit circuitry during high voltage transmit events. After the transmit event the switches change position and the received signals go through the low noise preamplifiers. These amplifiers need not have high amplification but should be low noise and be able to drive the low impedance of the cable and the system front end [55]. Such preamplifiers have already been implemented on standard US front-end chip sets [56]. To accommodate the high input impedance of the CMUT elements, high input impedance preamplifiers can be used. When accompanied with buffers high input impedance preamplifiers reduce signal loss due to the loading of the system cables. However, these preamplifiers are still susceptible to parasitic capacitances between the preamplifier and the transducer element. In case of high parasitic capacitance in the CMUT element and between the CMUT element and the preamplifier, transimpedance amplifiers (aka resistive feedback amplifiers) provide an elegant solution by creating a low impedance node at the preamplifier input which essentially shunts the parasitic capacitance. Both these approaches provide good solutions with some gain and wide bandwidth. Another approach is to use capacitive feedback preamplifiers. These amplifiers are similar to transimpedance amplifiers where the feedback resistor is replaced by a feedback capacitor. Because the impedance of the capacitor drops with frequency, these amplifier show low-pass behavior and are somewhat band-limited. On the other hand, because the feedback resistor is eliminated, capacitive feedback amplifiers show excellent noise performance [57].

4.2. Row-Column Addressing

Row-column addressed CMUTs have found a renewed interest in recent years. The row-column addressing allows the fabrication of 2D CMUT arrays relatively easily with reduced number of interconnects [46,58,59]. In this type of array, the bottom electrode is divided into lines (as opposed to making the whole silicon substrate a single electrode which is typically the case for 1D arrays). The top electrode on the other hand is also divided into lines that are perpendicular to the bottom electrode lines. The intersection of these perpendicular lines, which we can refer to as azimuth and elevation lines, constitute an element of the 2D array. Each element in the array is accessed by accessing the corresponding row and column electrodes. Hence, only $2N$ connections are required, rather than N^2 to access all the elements. The electronics associated with row-column addressed CMUTs can be somewhat more complicated than the front-end electronics for one-dimensional arrays depending on how they are implemented, but they are a lot simpler than that of fully addressable 2D arrays and produce volumetric images. Hence, row-column addressed 2D CMUT arrays present a very attractive alternative to fully addressable 2D arrays. A row-column addressed 2D array can be used as a synthetic 1D array whose elevation aperture is dynamically changed and electronically scanned in the elevation direction. In this scenario the azimuth lines are connected to the system channels directly whereas the elevation lines are connected to the bias voltage(s) through switches. By electronically turning on and off the switches the elevation aperture is adjusted for each firing [60–62]. Another approach is to switch the elevation and azimuth apertures between transmit and receive events while applying Fresnel focusing in the elevation direction, which provides isotropic resolution in azimuth and elevation directions [46]. In such systems, a switch matrix is used to selectively connect each azimuth and elevation line to a system channel, to the bias voltage or to ground. Such a switch matrix can be integrated in any one of the ways described above.

4.3. Catheter Based Imaging Systems

CMUTs have catalyzed considerable progress in catheter based imaging applications where array size and channel count are severely limited due to physical constraints such as blood vessel diameter. CMUTs offer elegant solutions to the array size problem. The fabrication flexibility allows manufacturing of small, high frequency, linear, ring shaped, cylindrical forward looking and side looking arrays. Small element size and the long cables associated with catheters warrant a higher level of electronic integration at the catheter tip even for piezoelectric transducers, and only more so for CMUTs. The electronic integration options discussed above along with fabrication simplicity makes CMUTs a better option for catheter based imaging systems. To overcome the parasitic capacitance that the cables present CMUTs are integrated with low noise amplifiers and buffers [21,24,63,64]. The size constraint also limits the number of cables that can run through a catheter. Hence, reducing the number of channels becomes a necessity. Analog multiplexing of the transducer channels and applying synthetic aperture imaging can reduce the number of connections to as low as two [65] with some compromise in the imaging quality and frame rate. A more efficient approach is to integrate TX beamformers and analog multiplexers with the CMUT array at the catheter tip to reduce the cable count without compromising the image quality [48,66,67].

4.4. Imaging System on a Chip

Developments in the electronics industry have opened up the way to building ultrasound imaging systems on a chip. Combined with post processing methods to fabricate CMUTs, it is now possible to build single chip ultrasound imaging systems. One caveat in this approach is that ultrasound imaging typically involves a very large dynamic range. Transmit voltages and CMUT DC bias voltages are typically high voltages (≈100 V), whereas received signals are very low voltages. Maintaining a high signal-to-noise ratio and frequency bandwidth is probably the most important objective in the receive chain. In addition, there is the digital component of the imaging system. Combining all of these in a single chip provides the best signal integrity but may compromise signal quality to some degree. However, HV-BCD processes seems to overcome such problems [57,67,68]. Building ultrasound imaging systems on a chip or even on multiple chips paves the way to very low cost, ultra portable ultrasound imaging systems. When combined with today's wireless communication capabilities and battery power technologies, such ultrasound systems turn into flexible, wearable, ingestible standalone ultrasound imaging systems. In our group we have developed and demonstrated the components of such a system which would go into an ingestible capsule form and provide the images of the gastrointestinal tract. This capsule combines an ultrasound imaging system with on-chip transmit and receive beamforming capability, with power management and wireless transfer circuitry [69,70]. The system acquires US images of the intestinal cross-section and wirelessly transmits them to a host computer Figure 13. In addition to the high dynamic range requirements, the form factor of an ingestible US imaging system forces a multichip approach for this integration problem.

4.5. Imaging and HIFU System Integration

CMUTs have two very distinctive advantages when it comes to high intensity focused ultrasound (HIFU) applications. One of them is the ability to do imaging and HIFU with the same transducer array given the inherent wide frequency band of the CMUT transducers. The other one is the lack of a self-heating mechanism in CMUTs (whereas for piezoelectric transducers self heating is the main issue). Therefore, CMUT transducer arrays are excellent candidates for dual mode operation. Dual mode operation usually requires specific electronic circuitry that interfaces the HIFU drivers with the transducer arrays. In HIFU operation long bursts of sinusoidal signals are used to excite the elements. The pulsers in the imaging circuitry are usually not efficient enough to generate such kind of long bursts without overheating, and therefore separate HIFU drivers are needed for dual mode operation. The HIFU driver is interfaced to the CMUT array and the imaging system with a switch matrix which switches from imaging to HIFU and back to imaging in a programmable manner to be able to ablate tissue and monitor the results in real time. In our group we have successfully developed and demonstrated such a dual mode imaging/HIFU system for ablation in shallow tissue that uses a 2D CMUT array which is flip-chip bonded to the electronic circuitry [71,72]. The 2D CMUT array consists of dedicated transmit and receive elements. The transmit elements are connected to a TX beamformer whereas the receive elements are connected to low noise receive amplifiers. To reduce power consumption in the ASIC, an off-chip, standalone, eight-channel HIFU driver is used. The ASIC includes high-voltage switches to switch the TX elements between imaging pulsers and HIFU channels Figure 14. With this integrated device, it is possible to do HIFU (up to 16 MPa peak to peak pressure at 1 cm focal depth at 5 MHz) and imaging with the same 2D array. As the level of electronic integration increases thermal management of the transducer array and electronics assembly start to become an important issue, especially in dual mode systems. For example, even though off-chip HIFU drivers are used the amount of power dissipation in the high-voltage switches in the ASIC is enough to increase the probe temperature to unacceptable levels (42 °C US probes). However, the thermal energy levels involved are modest and is easily managed by basic thermal design considerations.

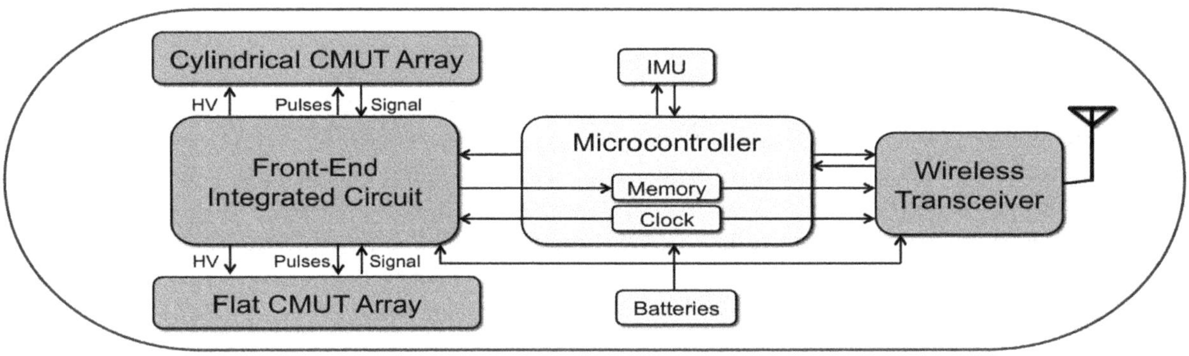

Figure 13. Capsule US imaging system.

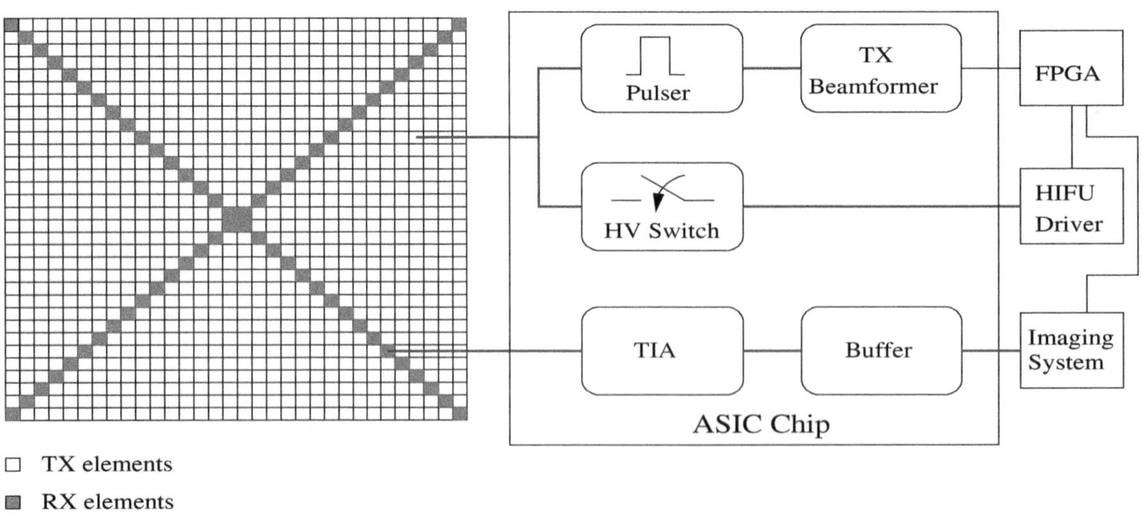

Figure 14. Dual-mode high intensity focused ultrasound (HIFU) and imaging system with 2D CMUT array and electronic circuitry (ASIC).

5. Applications

As there have already been many applications of CMUTs, we cannot present them all here. Instead, we have selected applications of particular interest from our own work.

5.1. Medical Ultrasound Imaging

Medical ultrasound imaging is non-ionizing, safe, and therefore broadly accepted for diagnostic use even for obstetrical applications. Compared to all other imaging modalities, ultrasound imaging is cheap and portable. These features have made ultrasound imaging a widely used imaging modality in medicine. We postulate that CMUTs can replace piezoelectric transducers in any medical ultrasound probe. Butterfly Network has recently released their first probe which is based on a 9000 element 2D CMUT array. The handheld device plugs directly into a smartphone and emulates both a phased array, convex array and linear array. A fetal scan carried out with their probe connected to a smartphone is shown in Figure 15.

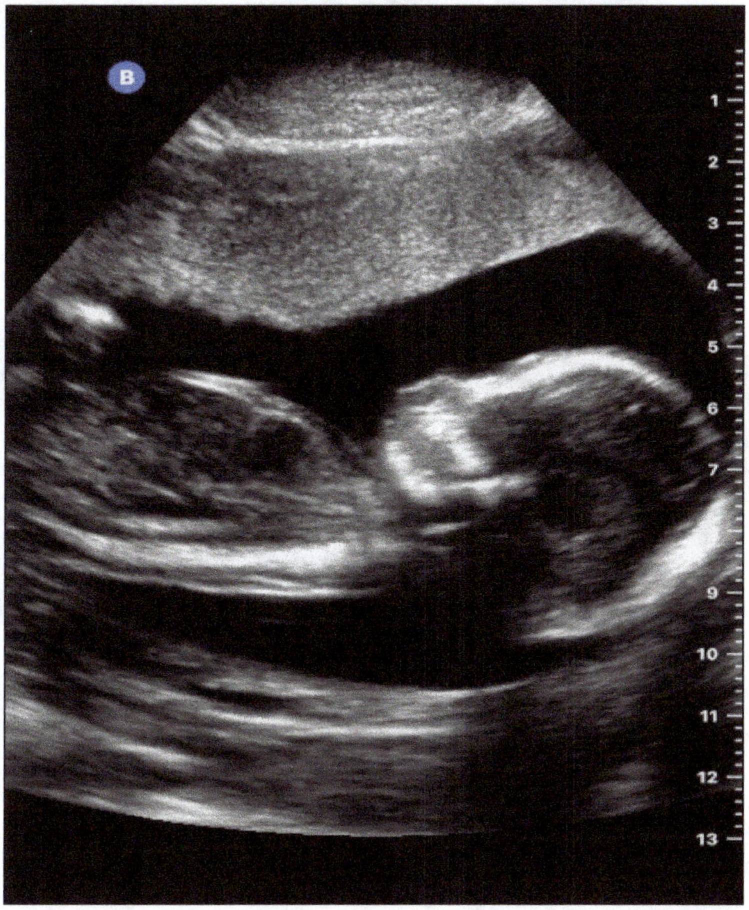

Figure 15. A fetal B-mode scanned with a CMUT transducer reproduced with permission from Butterfly Network [73].

5.2. Dual-Mode: HIFU and Imaging with the Same Transducer Array

High-intensity focused ultrasound (HIFU) is a minimally invasive, FDA-approved procedure to ablate tissue without damaging the surrounding tissue especially closer to the transducer [74]. Well-known examples of HIFU include targeted ultrasound drug delivery, treatment of uterine fibroids, neurological disorders, prostate cancer, and other types of cancers [75,76]. For a successful HIFU treatment it is required to guide the procedure with an imaging modality like ultrasound imaging or MRI. Normally both imaging modalities are separate from the HIFU system which makes it an engineering task to design a system that guarantees co-registration between the HIFU delivery location with the imaging. Here we present a device where we have combined the imaging and HIFU system into one integrated circuit (IC) that operates on one 32 × 32 element 2D CMUT array and the co-registration is therefore an integral part of the system. The IC can switch between HIFU mode and imaging mode on a millisecond scale giving the illusion to the user that the HIFU ablation and imaging is taking place at the same time. The switching time is limited by the speed of the DC power supplies. The dual-mode device is shown in Figure 16.

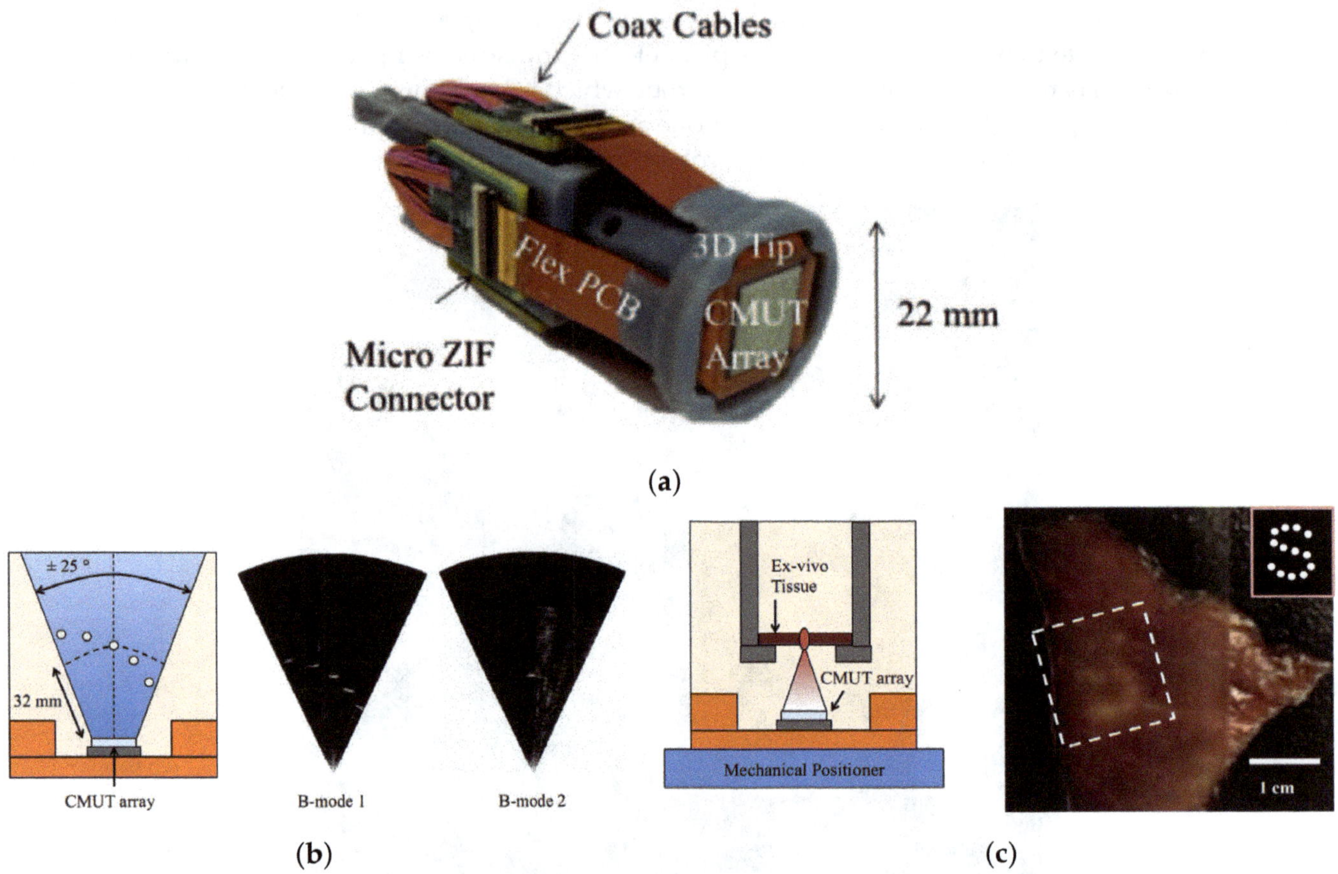

Figure 16. (**a**) The integrated CMUT, IC and flexible printed circuit board (flex PCB) prior to PDMS casting. (**b**) 3D imaging result of a wire phantom. (**c**) HIFU ablation of a piece of ex-vivo tissue. All images from [71]. Reproduced with permission from Jang, J.H. et al., 2015 IEEE International Ultrasonics Symposium (IUS); published by IEEE Xplore, 2015 [72]. Reproduced with permission from Jang, J.H. et al., 2017 IEEE International Ultrasonics Symposium (IUS).

5.3. Catheter Based Ultrasound Imaging

An alternative to an imaging and HIFU system that operates as one, is to have a system that eases the coupling between the two systems and therefore also the co-registration. We present here a CMUT ring array that has been fully integrated into a catheter assembly with a 12.5 mm OD and 4 mm ID. The circular catheter form-factor makes it easy to couple and co-register the imaging array with a center-piece, see Figure 17a, HIFU system or optical fibers for photoacoustic imaging. The catheter is shown in Figure 17.

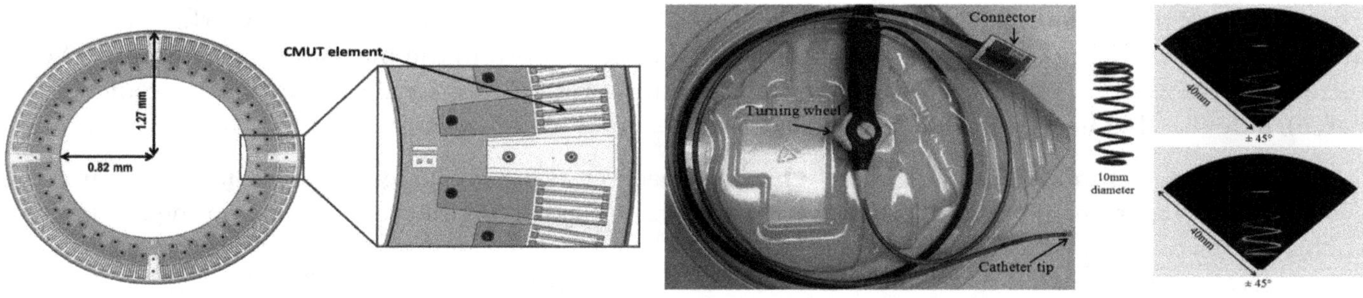

(a) (b) (c)

Figure 17. (**a**) CMUT ring array. (**b**) CMUT ring array integrated into a endoscopic assembly. (**c**) 3D imaging results of a spring. Images from [24]. Reproduced with permission from Moini, A. et al., 2016 IEEE International Ultrasonics Symposium (IUS); published by IEEE Xplore, 2016 [66]. Reproduced with permission from Moini, A. et al., ASME 2015 International Technical Conference and Exhibition on Packaging and Integration of Electronic and Photonic Microsystems collocated with the ASME 2015 13th International Conference on Nanochannels, Microchannels, and Minichannels; published by ASME, 2015 [77]. Reproduced with permission from Choe, J.W. et al., IEEE Transactions on Ultrasonics, Ferroelectrics, and Frequency Control.

6. Industrialization

Given the obvious advantage of manufacturing CMUTs using silicon integrated circuits processing technologies, commercialization was considered to be a short distance away from invention. In retrospect, it has been a fairly rapid path to full industrial products and volume production. The following will mention a subset of the industrialization effort with no intention of short-changing efforts that are unknown to the authors.

The first foray into industrialization was Sensant which was founded in 1998 and was eventually acquired by Siemens in 2005. Sensant started trying to commercialize CMUTs for flow gas metering, and eventually got into medical imaging. However, no product ever reached the market out of this effort. In 1998 the ACULAB laboratory at University of Roma Tre started an effort in CMUTs and is providing their technology for commercialization.

Hitachi Medico succeeded in the development and put into practical use a probe named "Mappie" that was attached to a system for detecting breast cancer. The system was introduced in 2008 at the 82nd Annual Scientific meeting of the Japan Society of Ultrasonic in Medicine at Tokyo, Japan. In 2017 Hitachi announced an updated system at the RSNA meeting in Chicago and introduced the product in the US market.

Around the same time frame of 2008, Vermon in Tours, France, introduced CMUT arrays for research purposes using the sacrificial release technology. These arrays were not available in the US till much later in time. In 2005, Kolo Technologies was formed and has continued in developing technology to commercialize CMUTs. Today, Kolo Medical (an outgrowth of Kolo Technologies) specializes in high frequency CMUT arrays (>25 MHz), and has a strong presence in the US and Suzhou, China.

Butterfly Network inc., a seven years old start-up, has made the most impact in successful commercialization of CMUTs. In the Fall of 2018, Butterfly announced the introduction of a handheld probe that plugs to an iPhone to make the full ultrasound imaging system. The system sells for less than $2000 and is FDA approved for 13 different examinations.

At the most recent IEEE Ultrasonics Symposium in Kobe, Japan, Philips announced that it is making available design and fabrication capability of CMUTs (operated in collapse mode) for end users. Philips has been working on CMUTs for a number of years and possesses an excellent technology base.

Similarly, the Fraunhofer Institute for Photonoic Microsystems (IPMS) has been working on CMUTs and is commercializing CMUTs for a number of applications both in the medical space and in airborne ultrasound. IPMS has a previous history in making vibrating ribbons for light modulation (silicon light valve), a device that is very similar to the CMUT in design and construction.

Another player in the space is Canon, which has been working on 3D real time photoacoustic imaging systems for breast screening using 2D arrays of CMUTs. It is expected that they will be on the market with such systems once they receive FDA approval.

Overall, it is estimated that there is a total of about 23 companies offering CMUT products.

7. Discussion

Since its inception 25 years ago, CMUT technology have seen significant developments, especially in the last decade. With the advance of the modern modeling tools, both analytical and numerical CMUT models have become accurate and reliable enough to make industrial quality designs possible both for normal mode and collapse mode of operation. Fabrication processes and electronic integration tools have also matured to the point that mass production of CMUT probes along with its accompanying electronics have become economically feasible. As a result, more and more ultrasound imaging companies have started to incorporate CMUT probes into their systems. The ease of miniaturization and variety of electronic integration options enabled low-cost, ultra-portable, wireless or with minimal wiring, wearable or ingestible complete ultrasound imaging systems possible.

CMUTs show distinctive advantages when it comes to high intensity focused ultrasound applications. The lack of self-heating mechanism and inherent wide frequency bandwidth make CMUTs an excellent candidate for HIFU and dual mode imaging/HIFU applications. Although this option hasn't seen a commercial application yet, primarily because it is an area that is being explored only recently, there has been successful demonstrations of dual mode operation with CMUTs. The future work on CMUTs is likely to include its therapeutic uses as well. Some imaging systems have already started including HIFU capability which should find commercial success in the coming years.

Acknowledgments: The authors would like to thank Soitec for kindly sponsoring SOI wafers used for CMUT fabrication in different projects by our group.

References

1. Haller, M.I.; Khuri-Yakub, B.T. A Surface Micromachined Electrostatic Ultrasonic Air Transducer. *IEEE Trans. Ultrason. Ferroelectr. Freq. Control* **1996**, *43*, 1–6. [CrossRef]
2. Soh, H.T.; Ladabaum, I.; Atalar, A.; Quate, C.F.; Khuri-Yakub, B.T. Silicon micromachined ultrasonic immersion transducers. *Appl. Phys. Lett.* **1996**, *69*, 3674–3676. [CrossRef]
3. Park, K.K.; Oralkan, O.; Khuri-Yakub, B. A comparison between conventional and collapse-mode capacitive micromachined ultrasonic transducers in 10-MHz 1-D arrays. *IEEE Trans. Ultrason. Ferroelectr. Freq. Control* **2013**, *60*, 1245–1255. [CrossRef] [PubMed]
4. Mason, W.P. *Electromechanical Transducers and Wave Filters*; D. Van Nostrand: New York, NY, USA, 1942.
5. Ladabaum, I.; Jin, X.; Soh, H.; Atalar, A.; Khuri-Yakub, B. Surface micromachined capacitive ultrasonic transducers. *IEEE Trans. Ultrason. Ferroelectr. Freq. Control* **1998**, *45*, 678–690. [CrossRef] [PubMed]
6. Khuri-yakub, B.T.; Cheng, C.H.; Degertekin, F.L.; Ergun, S.; Hansen, S.; Jin, X.; Oralkan, O. Silicon Micromachined Ultrasonic Transducers. *Jpn. J. Appl. Phys.* **2000**, *39*, 2883–2887. [CrossRef]

7. Nikoozadeh, A.; Bayram, B.; Yaralioglu, G.; Khuri-Yakub, B. Analytical calculation of collapse voltage of CMUT membrane. In Proceedings of the IEEE Ultrasonics Symposium, Montreal, QC, Canada, 23–27 August 2004; Volume 1, pp. 256–259. [CrossRef]
8. Lohfink, A.; Eccardt, P.C.; Benecke, W.; Meixner, H. Derivation of a 1D CMUT model from FEM results for linear and nonlinear equivalent circuit simulation. In Proceedings of the IEEE Symposium on Ultrasonics, Honolulu, HI, USA, 5–8 October 2003; pp. 465–468. [CrossRef]
9. Lohfink, A.; Eccardt, P.C. Linear and nonlinear equivalent circuit modeling of CMUTs. *IEEE Trans. Ultrason. Ferroelectr. Freq. Control* **2005**, *52*, 2163–2172. [CrossRef] [PubMed]
10. Morse, P.M.P.M.; Ingard, K.U. *Theoretical Acoustics*; Princeton University Press: Princeton, NJ, USA, 1986; p. 927.
11. Yaralioglu, G.; Ergun, S.; Khuri-Yakub, B. Finite-element analysis of capacitive micromachined ultrasonic transducers. *IEEE Trans. Ultrason. Ferroelectr. Freq. Control* **2005**, *52*, 2185–2198. [CrossRef] [PubMed]
12. Kupnik, M.; Wygant, I.O.; Khuri-Yakub, B.T. Finite element analysis of stress stiffening effects in CMUTS. In Proceedings of the 2008 IEEE Ultrasonics Symposium, Beijing, China, 2–5 November 2008; pp. 487–490. [CrossRef]
13. Bayram, B.; Yaralioglu, G.; Kupnik, M.; Ergun, A.; Oralkan, O.; Nikoozadeh, A.; Khuri-Yakub, B. Dynamic analysis of capacitive micromachined ultrasonic transducers. *IEEE Trans. Ultrason. Ferroelectr. Freq. Control* **2005**, *52*, 2270–2275. [CrossRef] [PubMed]
14. Khuri-Yakub, B.T.; Yaralioglu, G.G.; Bayram, B. 5F-3 Finite Element Analysis of CMUTS: Conventional vs. Collapse Operation Modes. In Proceedings of the 2006 IEEE Ultrasonics Symposium, Vancouver, BC, Canada, 2–6 October 2006; pp. 586–589. [CrossRef]
15. Jackson, J.D. *Classical Electrodynamics*, 3rd ed.; Wiley: Hoboken, NJ, USA, 1999; p. 808.
16. Apte, N.; Park, K.K.; Khuri-Yakub, B.T. Finite element analysis of CMUTs with pressurized cavities. In Proceedings of the 2012 IEEE International Ultrasonics Symposium, Dresden, Germany, 7–10 October 2012; pp. 979–982. [CrossRef]
17. Apte, N.; Park, K.K.; Nikoozadeh, A.; Khuri-Yakub, B.T. Bandwidth and sensitivity optimization in CMUTs for airborne applications. In Proceedings of the 2014 IEEE International Ultrasonics Symposium, Chicago, IL, USA, 3–6 September 2014; pp. 166–169. [CrossRef]
18. Ma, B.; Chang, C.; Oguz, H.K.; Firouzi, K.; Khuri-Yakub, B.T.; Lab, E.L.G. Multi-parameter optimization of vented CMUTs for airborne applications. In Proceedings of the 2017 IEEE International Ultrasonics Symposium (IUS), Washington, DC, USA, 6–9 September 2017; pp. 1–4. [CrossRef]
19. Lin, D.S.; Zhuang, X.; Wong, S.H.; Ergun, A.S.; Kupnik, M.; Khuri-Yakub, B.T. Characterization of fabrication related gap-height variations in capacitive micromachined ultrasonic transducers. In Proceedings of the IEEE Ultrasonics Symposium, New York, NY, USA, 28–31 October 2007. [CrossRef]
20. Knight, J.; McLean, J.; Degertekin, F.L. Low temperature fabrication of immersion capacitive micromachined ultrasonic transducers on silicon and dielectric substrates. *IEEE Trans. Ultrason. Ferroelectr. Freq. Control* **2004**, *51*, 1324–1333. [CrossRef]
21. Zahorian, J.; Hochman, M.; Xu, T.; Satir, S.; Gurun, G.; Karaman, M.; Degertekin, F.L. Monolithic CMUT-on-CMOS integration for intravascular ultrasound applications. *IEEE Trans. Ultrason. Ferroelectr. Freq. Control* **2011**, *58*, 2659–2667. [CrossRef] [PubMed]
22. Cheng, C.H.; Chow, E.M.; Jin, X.; Ergun, S.; Khuri-Yakub, B.T. An Efficient Electrical Addressing Method Using Through-Wafer Vias for Two-Dimensional Ultrasonic Arrays. In Proceedings of the IEEE International Ultrasonics Symposium (IUS), San Juan, PR, USA, 22–25 October 2000; pp. 1179–1182.
23. Wygant, I.O.; Zhuang, X.; Yeh, D.T.; Oralkan, O.; Ergun, A.S.; Karaman, M.; Khuri-Yakub, B.T. Integration of 2D CMUT arrays with front-end electronics for volumetric ultrasound imaging. *IEEE Trans. Ultrason. Ferroelectr. Freq. Control* **2008**, *55*, 327–342. [CrossRef] [PubMed]
24. Moini, A.; Nikoozadeh, A.; Choe, J.W.; Chang, C.; Stephens, D.N.; Sahn, D.J.; Khuri-Yakub, P.T. Fully integrated 2D CMUT ring arrays for endoscopic ultrasound. In Proceedings of the IEEE International Ultrasonics Symposium (IUS), Tours, France, 18–21 September 2016; pp. 3–6. [CrossRef]

25. Moini, A. Capacitive Micromachined Ultrasonic Transducer (CMUT) Arrays for Endoscopic Ultrasound. Ph.D. Thesis, Stanford University, Stanford, CA, USA, 2016.
26. Huang, Y.; Ergun, A.S.; Haeggstrom, E.; Khuri-Yakub, B.T. Fabrication of Capacitive Micromachined Ultrasonic Transducers (CMUTs) Using Wafer Bonding Technology for Low Frequency (10 kHz–150 kHz) Sonar Applications. In Proceedings of the IEEE Oceans, Biloxi, MI, USA, 29–31 October 2002; pp. 2322–2327.
27. Sarioglu, A.F.; Kupnik, M.; Vaithilingam, S.; Khuri-Yakub, B.T. Nanoscale Topography of Thermally-Grown Oxide Films at Right-Angled Convex Corners of Silicon. *J. Electrochem. Soc.* **2011**, *159*, H79–H84. [CrossRef]
28. Miki, N.; Spearing, S.M. Effect of nanoscale surface roughness on the bonding energy of direct-bonded silicon wafers. *J. Appl. Phys.* **2003**, *94*, 6800–6806. [CrossRef]
29. Logan, A.; Yeow, J.T.W. Fabricating capacitive micromachined ultrasonic transducers with a novel silicon-nitride-Based wafer bonding process. *IEEE Trans. Ultrason. Ferroelectr. Freq. Control* **2009**, *56*, 1074–1084. [CrossRef] [PubMed]
30. Park, K.K.; Lee, H.; Kupnik, M.; Khuri-Yakub, B.T. Fabrication of capacitive micromachined ultrasonic transducers via local oxidation and direct wafer bonding. *J. Microelectromech. Syst.* **2011**, *20*, 95–103. [CrossRef]
31. Molgaard, M.J.; Hansen, J.M.; Jakobsen, M.H.; Thomsen, E.V. Sensitivity Optimization of Wafer Bonded Gravimetric CMUT Sensors. *J. Microelectromech. Syst.* **2018**, *7*, 1089–1096. [CrossRef]
32. Kupnik, M.; Vaithilingam, S.; Torashima, K.; Wygant, I.O.; Khuri-Yakub, B.T. CMUT fabrication based on a thick buried oxide layer. In Proceedings of the IEEE Ultrasonics Symposium, San Diego, CA, USA, 11–14 October 2010. [CrossRef]
33. Ho, M.C.; Kupnik, M.; Park, K.K.; Khuri-Yakub, B.T. Long-term measurement results of pre-charged CMUTs with zero external bias operation. In Proceedings of the IEEE International Ultrasonics Symposium (IUS), Dresden, Germany, 7–10 October 2012. [CrossRef]
34. Xu, T.; Tekes, C.; Degertekin, F. CMUTs with high-K atomic layer deposition dielectric material insulation layer. *IEEE Trans. Ultrason. Ferroelectr. Freq. Control* **2014**, *61*, 2121–2131. [CrossRef] [PubMed]
35. Yamaner, F.Y.; Zhang, X.; Oralkan, O. A three-mask process for fabricating vacuum-sealed capacitive micromachined ultrasonic transducers using anodic bonding. *IEEE Trans. Ultrason. Ferroelectr. Freq. Control* **2015**, *62*, 972–982. [CrossRef] [PubMed]
36. Zhang, X.; Adelegan, O.; Yamaner, F.Y.; Oralkan, O. CMUTs on glass with ITO bottom electrodes for improved transparency. In Proceedings of the IEEE International Ultrasonics Symposium (IUS), Tours, France, 18–21 September 2016. [CrossRef]
37. Gerardo, C.D.; Cretu, E.; Rohling, R. Fabrication and testing of polymer-based capacitive micromachined ultrasound transducers for medical imaging. *Microsyst. Nanoeng.* **2018**, *4*, 19. [CrossRef]
38. Pang, D.C.; Chang, C.M. Development of a novel transparent flexible capacitive micromachined ultrasonic transducer. *Sensors* **2017**, *17*, 1443. [CrossRef] [PubMed]
39. Zhuang, X.; Lin, D.S.; Oralkan, O.; Khuri-Yakub, B.T. Fabrication of flexible transducer arrays with through-wafer electrical interconnects based on trench refilling with PDMS. *J. Microelectromechan. Syst.* **2008**, *17*, 446–452. [CrossRef]
40. Wang, J.; Memon, F.; Touma, G.; Baltsavias, S.; Jang, J.H.; Chang, C.; Rasmussen, M.F.; Olcott, E.; Jeffrey, R.B.; Arbabian, A.; et al. Capsule ultrasound device: Characterization and testing results. In Proceedings of the 2017 IEEE International Ultrasonics Symposium (IUS), Washington, DC, USA, 6–9 September 2017; pp. 1–4. [CrossRef]
41. Wygant, I.O.; Kupnik, M.; Khuri-Yakub, B.T. Analytically Calculating Membrane Displacement and the Equivalent Circuit Model of a Circular CMUT Cell. In Proceedings of the IEEE International Ultrasonics Symposium (IUS), Beijing, China, 2–5 November 2008; pp. 2111–2114.
42. Huang, Y.; Zhuang, X.; Hæggstrom, E.O.; Ergun, A.S.; Cheng, C.H.; Khuri-Yakub, B. Capacitive micromachined ultrasonic transducers with piston-shaped membranes: Fabrication and experimental characterization. *IEEE Trans. Ultrason. Ferroelectr. Freq. Control* **2009**, *56*, 136–145. [CrossRef] [PubMed]

43. Yoon, H.S.; Ho, M.C.; Apte, N.; Cristman, P.; Vaithilingam, S.; Kupnik, M.; Butts-Pauly, K.; Khuri-Yakub, B.T. Fabrication of CMUT cells with gold center mass for higher output pressure. *AIP Conf. Proc.* **2011**, *1359*, 183. [CrossRef]
44. Nikoozadeh, A.; Khuri-Yakub, B. CMUT with substrate-embedded springs for non-flexural plate movement. In Proceedings of the IEEE Ultrasonics Symposium, San Diego, CA, USA, 11–14 October 2010. [CrossRef]
45. Lee, B.C.; Nikoozadeh, A.; Park, K.K.; Khuri-Yakub, B.T. Non- flexural parallel piston movement across CMUT with substrate-embedded springs. In Proceedings of the IEEE International Ultrasonics Symposium, Chicago, IL, USA, 3–6 September 2014; pp. 591–594. [CrossRef]
46. Daft, C.; Wagner, P.; Panda, S.; Ladabaum, I. Elevation beam profile control with bias polarity patterns applied to microfabricated ultrasound transducers. In Proceedings of the IEEE Symposium on Ultrasonics, Honolulu, HI, USA, 5–8 October 2003; pp. 1578–1581. [CrossRef]
47. Gurun, G.; Hasler, P.; Degertekin, F.L. Front-end receiver electronics for high-frequency monolithic CMUT-on-CMOS imaging arrays. *IEEE Trans. Ultrason. Ferroelectr. Freq. Control* **2011**, *58*, 1658–1668. [CrossRef] [PubMed]
48. Gurun, G.; Tekes, C.; Zahorian, J.; Xu, T.; Satir, S.; Karaman, M.; Hasler, J.; Degertekin, F.L. Single-Chip CMUT-on-CMOS Front-End System for Real-Time Volumetric IVUS and ICE Imaging. *IEEE Trans. Ultrason. Ferroelectr. Freq. Control* **2014**, *61*, 239–250. [CrossRef] [PubMed]
49. Lu, Y.; Tang, H.; Fung, S.; Wang, Q.; Tsai, J.M.; Daneman, M.; Boser, B.E.; Horsley, D.A. Ultrasonic fingerprint sensor using a piezoelectric micromachined ultrasonic transducer array integrated with complementary metal oxide semiconductor electronics. *Appl. Phys. Lett.* **2015**, *106*, 263503. [CrossRef]
50. Jiang, X.; Lu, Y.; Tang, H.Y.; Tsai, J.M.; Ng, E.J.; Daneman, M.J.; Boser, B.E.; Horsley, D.A. Monolithic ultrasound fingerprint sensor. *Microsyst. Nanoeng.* **2017**, *3*, 17059. [CrossRef]
51. Tsuji, Y.; Kupnik, M.; Khuri-Yakub, B.T. Low temperature process for CMUT fabrication with wafer bonding technique. In Proceedings of the IEEE Ultrasonics Symposium, San Diego, CA, USA, 11–14 October 2010; pp. 551–554. [CrossRef]
52. Oralkan, O.; Ergun, A.S.; Cheng, C.H.; Johnson, J.A.; Karaman, M.; Lee, T.H.; Khuri-Yakub, B.T. Volumetric ultrasound imaging using 2-D CMUT arrays. *IEEE Trans. Ultrason. Ferroelectr. Freq. Control* **2003**, *50*, 1581–1594. [CrossRef] [PubMed]
53. Wildes, D.; Lee, W.; Haider, B.; Cogan, S.; Sundaresan, K.; Mills, D.M.; Yetter, C.; Hart, P.H.; Haun, C.R.; Concepcion, M.; et al. 4-D ICE: A 2-D Array Transducer with Integrated ASIC in a 10-Fr Catheter for Real-Time 3-D Intracardiac Echocardiography. *IEEE Trans. Ultrason. Ferroelectr. Freq. Control* **2016**, *63*, 2159–2173. [CrossRef] [PubMed]
54. Chen, C.; Chen, Z.; Bera, D.; Raghunathan, S.B.; Shabanimotlagh, M.; Noothout, E.; Chang, Z.Y.; Ponte, J.; Prins, C.; Vos, H.J.; et al. A Front-End ASIC with Receive Sub-array Beamforming Integrated with a 32 × 32 PZT Matrix Transducer for 3-D Transesophageal Echocardiography. *IEEE J. Solid-State Circuits* **2017**, *52*, 994–1006. [CrossRef]
55. Savoia, A.S.; Caliano, G.; Pappalardo, M. A CMUT probe for medical ultrasonography: From microfabrication to system integration. *IEEE Trans. Ultrason. Ferroelectr. Freq. Control* **2012**, *59*, 1127–1138. [CrossRef] [PubMed]
56. Maxim Integrated. MAX4805 Octal High-Voltage-Protected, Low-Power, Low-Noise Operational Amplifiers. 2010. Available online: https://datasheets.maximintegrated.com/en/ds/MAX4805-MAX4805A.pdf (accessed on 11 January 2019).
57. Sautto, M.; Savoia, A.S.; Quaglia, F.; Caliano, G.; Mazzanti, A. A comparative analysis of CMUT receiving architectures for the design optimization of integrated transceiver front ends. *IEEE Trans. Ultrason. Ferroelectr. Freq. Control* **2017**, *64*, 826–838. [CrossRef] [PubMed]
58. Sampaleanu, A.; Zhang, P.; Kshirsagar, A.; Moussa, W.; Zemp, J. Top-Orthogonal-to-Bottom-Electrode (TOBE) CMUT Arrays for 3-D Ultrasound Imaging. *IEEE Trans. Ultrason. Ferroelectr. Freq. Control* **2014**, *61*, 885–3010. [CrossRef] [PubMed]

59. Christiansen, T.L.; Rasmussen, M.F.; Bagge, J.P.; Moesner, L.N.; Jensen, J.A.; Thomsen, E.V. 3-D imaging using row-column-addressed arrays with integrated apodization-part ii: Transducer fabrication and experimental results. *IEEE Trans. Ultrason. Ferroelectr. Freq. Control* **2015**, *62*, 959–971. [CrossRef] [PubMed]
60. Seo, C.H.; Yen, J.T. A 256 × 256 2-D array transducer with row-column addressing for 3-D rectilinear imaging. *IEEE Trans. Ultrason. Ferroelectr. Freq. Control* **2009**, *56*, 837–847. [CrossRef] [PubMed]
61. Yen, J.T.; Seo, C.H.; Awad, S.I.; Jeong, J.S. A dual-layer transducer array for 3-D rectilinear imaging. *IEEE Trans. Ultrason. Ferroelectr. Freq. Control* **2009**, *56*, 204–212. [CrossRef] [PubMed]
62. Logan, A.S.; Wong, L.L.P.; Chen, A.I.H.; Yeow, J.T.W. A 32 × 32 element row-column addressed capacitive micromachined ultrasonic transducer. *IEEE Trans. Ultrason. Ferroelectr. Freq. Control* **2011**, *58*, 1266–1271. [CrossRef] [PubMed]
63. Nikoozadeh, A.; Choe, J.W.; Kothapalli, S.r.; Moini, A.; Sanjani, S.S.; Kamaya, A.; Gambhir, S.S.; Khuri-yakub, P.T. Photoacoustic Imaging Using a 9F MicroLinear CMUT ICE Catheter. In Proceedings of the IEEE International Ultrasonics Symposium, Dresden, Germany, 7–10 October 2012.
64. Stephens, D.N.; Truong, U.T.; Nikoozadeh, A.; Oralkan, O.; Seo, C.H.; Cannata, J.; Dentinger, A.; Thomenius, K.; Rama, A.d.l.; Nguyen, T.; et al. First In Vivo Use of a Capacitive Micromachined Ultrasound Transducer Array—Based Imaging. *J. Ultrasound Med.* **2012**, *31*, 247–256. [CrossRef] [PubMed]
65. Lim, J.; Tekes, C.; Degertekin, F.L.; Ghovanloo, M. Towards a Reduced-Wire Interface for CMUT-Based Intravascular Ultrasound Imaging Systems. *IEEE Trans. Biomed. Circuits Syst.* **2017**, *11*, 400–410. [CrossRef] [PubMed]
66. Moini, A.; Nikoozadeh, A.; Choe, J.W.; Khuri-Yakub, B.T.; Chang, C.; Stephens, D.; Smith, L.S.; Sahn, D. Fabrication, Packaging, and Catheter Assembly of 2D CMUT Arrays for Endoscopic Ultrasound and Cardiac Imaging. In Proceedings of the ASME 2015 International Technical Conference, San Francisco, CA, USA, 6–9 July 2015; p. V003T07A008. [CrossRef]
67. Jung, G.; Tekes, C.; Rashid, M.W.; Carpenter, T.; Cowell, D.; Freear, S.; Degertekin, L.; Ghovanloo, M. A Reduced-Wire ICE Catheter ASIC with Tx Beamforming and Rx Time-Division Multiplexing. *IEEE Trans. Biomed. Circuits Syst.* **2018**, *12*, 1246–1255. [CrossRef] [PubMed]
68. Chen, K.; Lee, H.S.; Chandrakasan, A.P.; Sodini, C.G. Ultrasonic imaging transceiver design for cmut: A three-level 30-vpp pulse-shaping pulser with improved efficiency and a noise-optimized receiver. *IEEE J. Solid-State Circuits* **2013**, *48*, 2734–2745. [CrossRef]
69. Memon, F.; Touma, G.; Wang, J.; Baltsavias, S.; Moini, A.; Chang, C.; Rasmussen, M.; Nikoozadeh, A.; Choe, J.; Arbabian, A.; et al. Capsule ultrasound device. In Proceedings of the 2015 IEEE International Ultrasonics Symposium (IUS 2015), Taipei, Taiwan, 21–24 October 2015. [CrossRef]
70. Memon, F.; Touma, G.; Wang, J.; Baltsavias, S.; Moini, A.; Chang, C.; Rasmussen, M.; Nikoozadeh, A.; Choe, J.; Olcott, E.; et al. Capsule ultrasound device: Further developments. In Proceedings of the IEEE International Ultrasonics Symposium (IUS), Tours, France, 18–21 September 2016. [CrossRef]
71. Jang, J.H.; Rasmussen, M.F.; Bhuyan, A.; Yoon, H.S.; Moini, A.; Chang, C.; Ronald, D.; Choe, J.W.; Nikoozadeh, A. Dual-Mode Integrated Circuit for Imaging and HIFU With 2-D CMUT Arrays. In Proceedings of the IEEE International Ultrasonics Symposium (IUS), Taipei, Taiwan, 21–24 October 2015; pp. 1–4.
72. Jang, J.H.; Chang, C.; Rasmussen, M.; Moini, A.; Brenner, K.; Stephens, D.; Oralkan, O.; Khuri-Yakub, B. Integration of a dual-mode catheter for ultrasound image guidance and HIFU ablation using a 2-D CMUT array. In Proceedings of the IEEE International Ultrasonics Symposium (IUS), Washington, DC, USA, 6–9 September 2017; pp. 1–4. [CrossRef]
73. Butterfly Network. 2019. Available online: www.butterflynetwork.com/clinical/ob (accessed on 11 January 2019).
74. Kennedy, J.E. High-intensity focused ultrasound in the treatment of solid tumours. *Nat. Rev. Cancer* **2005**, *5*, 321. [CrossRef] [PubMed]
75. Dubinsky, T.J.; Cuevas, C.; Dighe, M.K.; Kolokythas, O.; Joo, H.H. High-intensity focused ultrasound: Current potential and oncologic applications. *Am. J. Roentgenol.* **2008**, *190*, 191–199. [CrossRef] [PubMed]

76. Sanghvi, N.T. Noninvasive surgery of prostate tissue by high-intensity focused ultrasound. *IEEE Trans. Ultrason. Ferroelectr. Freq. Control* **1996**, *43*, 1099–1110. [CrossRef]
77. Choe, J.W.; Oralkan, O.; Nikoozadeh, A.; Gencel, M.; Stephens, D.N.; O'Donnell, M.; Sahn, D.J.; Khuri-Yakub, B.T. Volumetric real-time imaging using a CMUT ring array. *IEEE Trans. Ultrason. Ferroelectr. Freq. Control* **2012**, *59*, 1201–1211. [CrossRef] [PubMed]

13

Design and Fabrication of a Push-Pull Electrostatic Actuated Cantilever Waveguide Scanner

Wei-Chih Wang [1,2,3,4,*], Kebin Gu [1] and ChiLeung Tsui [2]

1. Department of Mechanical Engineering, University of Washington, Seattle, WA 98185, USA
2. Department of Electrical and Computer Engineering, University of Washington, Seattle, WA 98185, USA
3. Institute of Nanoengineering and Microsystems, National Tsinghua University, Hsinchu 300, Taiwan
4. Department of Power Mechanical Engineering, National Tsinghua University, Hsinchu 300, Taiwan

* Correspondence: abong@u.washington.edu

Abstract: The paper presents a novel fully integrated MEMS-based non-resonating operated 2D mechanical scanning system using a 1D push-pull actuator. Details of the design, fabrication and tests performed are presented. The current design utilizes an integrated electrostatic push-pull actuator and a SU-8 rib waveguide with a large core cross section (4 μm in height and 20 μm in width) in broadband single mode operation (λ = 0.4 μm to 0.65 μm). We have successfully demonstrated a 2D scanning motion using non- resonating operation with 201 Hz in vertical direction and 20 Hz in horizontal direction. This non-resonating scanner system has achieved a field of view (FOV) of 0.019 to 0.072 radians in vertical and horizontal directions, with the advantage of overcoming its frequency shift caused by fabrication uncertainties. In addition, we observed two fundamental resonances at 201 and 536 Hz in the vertical and horizontal directions with corresponding displacements of 130 and 19 μm, or 0.072 and 0.0105 radian field of view operating at a +150 V input. A gradient index (GRIN) lens is placed at the end of the waveguide to focus the diverging beam output from the waveguide and a 20 μm beam diameter is observed at the focal plane. The transmission efficiency of the waveguide is slightly low (~10%) and slight tensile residual stress can be observed at the cantilever portion of the waveguide due to inherent imperfections in the fabrication process.

Keywords: cantilever waveguide; electrostatic actuator; non-resonating scanner; optical scanner; push-pull actuator; rib waveguide

---

1. Introduction

Modern day micro-scale imaging and display systems utilizes miniature scanner technologies for capturing images and displaying high density information in a small working environment. Advanced imaging systems, such as scanning confocal microscopy use micro scale scanners for real-time sub-cellular resolution imaging [1–4]. Portable video projection systems use miniature scanners for displaying high resolution contents with a light-weight form factor and low power requirement. [5–9]. Virtual displays found in head-mounted displays (HMD) systems uses scanners to display large amount of information in a small display area for augmented reality/virtual reality applications [10–14]. Most of the miniature scanner system utilizes MEMS scanning mirrors, which requires the mirrors and the deflecting components to be significantly larger than the input beam diameter to avoid clipping or creating additional diffractions at the output. Furthermore, the size of the conventional display system is proportional to the resolution and/or the field of view (FOV) of the device, which severely limits the possibility of reducing system footprint without making a compromise on the device specification.

To overcome the minimum size restrictions of mirror-based scanner systems without sacrificing resolution and FOV, an optical scanner based on an electromechanically deflected micro-fabricated waveguide has been previously developed by our research team [15–20]. A pair of commercially available lead zirconate titanate (Pb[Zr(x)Ti(1-x)]O3) (PZT) actuators drives the 2D motion of the waveguide. The design is able to steer the coupled optical beam via the deflection of the waveguide; however, the design still has a relatively large footprint (each actuator is 20 mm × 4.8 mm × 0.6 mm and they are arranged perpendicularly) compared to its output beam deflection angle. Also, the assembly process is challenging, time consuming, and inconsistent due to the combined use of off-the-shelf parts and micro-fabricated waveguide. The output of the scanner is also inconsistent after each system reset due to the assembly process.

In this paper, design improvements to the micro-fabricated waveguide system is presented (Figure 1). To increase the robustness of the scanner system in the new design, a MEMS-based push-pull actuator is fully integrated with the micro-fabricated waveguide. The integrated actuator reduces the rigid length of the device and increases the flexibility of the overall system, allowing it to work in tight spaces without invading the surroundings. The new design also allows the incorporation of the light source and the scanner probe in a single package, thus reducing the overall system size. Compared to off-the-shelf actuators, the MEMS-based push-pull actuator provides a better signal to noise ratio and consumes relatively lower power during operations. Finally, the push-pull actuator mechanism will be able to provide a 2D scanning motion via 1D actuation, which reduces the complexity of the scanner and the footprint of the entire system.

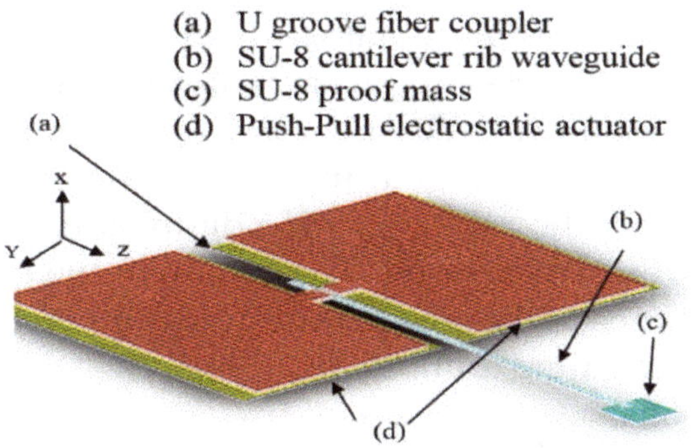

Figure 1. Schematic of the electrostatic MEMS scanner.

Most of the resonant scanner designs reported so far, including our previous designs, operate at resonance to achieve high line resolution and high FOV [15–22]. However, this design presents several challenges, such as achieving a large frequency difference between the two resonant operating frequencies. A larger deflection angle of the high-frequency mode is usually harder to achieve due to damping in the system. In addition, reducing the frequency of the low-frequency mode would require altering materials or geometry of the scanner. Thus, frequency reduction can only be achieved by sacrificing the device compactness [15]. Furthermore, the final frequency of operation is highly dependent on the fabrication process.

In this paper, we report a new driving scheme that can potentially overcome the above issues by operating one of the two directions at an extremely low non-resonant frequency (>20 fps) while maintaining a high resonant frequency in the other direction. The non-resonant frequency operation relaxes the restriction of the lower operating frequency and further improves the operating condition. The high resolution of the device can then be obtained through the large difference of the two operation frequencies. The deflection angle or FOV can also be optimized. In the following section, we will first examine the design and operational principles of this novel scanner through finite element analysis (FEA) using ANSYS (ANSYS, Canonsburg, PA., USA), CoventorWare and Rsoft (RSoft Design Group, Inc., Ossining, NY, USA) followed by a description of the fabrication process and results from the optical performance.

2. Design and Operation Principles

2.1. Operation Principles

The design of the scanner uses the 1D actuation of a pair of "push–pull" actuators to generate 2D scanning motion on a micro-fabricated cantilever waveguide (Figure 1). For image acquisition, the same scanning waveguide is used to capture and channel the backscattered to a photodetector. For display operation, this step is not needed. A long, slender SU-8 structure is placed between the two actuators to serve as the waveguide for the scanner. A coupler is placed at the input end of the SU-8 waveguide to couple the light from an optical fiber to the cantilever waveguide. The optical fiber is placed in a U-shape fiber groove to properly align it with the coupler. A proof mass is attached at the output end of the SU-8 waveguide for reducing the tip displacement of the microfabricated SU-8 waveguide without affecting the output beam deflection angle. The waveguide structure is connected to the actuators by the rotating arm. The two ends (in the z-direction) of rectangular-shaped actuating pads in Figure 1 are anchored to the substrate leaving the middle of the actuator suspended and connected to the rotating arm. This push-pull actuator configuration can be used with piezoelectric, electrostatic, electromagnetic, or magnetostrictive actuation methods. In this paper, a parallel-plate MEMS electrostatic actuator is presented.

The basic operating principle of this 2D scanner is shown in Figure 2 [22]. The scanner motion is generated by the pair of push-pull electrostatic actuators. The out-of-plane buckling of the four actuating pads generates bending and twisting motion on the rotating arm. The resulting bending and twisting on the rotating arm causes the attached waveguide to move in or out of plane. For out-of-plane waveguide motion (Figure 2a), actuator pads 1 and 2 (or actuator pads 3 and 4) must be actuated in the same direction, magnitude and phase. This will create vertical motion at the rotating arm due to the actuators hinging on the fixed ends. For horizontal waveguide motion (Figure 2b), actuator pads 1 and 3 (or actuator pad 2 and 4) must be driven in the same direction, magnitude and phase. This will produce rock the rotating arm side to side, causing the waveguide to move horizontally. The simultaneous excitation of the waveguide in the horizontal and vertical direction with the superposition of waveforms at the correctly designed frequencies and/or phase will drive the waveguide in Lissajou or raster scanning motion.

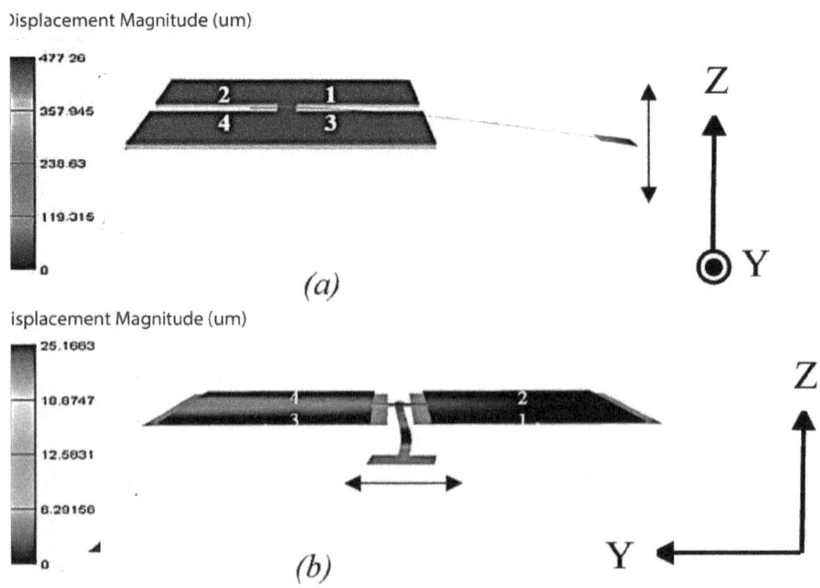

Figure 2. ANSYS harmonic virtualization of a mechanical resonating scanner. (**a**) Low-frequency motion under the excitation of the first mode along the z-axis, and (**b**) high-frequency motion under the excitation of the second mode along the y-axis.

Lissajou and raster scanning pattern is used instead of spiral scanning pattern due to the geometry of the micro-fabricated waveguide. The high aspect ratio of the rectangular cross-sectioned beam (cross-section width is ~5 times its thickness) makes it difficult to achieve spiral scanning motion. For spiral scanning pattern, a circular cladded waveguide is the preferred geometry, which is challenging to fabricated using the planar process in typical micro-fabrication. Additionally, a comparative large cladding (>50 μm) is required to confine the wave and maintains a single mode operation at the require geometry (~few μm for the core) in a waveguide with uniform cladding. Thus, to eliminate the need of a large cladding to create a waveguide core that has similar size to an optical fiber core, the rib waveguide geometry is employed in our design. The rib waveguide is a two-layer waveguide structure that consists of a rib layer on top of a wider slab layer, and the careful optimization of the geometric ratio between the two layer is necessary to achieve the desirable mechanical performance and optical output.

2.2. Mechanical Design and Simulation

The scanning FOV and line resolution are two critical parameters that needs to be studied to optimize the scanner system performance. A large FOV can be obtained when the displacement and the angle of rotation for the waveguide is maximized at its resonant frequencies and higher line resolution can be achieved by increasing the ratio of the horizontal and vertical operating frequencies. Thus, the design of the scanner needs to allow the system to operate at two distinctly different resonant frequencies in the horizontal and vertical directions.

The components of the system were analyzed individually to obtain optimized dimensions for achieving the best line resolution and FOV. The critical parameters that needed to be analyzed were (1) length, width, and height of the proof mass, (2) the width, thickness, and length of the waveguide, and (3) the geometry, layout, and input voltage of the actuator. Both analytical and numerical analyses were performed and compared.

The modified parallel plate actuator was used in the scanner design. The conventional capacitive actuator was either a set of parallel plates or a set of comb drives [23]. However, the driving force was dominant in one direction and negligible in the other two directions. Figure 3 shows the modified actuator design with the extended bottom electrode. The non-equivalent electrodes increase the utilization of electrostatic fringe effect. Therefore, a larger in-plane electrostatic force was generated in the y direction. The FEM results show that an input of 20 V to the modified actuator results in a 27.66 μN out-of-plane reaction force (Fz). In the two in-plane directions, Fy was 8.64×10^{-2} μN, which was over two orders of magnitude larger than Fx of 1.92×10^{-4} μN. The model used slightly different dimensions to generate the subsequent FEM harmonic response of the scanner.

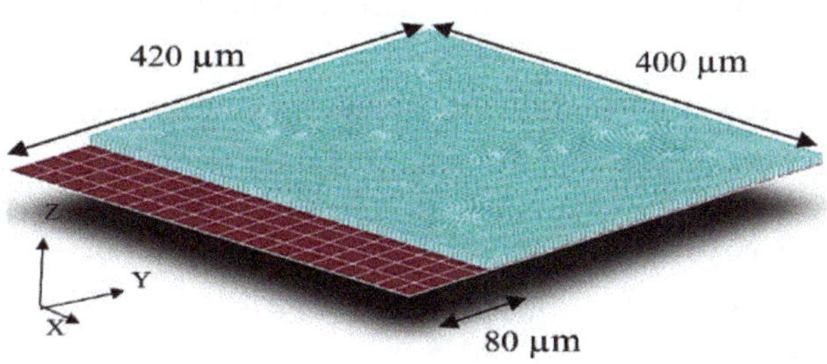

Figure 3. The modified parallel plate actuator. The bottom electrode is expanded along the y-axis so that the fringe effect causes larger electrostatic force in the y direction than in the x direction.

For the cantilever waveguide mechanical model, both analytical and numerical analyses were performed. The analytical model uses the Timoshenko beam model to estimate the deflection angle of the cantilever waveguide (Figure 4a). Figure 4b shows the free-body diagram of an element of a beam, where M(x,t) is the bending moment; V(x,t) is the shear force; w(x,t) is the displacement of the vibration; and f(x,t) is the external force per unit length.

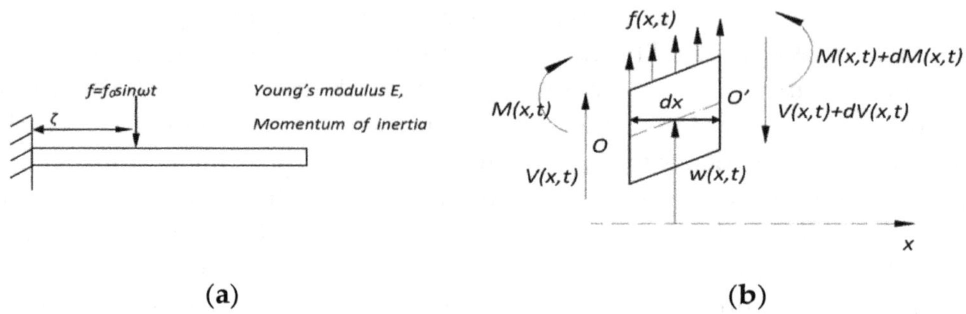

Figure 4. (**a**) A beam is subject to the external force f and (**b**) free-body diagram of an element of a beam.

The displacement of the beam can be determined using the mode superposition principle and is written as [24]:

$$w(x,t) = \sum_{n=1}^{\infty} W_n(x) q_n(t), \tag{1}$$

where $W_n(x)$ is the n-th normalized mode shape and $q_n(t)$ is the generalized coordinate in the n-th mode. For the fixed-free boundary condition as shown in Figure 4a, $W_n(x)$ and $q_n(t)$ can be calculated in (2) and (3), respectively [24]:

$$W_n(x) = C_n[\sin\beta_n x - \sinh\beta_n x - \alpha_n(\cos\beta_n x - \cosh\beta_n x)] \tag{2}$$

$$\begin{aligned} \frac{d^2 q_n(t)}{dt^2} + {\omega_n}^2 q_n(t) &= \int f_0 \delta(x-\zeta) \sin\omega t W_n(x) dx \\ &= f_0 \sin\omega t W_n(\zeta) \end{aligned}, \tag{3}$$

where

$$\beta_n{}^4 = \frac{{\omega_n}^2}{c^2} = \frac{\rho A {\omega_n}^2}{EI}$$

$$\alpha_n = \frac{\sin\beta_n l + \sinh\beta_n l}{\cos\beta_n l + \cosh\beta_n l}.$$

$W_n(x)$ is determined by boundary conditions, material properties and resonant frequencies. $q_n(t)$ is subject to the change of the external force f and $W_n(\zeta)$. To achieve large deflection angle which is proportional to $dw(x,t)/dx$, the most straightforward strategy is to increase f_0 and $W_n(\zeta)$:

1. f_o can be increased by increasing the driving electrostatic force.
2. To increase $W_n(\zeta)$, if the device is operating at the first resonance frequency, $W(x)$ increases as x increases. ζ should be far away the fixed end to increase $W_n(\zeta)$. However, due to the limitation of the overall length of the MEMS device, ζ cannot be too far from the fixed end. If the device is operating at the higher resonant frequency, the force should not be applied to the nodal point, where $W_n(\zeta)$ is equal to zero.

The overall scanner design was also analyzed numerically using Architect3D in CoventorWare for optimization. The system-level model method can significantly reduce the simulation time compared to traditional finite element methods (FEM) while maintaining relatively high accuracy. The schematic layout modeled in Architect3D and the corresponding 3D model is shown in Figure 5, it included components such as beams, beams with electrodes, rigid plate, anchors, bus connectors, reference frames and signal sources. These components modeled the mechanical and electrical behaviors of the scanner during the optimization process.

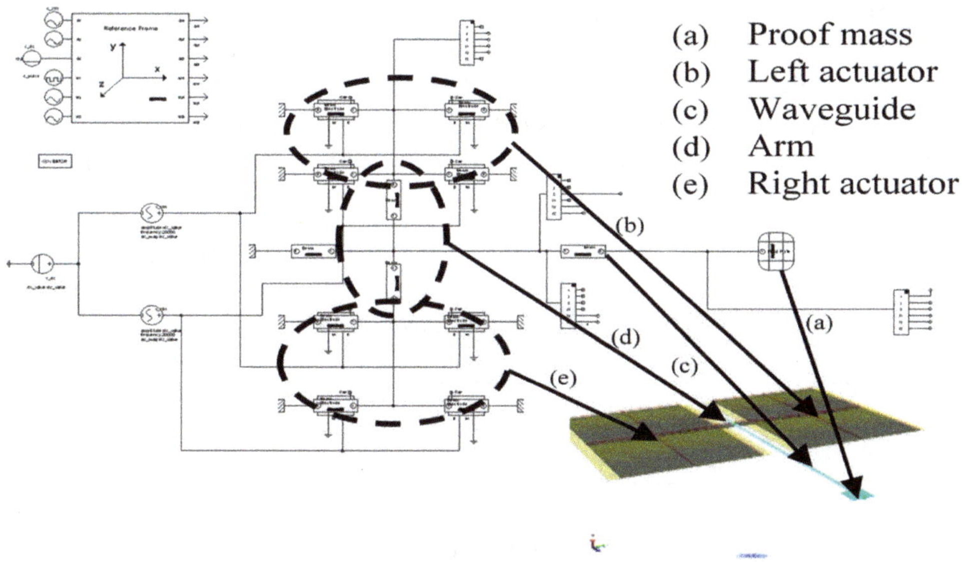

Figure 5. The 3D physical geometry of the scanner mapped to the corresponding behavior symbols.

The optimization of the scanner involved tuning the devices parameters so that the FOV and the line resolution of the scanners are optimized. The line resolution of the device is maximized by increasing the difference between the two operation frequencies.

The resonant frequency of the high-frequency mode was designed so that it was 200 times larger than the resonant frequency of the low-frequency mode in order to obtain the highest scanning resolution. In our current experimental setup, it was difficult to drive a device above 20 kHz. Therefore, resonant frequency of the low-frequency mode was limited to less than 100 Hz. The field of view was maximized for the scanning direction that operates at the lower resonant frequency.

The resonant frequency of a cantilever beam is a function of its mass and spring constant, thus the operating frequency can be reduced by increasing the length of the waveguide or by incorporating a large proof mass. However, a waveguide design with excessive length is going to compromise the compactness of the device. Therefore, the final design for the length and width of the waveguide is 2250 μm and 55 μm, respectively, and the size of proof mass is 300 μm × 300 μm × 24 μm. The thickness of the slab and the ridge are both 2 μm. The modal analysis results obtained from Architect are verified by FEM and analytical results (Table 1) and the rotational angle for each of the obtained modes is optimized.

Table 1. Resonant frequencies obtained by analytical estimation, finite element methods (FEM), and Architect3D.

		Analytical	**FEM**	**Architect3D**
X-axis	1st	58.5	58.3	55.9
	2nd	743	630	707
Y-axis	1st	1113	1103	1062

Unit for frequency measurements is in Hz.

The harmonic response of the scanner design is studied by applying electrostatic actuation to excite vertical (at lower operating frequency) and horizontal motion (at higher operating frequency) in the waveguide as shown in Figure 2. Air damping factor is also applied to the simulation based on the measurement from a fiber viscometer [25]. The rotational angle response for the waveguide motion in both directions are shown in Figure 6. For vertical motion (the top trace), two rotational angle peaks are observed. To maximize the FOV, the lower frequency (55.9 Hz) is chosen as the designed operating frequency with a rotational angle of 0.44 rad. In the vertical direction, two peaks are also observed in the response (the middle trace) and the 12,775 Hz peak is chosen as the high-frequency mode (rotational angle is 0.089 rad) to maximize the line resolution. The bottom trace shows the deflection response of the electrodes and it can be observed that the electrodes achieves a maximum of 4.27 μm at the high frequency operation mode. This means that the actuators are able to operate without interference with the designed gap space (20 μm) between the parallel plates.

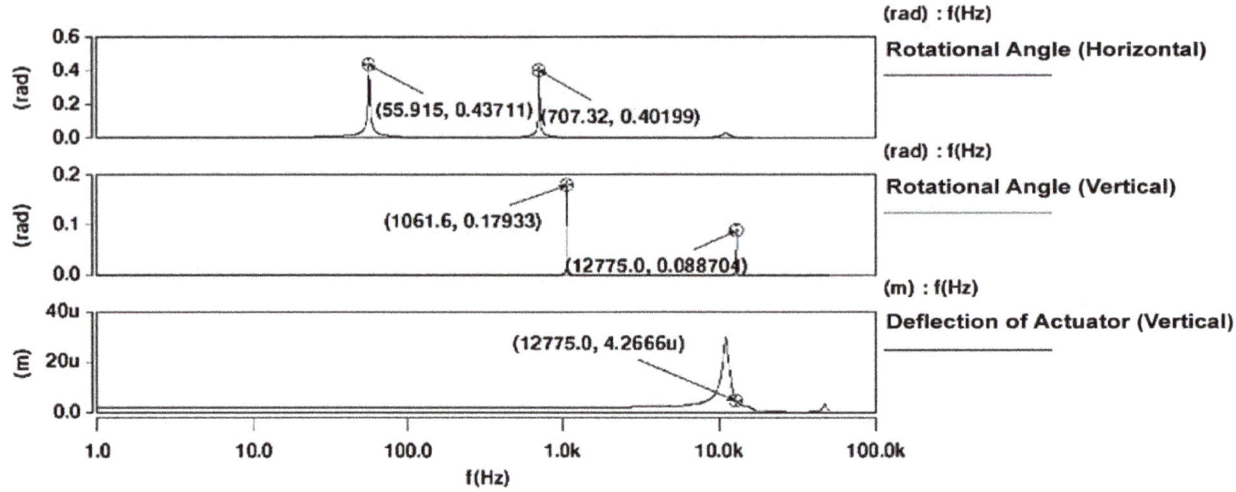

Figure 6. Architect3D in CoventorWare simulation results: (**top** and **middle**): deflection angle as a function of frequency and (**bottom**): deflection response of the actuator.

Although the simulation shows promising line resolution and FOV, there were challenges found in fabrication and in tests performed of the resonating design. The main obstacle is apparently on overcoming the weight of the proof mass at the tip of the cantilever. It was found later that SU-8 cantilever is much softer than the model based on the published material properties. Several design changes were made including the proof mass thickness and the no-resonating design to further simplify the fabrication and operation.

For the non-resonating scanner design, the same parametric study to optimize the design was also performed using Architect3D in CoventorWare. The modified actuator shown in Figure 7 is used to increase the in-plane electrostatic force, leading to a larger FOV. When the device is in operation, Electrode 1 and 3 are applied with the same waveform function of $V_0 sin\omega t$ and Electrode 2 and 4 are applied with a $V_0 cos\omega t$, where ω is the resonant frequency of the high-frequency mode and V_o is the amplitude of the input voltage. For low frequency direction, all electrodes were driven by a same wave function with lower frequency. Suppose the waveguide is simultaneously driven at the above two frequencies, a raster scanning motion will appear at the distal end.

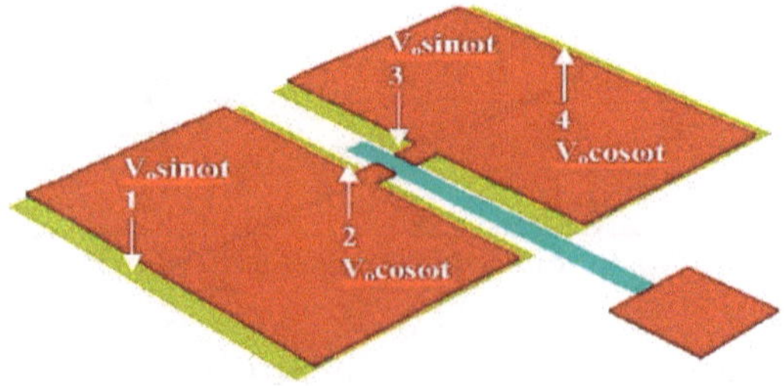

Figure 7. The optimized scanner design with a proof mass of 60 μm × 60 μm × 4 μm, waveguide length of 1820 μm and a width of the slab of 20 μm.

The result of the deflection angles of the optimized scanner is shown in Figure 8. The simulation shows that when the device is operating at 10 Hz in the non-resonant frequency direction (vertical direction) and 1.343 kHz in the resonant frequency direction (horizontal direction), the FOV are 16 and 15 mrad, respectively and a 130-line resolution at 0.08 Rayleigh damping and ±20 V input.

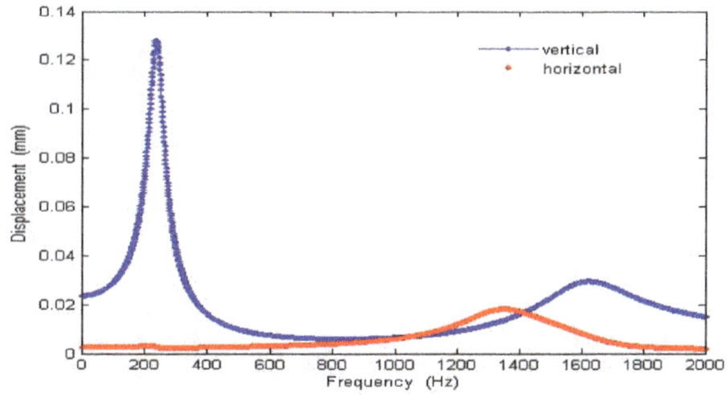

Figure 8. ANSYS Workbench harmonic responses of the optimized design with 60 μm × 60 μm × 4 μm proof mass, 1820 μm waveguide length and 20 μm slab width.

The reduction in the proof mass from 300 μm × 300 μm × 24 μm in resonating design to 60 μm × 60 μm × 4 μm in non-resonating design was needed to simplify the fabrication and also to prevent the cantilever from bending too much due to the additional weight (Figure 19a). The width of the waveguide was also reduced from 55 to 20 μm to increase vibration in the horizontal direction.

In the parametric study, the geometry of the waveguide (the cross section and the length) dominated the line resolution of the scanner; the resolution increased with a flatter and shorter waveguide. The rib waveguide had a very similar resonant frequency response as long as the dimensions of the width of the ridge section were kept relatively small compared to the width of the slab section (<4×). All other geometric parameters did not appear to affect the line resolution significantly. In the analyses for the actuator and arm geometries, larger actuator pads allowed larger actuation; however, the sizes of the pads are limited by the design footprint (3 mm × 3 mm) defined for the previous endoscopic application. The largest angle of rotation achieved by the investigated push–pull designs was ~0.44 and 0.089 rad in vertical and horizontal direction respectively (for the resonating design) and 71 and 15 mrad, for the non-resonating design A shorter rotating arm appears to provide a larger angle of rotation. These findings suggest that the waveguide and the actuator layout can be considered separately to optimize the line resolution and scanning magnitude as we have shown in the analysis.

2.3. Optical Analysis

To optimize the light transmission and coupling between the tip of the input fiber and the cantilever beam requires modal analysis and investigation of the system's coupling efficiency. The waveguide for the scanner has a rib waveguide feature (Figure 9), and it is made of an epoxy-based SU-8 negative-tone photoresist. The wavelength range required for the proposed display application is 400 to 650 nm. The final dimension of the waveguide structure was slightly different from the mechanical simulation. The slab was reduced to 20 microns and the proof mass also reduced to 60 μm × 60 μm × 4 μm to simplify the fabrication and improve dynamic performance of the cantilever vibration. One way to predict the dimensions of the rib waveguide structure was based on the single mode conditions proposed by Soref [26].

$$\frac{H}{\lambda}\sqrt{n_f^2 - n_s^2} \geq 1 \tag{4}$$

$$0.5 \leq r \equiv \frac{h}{H} < 1 \tag{5}$$

$$\frac{a}{b} = \frac{W}{H} \leq \left(\frac{q + 4\pi b}{4\pi b}\right)\frac{1 + 0.3\sqrt{\left(\frac{q+4\pi b}{q+4\pi rb}\right)^2 - 1}}{\sqrt{\left(\frac{q+4\pi b}{q+4\pi rb}\right)^2 - 1}}, \tag{6}$$

where q is defined as:

$$q = \frac{\gamma_c}{\sqrt{n_f^2 - n_c^2}} + \frac{\gamma_s}{\sqrt{n_f^2 - n_s^2}}, \tag{7}$$

where $\gamma_c = \gamma_s = 1$ for transverse electric (TE) modes and $\gamma_c = \frac{n_c^2}{n_f^2}$ and $\gamma_s = \frac{n_s^2}{n_f^2}$ for TM modes.

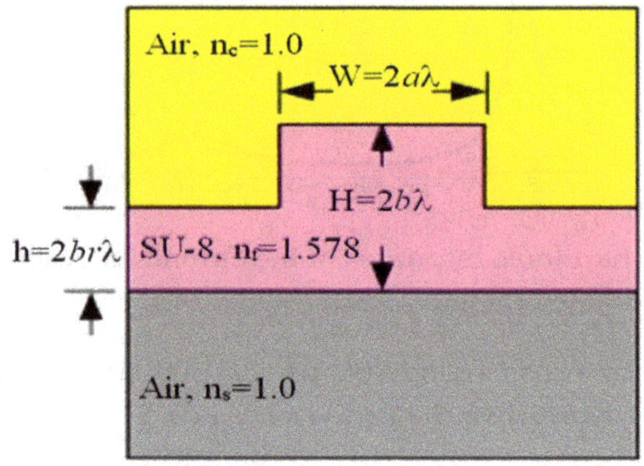

Figure 9. Cross section of the waveguide structure showing the geometric parameters and optical properties of the materials in each layer.

It can be seen from equation 4 that $H \geq \frac{\lambda}{\sqrt{n_f^2 - n_s^2}}$ for single mode operation. Therefore, H ≥ 0.314 µm at λ = 400 nm and H ≥ 0.531 µm at λ = 650 nm.

To maintain a single mode operation based on the above condition in TE polarization for any given H, the rib width W must be designed and operated less than or equal to the value on the curve (Figure 10). By fixing the ratio (r) between the overall height (H) and the slab height (h) to 0.5, we generate a list of waveguide dimensions that we can use for the scanner design (Figure 6 and Table 2. In case 1, the cross section of the rib waveguide has dimensions relative to the core diameter of a single mode fiber (2.9 to 3.9 µm mode field diameter for 400 to 600 nm wavelengths), which is an ideal geometry for the proposed end-butted coupling design. Assuming the same input applies at the center of the rib waveguide, the output power for different waveguide geometries is summarized in Table 2.

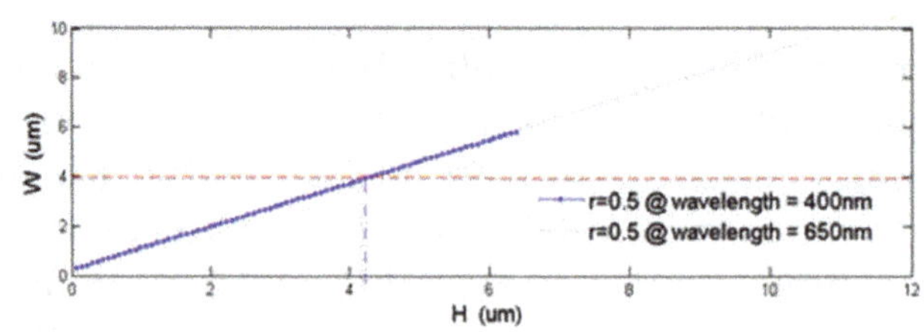

(**a**)

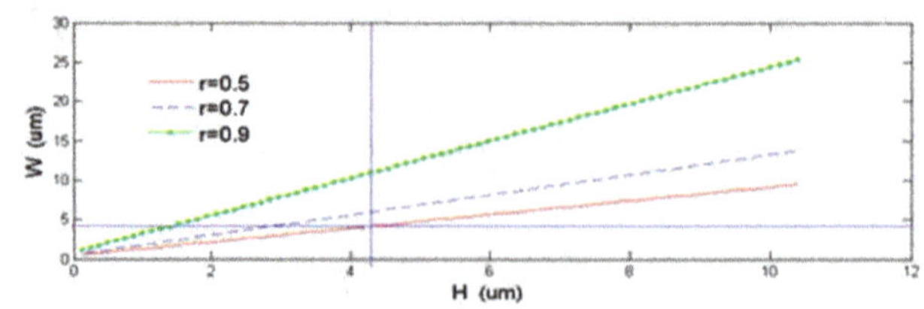

(**b**)

Figure 10. Waveguide width as a function of waveguide height at (**a**) λ = 400 and 650 nm and (**b**) at different r values at λ = 650 nm.

Table 2. Comparison of output power as a function of input beam position and waveguide geometry.

	r	W	H	h	Center of Input	Output Power
Case 1	0.5	4.045	4.290	2.145	X = 0, Y= 2.0	94.2%
Case 2	0.5	6.097	6.630	3.315	X = 0, Y = 3.0	90%
Case 3	0.5	8.036	8.840	4.420	X = 0, Y = 4.0	77%
Case 4	0.7	5.851	4.290	2.145	X = 0, Y = 2	95%
Case 5	0.9	10.755	4.290	2.145	X = 0, Y = 2	96%
Case 6	0.5	4.045	4.290	2.145	X = 0, Y = 1	77%
Case 7	0.5	4.045	4.290	2.145	X = 0, Y = 3	76%
Case 8	0.5	4.045	4.290	2.145	X = 0, Y = 4	46%
Case 9	0.5	4.045	4.290	2.145	X = 1, Y = 3	60%
Case 10	0.5	4.045	4.290	2.145	X = 2, Y = 3	33%
Case 11	0.5	4.045	4.290	2.145	X = 20, Y = 1	0.5%
Case 12	0.5	4.026	4.40	2.20	X = 0, Y = 2.0	93.8%

Case 1 to 11 are waveguide geometry and corresponding output power at 650 nm. Case 12 is operating at 400 nm (unit: μm).

Using modal analysis, based on a SU-8 (n = 1.578 at λ = 650 nm and n = 1.624 at λ = 400 nm [27]) rib waveguide structure with a rib width (*W*): waveguide height (*H*): slab height (*h*) ratio as shown in Table 2, the result confirms single mode operation for TE mode input with wavelengths between 400 to 650 nm. Figure 11 shows the index and modal profile of all three cases observed at 1.282 mm from the coupling end at λ = 650 nm (Figure 11b–d). The profile is similar at 400 nm (Figure 11a). Fields all appear confined and single mode.

An optical simulation using Rsoft beam propagation program (BMP) software was performed to analyze the coupling efficiency. In order to simplify the analysis, scattering and absorption were neglected and it is assumed that the input to the waveguide is a single mode Gaussian beam. The numerical simulation is based on a SU-8 rib waveguide structure with a rib width: waveguide height: slab height ratio of 4:4:2. The results confirmed single mode operation for TE mode input with wavelengths between 400 and 650 nm. As shown in Figure 12, a very low light loss for wavelengths operates between 0.4 and 0.65 μm if center of the input mode field aligns with the center core of the waveguide (X = 0, Y = 2). For an input with a Gaussian profile, the coupling efficiency for both wavelengths was around 96.5% and 97% for λ = 400 nm and λ = 0.65 μm, respectively. Minimum light attenuation was observed along the taper and cantilever waveguide sections. The light throughput is roughly the same as the initial coupling efficiency (93.8% and 94.2% respectively). The same coupling efficiency and throughput was also observed if the input was a zeroth order mode. However, the alignment of the input with respect to the core of the rib waveguide greatly affects the coupling efficiency. Table 2 summarizes the output power as a function of input position operating at 650 nm wavelength. When fiber is vertical lateral displacement (y direction), the coupling loss was less significant than the horizontal displacement (x direction) as long as the beam was confined inside the waveguide. This is most likely the main contribution to the observed low coupling efficiency in the measurement. It is also shown in our previous multimode 100 μm × 85 μm × 2100 μm SU-8 rectangular waveguide that combine loss stem from mode coupling, scattering and absorption is around 28.6% [17,18]. The simulation also shows that the shape of the proof mass does not matter in the optical simulation, because as long as the input beam is confined inside the ridge area of the waveguide, single mode propagation is maintained. As shown in Figure 12a,b, both output fields at 400 and 650 nm appear to be single mode and nicely confined inside the waveguide. The far field intensity profile is also generated and match quite closely to the experiment result with ~ 0.22° in x direction and 8.8° in y direction FWHM at $\lambda = 400$ and 650 nm (Figure 8). As expected, the FWHM for 400 nm is slightly smaller than 650 nm.

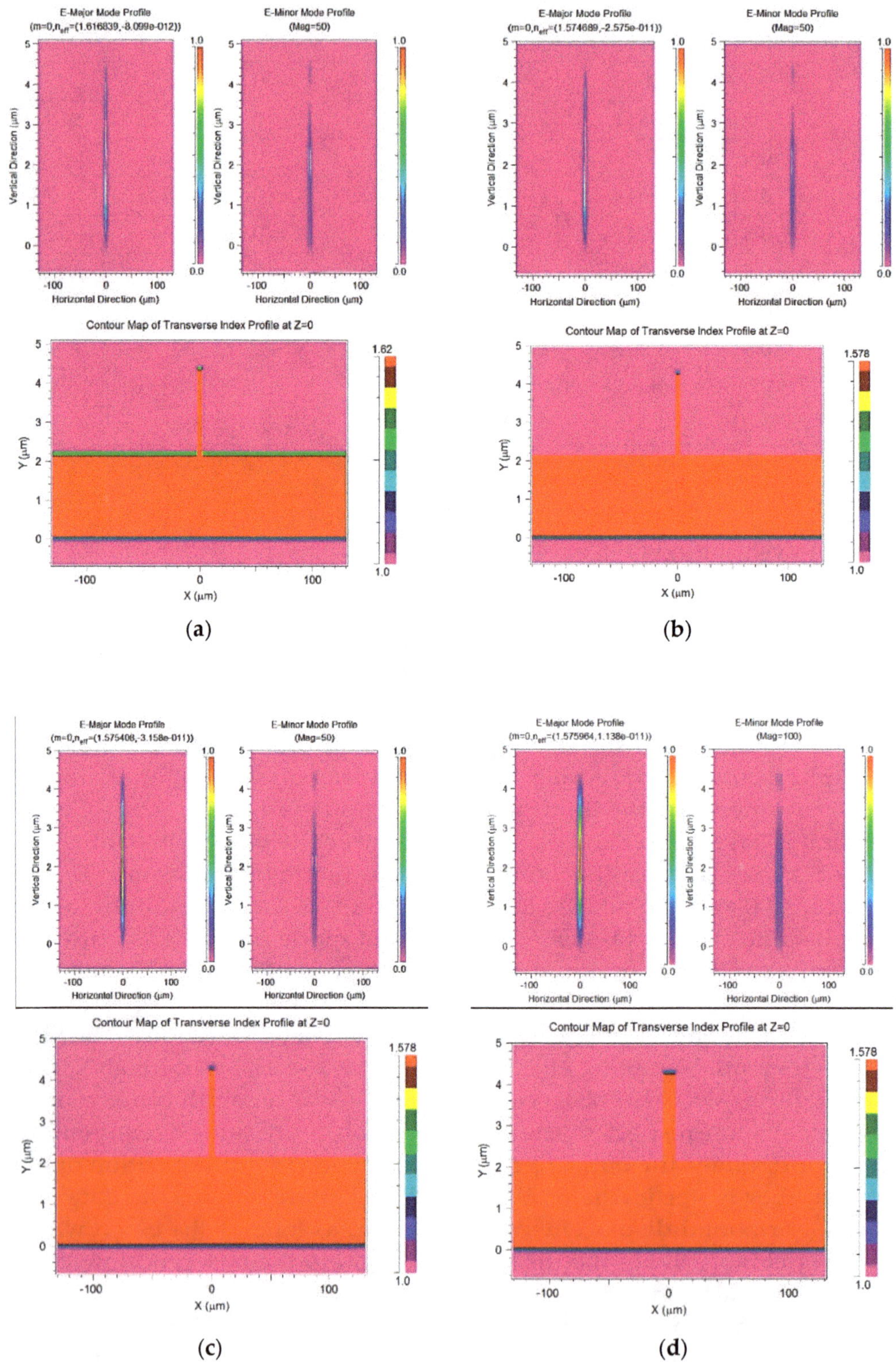

Figure 11. Index and modal profile of the proposed rib waveguide at $\lambda =$ (**a**) 400 and (**b**) 650 nm with r = 0.5 and at 650 nm with (**c**) r = 0.7 (**d**) and r = 0.9 respectively.

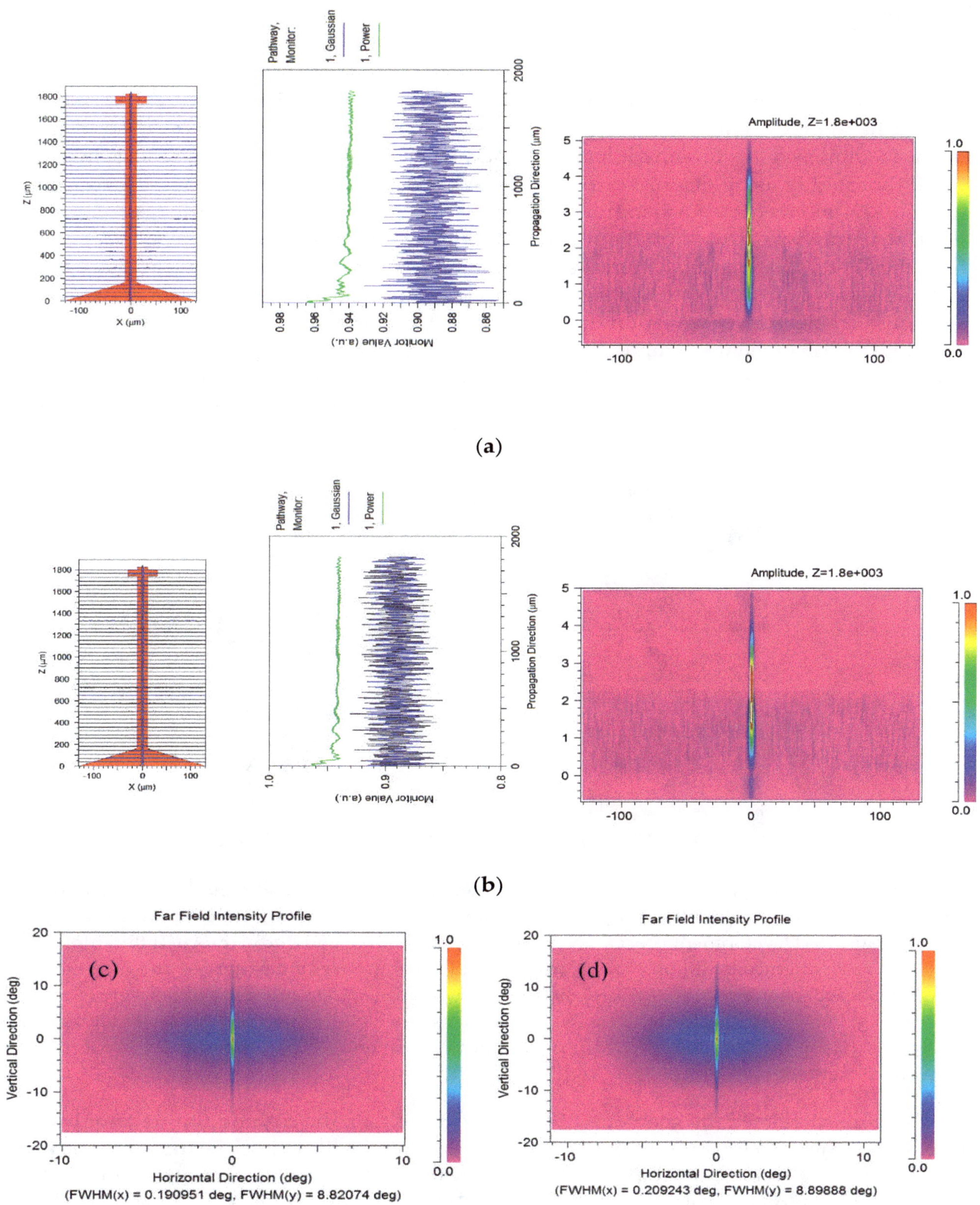

Figure 12. Wave propagation along the waveguide using a Gaussian beam profile for the 4 μm core input fiber (**a**) operating at 0.4 μm, (**b**) operating at 0.65 μm, middle figure showing field amplitude profile at z = 1800 μm (near the tip of the cantilever waveguide), (**c**) far field beam profile at λ = 400 nm and (**d**) 650 nm.

3. Fabrication

3.1. Scanner Fabrication Process

The fabrication procedure of the electrostatic scanner is shown in Figure 13 [22]. A 4-inch silicon wafer with a standard thickness of 525 ± 25 µm served as the substrate for the device fabrication. The substrate was immersed in a Piranha solution (H2SO4:H2O2 = 4:1) to clean off organic residues and it was rinsed thoroughly using deionized (DI) water. After rinsing, the substrate was dried using spin rinse dryer (SRD) and then it is further dried on a hotplate at 200 °C for 10 min. After cleaning, a double layer SU-8 structure was created on the substrate using photo-lithography process. A 2 µm layer of SU-8 5 (MicroChem, MA) was first spun coat onto the silicon substrate to form the actuator body and slab part of the waveguide following instructions provided by the MicroChem Corp. An additional layer of 2 µm-thick SU-8 layer was spun and exposed on top of the first layer after post-exposure bake (PEB) to create the rib of the waveguide. During pre-baking, the temperature was first held at 70 °C for one minute before ramping from 70 °C to 105 °C at a rate of 3 °C/min to reduce the extrinsic stress of the SU-8. Finally, the sample was held at 105 °C for 15 min before cooling down to room temperature at a rate of 2 °C/min.

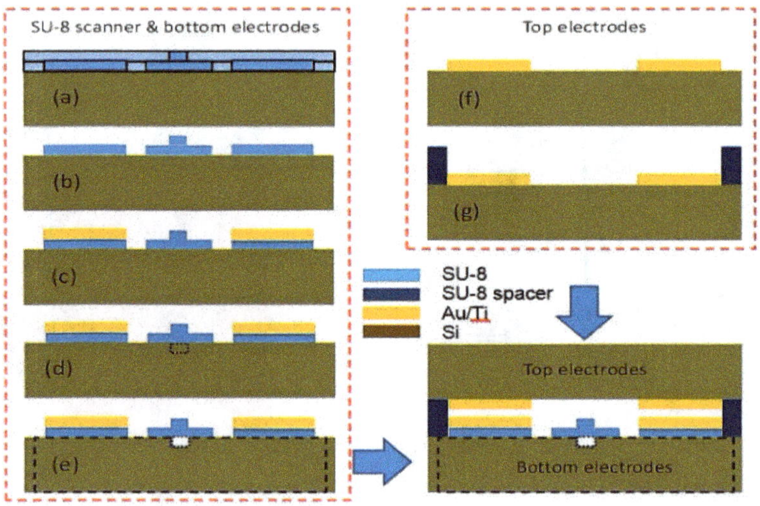

Figure 13. Fabrication process of electrostatic scanner. (**a–e**): scanner body and bottom electrodes (**f,g**): top electrodes. (**a**) Double-layer photolithography process to define rib shape waveguide and scanner pads; (**b**) Development process to create SU-8 waveguide and body; (**c**) Au/Ti thin films are deposited and patterned by lift-off process; (**d**) Front side fiber grooves are patterned and deep etched using deep reactive-ion etching (DRIE); (**e**) the scanner (bottom electrode and waveguide) were released by DRIE again from the backside of the wafer; (**e**) Backside etch-through to release actuators and waveguide; (**f**) top electrode is deposited and patterned on a second silicon wafer; (**g**) SU-8 spacers are spun and patterned.

Using a contact aligner, the geometry of the waveguide slab, the rib, and the actuator body were transferred from the soda lime masks onto the double-layer SU-8 film via UV exposure. The exposed film underwent the post exposure bake (PEB) to cross-linked the defined geometry. During PEB, the wafer was first placed on a hotplate for 1 min. at 70 °C. The temperature was held for 1 min, and then it was ramped from 70 °C to 105 °C at a rate of 3 °C/min. The hotplate was held at 105 °C for 1 min, and then it was cooled to room temperature over a 30-min period (a longer cooling period compared to manufacture specification). After the sample was cooled down to room temperature, the double-layer SU-8 film was then developed in PMGEA (an ethyl lactate and diacetone alcohol, MicroChem Corp., Westborough, MA, USA) for 1 min with mild agitation. The wafer was rinsed thoroughly in isopropyl alcohol (IPA) for another 1 min and then it was dried using SRD. The 20 nm Ti with 200 nm Au metal electrodes were made using E-beam deposition and lift-off process. Prior to metal deposition, a layer of negative photoresist NR9-3000PY (Futurrex Inc, Franklin, NJ, USA) was spun onto the SU-8 layer. The pattern was then transferred from a soda lime mask to the resist to define the electrode area. Similar to the previous process, the fiber groove was formed through subsequent photolithography and DRIE. Finally, the device (scanner and bottom electrodes) were released from backside via bulk silicon etching using DRIE.

The 20 nm Ti with 200 nm Au metal electrodes were made using E-beam deposition and lift-off process. A layer of negative photoresist NR9-3000PY (Futurrex Inc) was spun onto the SU-8 layer before the metal deposition. The pattern was then transferred from a soda lime mask to the photoresist to define the electrode area. Similar to the previous process, the fiber groove was formed through subsequent photolithography and DRIE. Finally, the device (scanner and bottom electrodes) was released from backside via bulk silicon etching using DRIE.

The fabrication process of the top electrode was a two-step micro-fabrication process. A second four-inch wafer was prepared as a substrate for SU-8 deposition as before. The top electrode area is defined using photolithography process, and an e-beam evaporator system is used to deposit the Titanium adhesion layer and the Au electrode. The metal thin films were then patterned by lift-off process. A SU-8 spacer was spun and patterned onto the electrode layer. With the aid of an extra packaging design, which will be introduced in the next section, the top electrodes were aligned with the scanner and the bottom electrodes.

3.2. Device Package

An 8.0 mm × 8.0 mm × 1.0 mm acrylic-based photopolymer holder was designed and fabricated using a multi-material three-dimensional printing system (X-axis: 600 dpi; Y-axis: 600 dpi; Z-axis: 1600 dpi, Connex350, Stratasys Ltd.) [22] to secure the MEMS device. A gradient index (GRIN) lens (4.85 mm length × 2 mm diameter GRIN lens rod by GRINTECH GmbH, Jena, Germany, working distance = 20 mm, beam width = 20 μm, view angle = ±30°, and NA = 0.5) was installed and secured in a tube structure formed by the assembly of the upper and the lower part of the holder as shown in Figure 14. Our proposed GRIN lens was fixed and placed at a predetermine distance beyond the end of the cantilever inside the holder to focus the diverging beams at the output of the waveguide to an object plane at a certain distance away. The estimated beam width at the focal plane was around 20 μm when the GRIN lens was placed at 0.4 mm away from the waveguide at the scanner designed wavelength of operation. The calculated angular deflection of the proposed scanning system was about 5° total (2.5° on each side), which minimizes aberrations and vignette at the output.

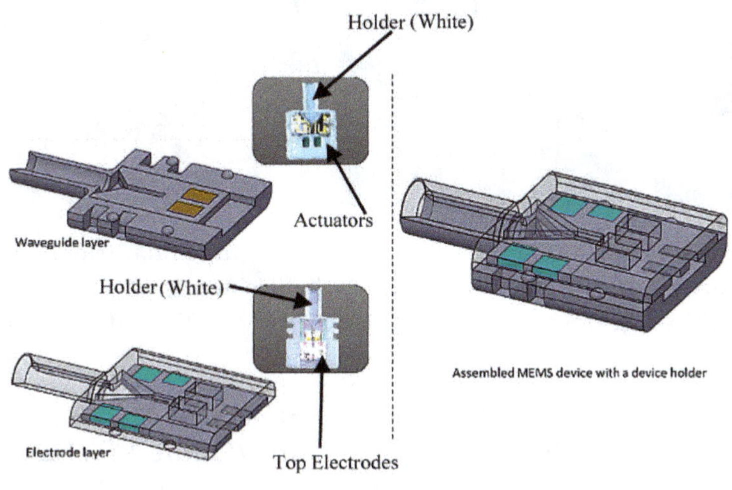

Figure 14. Schematics of assembled MEMS device, including top electrode, scanner, bottom electrodes, and gradient index (GRIN) lens with the device holder.

4. Results and Discussions

The device was successfully fabricated (Figure 15a,c) [22]. Initially, due to its large aspect ratio and residual stress, the cantilever waveguide appeared bent (Figure 15b) [22]. This problem was quickly resolved by carefully controlling the baking procedure. Using more gradual heating and cooling and different baking temperatures, we were able to obtain a straighter beam (Figure 19a) [22]. To resolve the adhesion problem (shown in Figure 16a) [22] between the SU-8 waveguide and the silicon nitride substrate, the soft bake temperature was increase from 65 °C to 70 °C (soft bake) and the post exposure bake (PEB) temperature was increased from 95 °C to 105 °C. The increase in temperature produced a smooth and laminated surface on the SU-8 layer (Figure 16b) [22]. The dimension of the waveguide was slightly reduced in thickness and width due to the double layer structure usually being produced much thinner.

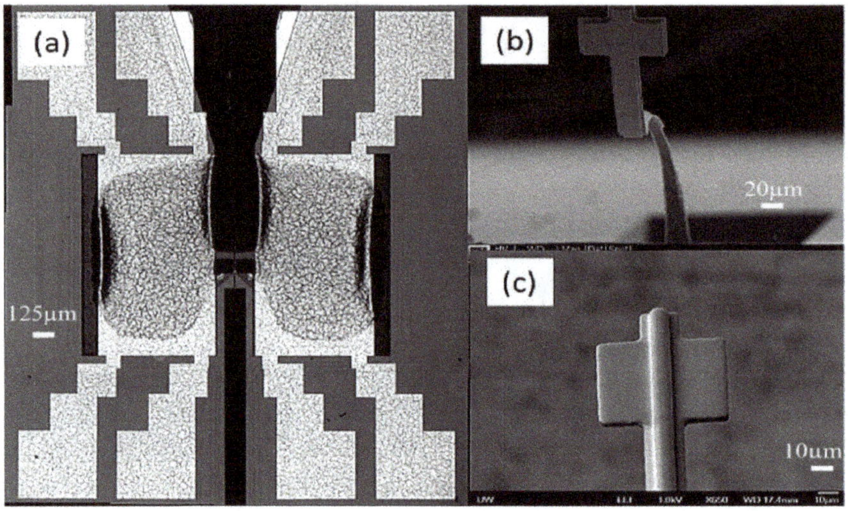

Figure 15. (**a**) MEMS scanner with push-pull actuators. (**b**) Bending waveguide due to large aspect ratio and residual stress. (**c**) SU-8 rib waveguide at the tip.

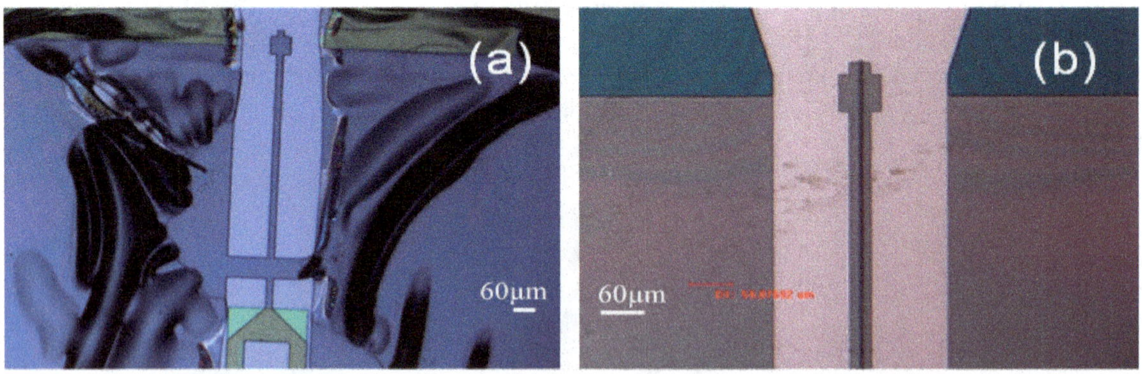

Figure 16. Lithographic result of double-layer SU-8 waveguide on nitride/silicon substrate. (**a**) Baking at lower temperature (65 °C /95 °C) where large SU8 film area such as actuators appear to peel from the nitride surface (**b**) when operates at higher temperature (70 °C/105 °C), SU8 film appears smooth and laminated.

The devices were released using backside deep reactive-ion etching (DRIE). However, it was harder to etch around the corner, leaving silicon residue (Figure 17a) [22]. When more etching cycles were added, the corners became clear, but some of the SU-8 waveguide did not survive (Figure 17b) [22]. In the future, we will revise the mask design so that SU-8 waveguides are better protected during the DRIE.

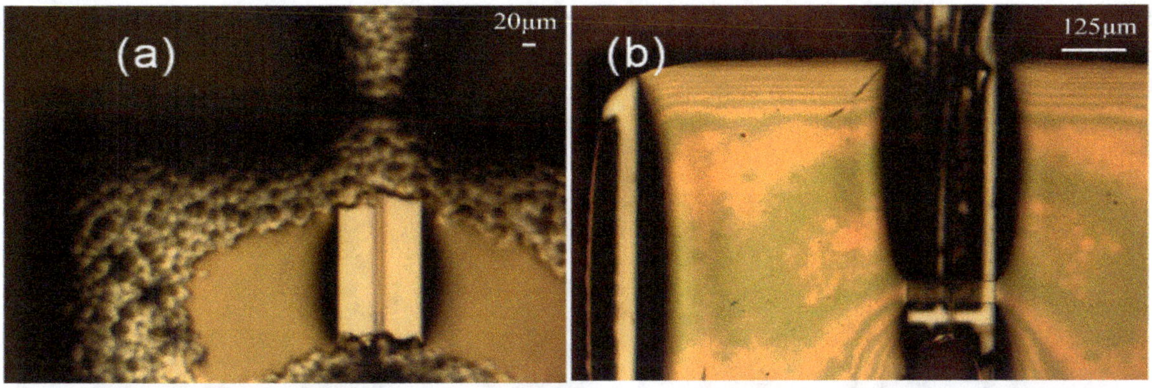

Figure 17. (**a**) The 750-deep reactive ion etching cycles were used to release the scanner (picture is taken from the backside), (**b**) 30 additional cycles were later added to further remove the Si residue around the edges of the window.

The scanner test sample setup is shown in Figure 18 [22]. The top and bottom layers of the scanner were secured inside the rapid-prototyped holder and larger external contact pads were built to allow easier access to the smaller device contacts (Figure 18a). A 10 mW He–Ne laser (λ = 632.8 nm) provides the input light to a single mode optical fiber (diameter = 4.3 μm). A XYZ positioning stage (incremental linear encoder with 100 nm resolution) provides the accurate light coupling between the light-carrying optical fiber to the SU-8 rib waveguide. Two cameras equipped with high power lenses (250× magnification) were used to aid the alignment of the optical fiber in the vertical and horizontal directions. A third camera, a microscope, is placed near the tip of the waveguide to observe the light emitted.

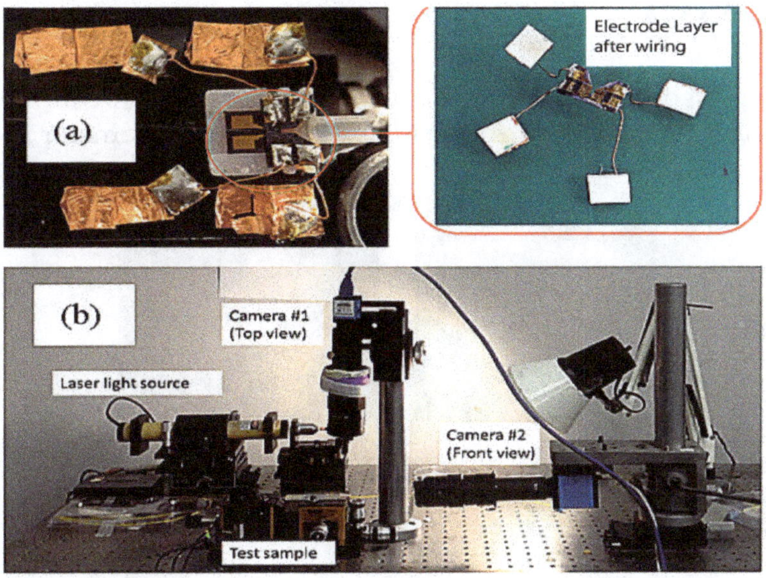

Figure 18. (**a**) MEMS device test sample: device in the red square shows the top electrode. The bottom electrode consists of the moving push-pull actuators and the cantilever waveguide (partially covered by the top electrode), (**b**) optical tests were taken by two cameras equipped with high power lenses (250× magnification).

After using the microscope and the cameras to align the fiber to the scanner, light can be observed at the tip of the waveguide (Figure 19), Figure 19a shows the aerial view of the light coupling from taper fiber to the rib waveguide. Light can be seen at the tip of the waveguide. Some coupling loss can be seen from the escaping light at the interface. Some dimmer escaping light can also be observed at the bending part of the waveguide. Despite the losses, Figure 19b shows that the optical beam is nicely confined by the core of the waveguide. The intensity of the light at the output of the waveguide and the light from the input fiber were measured. The average coupling (or transmission) efficiency was measured to be around 10% (Table 3). The low coupling efficiency was mainly due to inherent process imperfections in making the fiber groove.

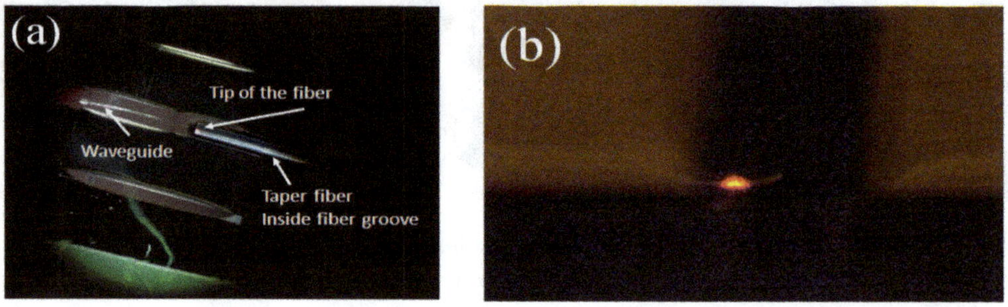

Figure 19. (**a**) Optical coupling from the taper fiber to the SU8 rib waveguide. (**b**) Light observed at the tip of the SU8 rib waveguide. Light appears nicely confined inside the core of the waveguide.

Table 3. Light coupling measurements.

	Intensity Measured at Input Fiber End (V)	Intensity Measured at Waveguide Output (V)
mean 1	0.077	0.014
mean 2	0.079	0.004
mean 3	0.075	0.006
Mean	0.077 ± 0.001	0.008 ± 0.001
Coupling efficiency (%)	N/A	10.390

The optical test was also performed on scanner to measure the beam profile coming from the GRIN lens coupled device package (Figure 20). A 20-micron beam diameter is observed at 2 cm focal length, matching the estimated beam width.

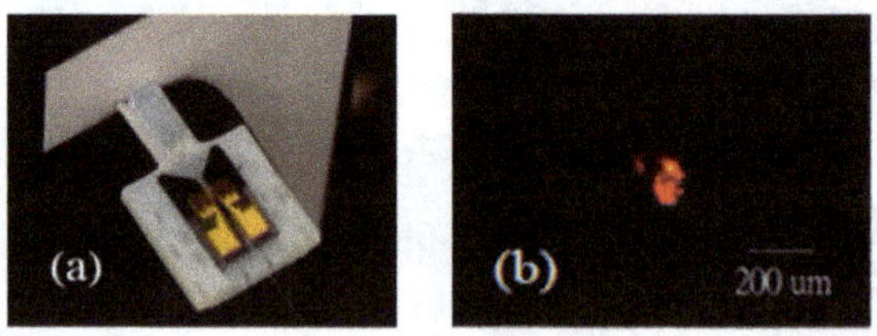

Figure 20. Pictures show (**a**) scanner coupled with optical fiber and GRIN lens. (**b**) direct observation of beam profile. Beam spot is the bright spot in the figure. Surround scattering red lights are from input fiber.

The performance of the device was evaluated by applying voltage according the patterns shown in Figure 2. Vertical scanning motion of the waveguide was accomplished by applying 100 VDC to the bottom electrodes and ±150 V AC voltage to all of the top electrode with synchronized phase. Horizontal scanning motion of the waveguide was achieved by driving actuators with the same voltage settings for generating vertical motion but with a 180° phase delay between the left and right top electrodes. The driving voltages were much larger than the estimated voltages due to the increase in gap space between top and bottom electrodes compared to the original design. To find the resonant frequencies for both directions of the waveguide motion, the operating frequency was swept from 1 to 10,000 Hz (1 to 6000 Hz is shown here) (Figure 21) and the displacement of the waveguide was measured. A vertical resonant mode was found at 201 Hz, which was slightly lower than the simulation result (240.07 Hz). A horizontal mode was found at 535 Hz, compared to 1343.82 Hz in the simulation. The amplitudes of vibration were 130 and 19.2 μm, respectively. The initial displacement measurement and actuation displacement of the scanner was smaller than expected, most likely due to inaccurate modelling of air damping and boundary condition, intrinsic stress in the cantilever and the under etched residual silicon around edges of the actuator (Figure 26).

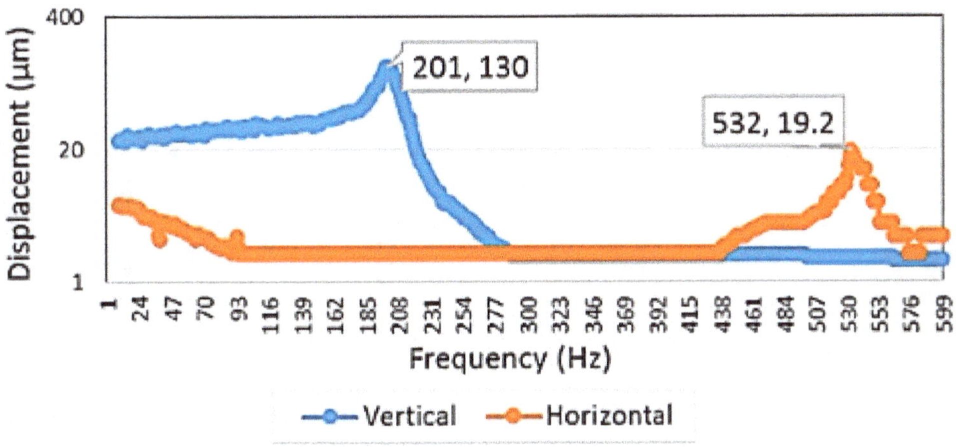

Figure 21. Waveguide mechanical frequency response. Both vertical and horizontal displacement were measured. Driving input voltages are 100 V DC applied at the bottom electrodes and +150 V AC at the top electrodes.

Due to larger air gap (compared to the simulation), additional DC voltage was added to reduce the input driving voltage. Figure 22 [22] shows the behavior of actuator membrane when various DC voltages were applied to the top electrode while bottom electrodes were grounded. The deformation of the actuator membrane can be observed visibly starting at 200 V.

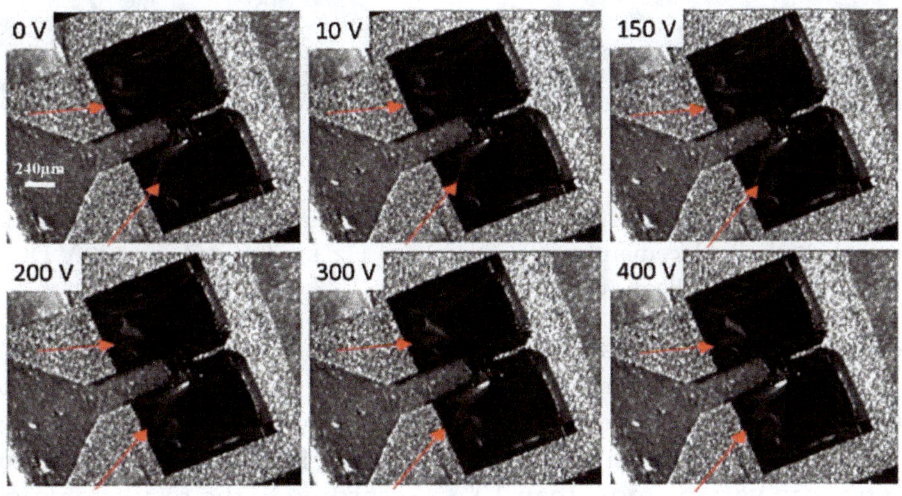

Figure 22. Actuator deformation under different DC applied voltages. Deformation can be observed by comparing the change in areas indicated by the red arrows.

To characterize the scanning performance, the tip displacement and the scanning angle of the waveguide were measured against input actuation voltages (Figure 23) [22]. The scanning angle was calculated as the inverse of the sine function of the tip displacement over the waveguide length, in this case, 1820 μm. An amplifier (30×) was used in order to create a large enough electric field for driving the device. A linear relation can be observed between the tip deflection/scanning angle and the driving voltage. A tip displacement of 111.8 μm (vertical) and 20 μm (horizontal) was observed at the maximum test voltage of 150V under 1 Hz driving frequency (Figure 24).

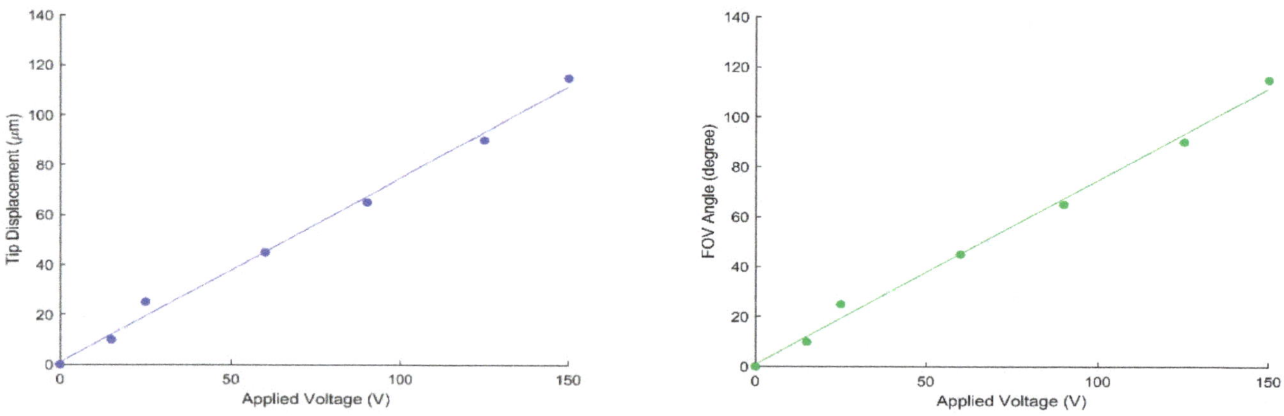

(a) (b)

Figure 23. (**a**) Waveguide tip displacement and (**b**) corresponding scanning angle vs. applied voltage at 1 Hz driving frequency.

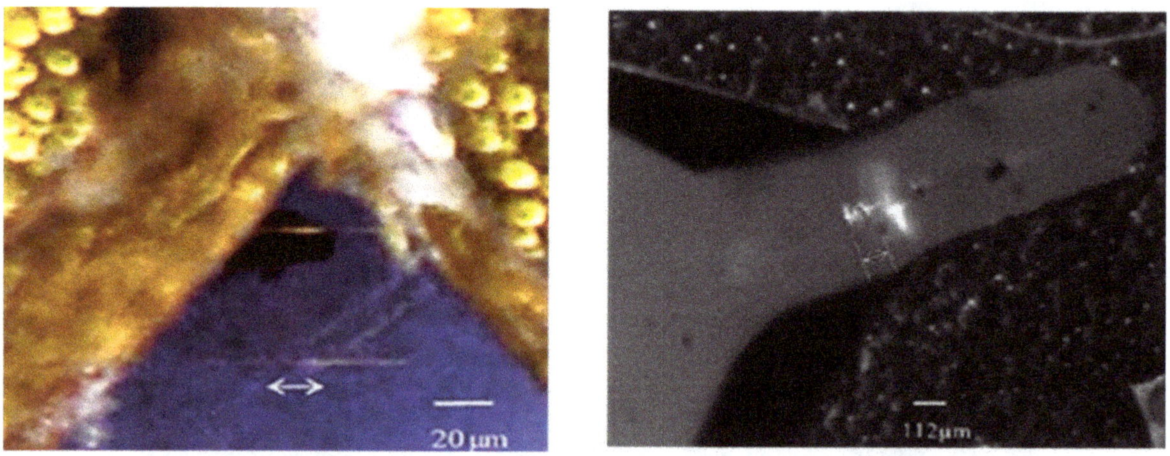

(a) (b)

Figure 24. Pictures show superimposition of waveguide's peak displacement in (**a**) horizontal and (**b**) vertical direction. Both displacements are operated at 1 Hz ± 150 V AC and 100 V DC. Black spot on proof mass in left image is the silicon residue.

The frequencies of the two lowest vertical and horizontal modes are 240.07 and 1343.8 Hz in non-resonating simulation, compared to 201 and 532 Hz in experimentation. (Figure 21). The discrepancies were most likely due to reduction in the overall geometry in the final device. Due to heat related shrinkage, with 10% deviation in the width and/or thickness, overexposure, and process errors, the resonant frequency can vary by more than 10%. According to the results obtained from our later ANSYS simulation, where by decreasing the slab width from 20 to 10 microns, the two lowest resonant frequencies then matched closely to the experiment results. In this case, the vertical and horizontal frequencies in the simulation were then 238.32 and 562.68 Hz, respectively (Figure 25).

The other factors could be stem from imperfections in the fabrication process. For example, varying thickness in the (optimally uniform thickness) SU-8 waveguides, additional under-etched silicon residues on the SU-8 after the DRIE backside etching (see the dark spot (silicon residue)) on the backside of the proof mass in Figure 24 and vibration reduction in actuators due to the silicon residue on the edges of the backside window in Figure 26.

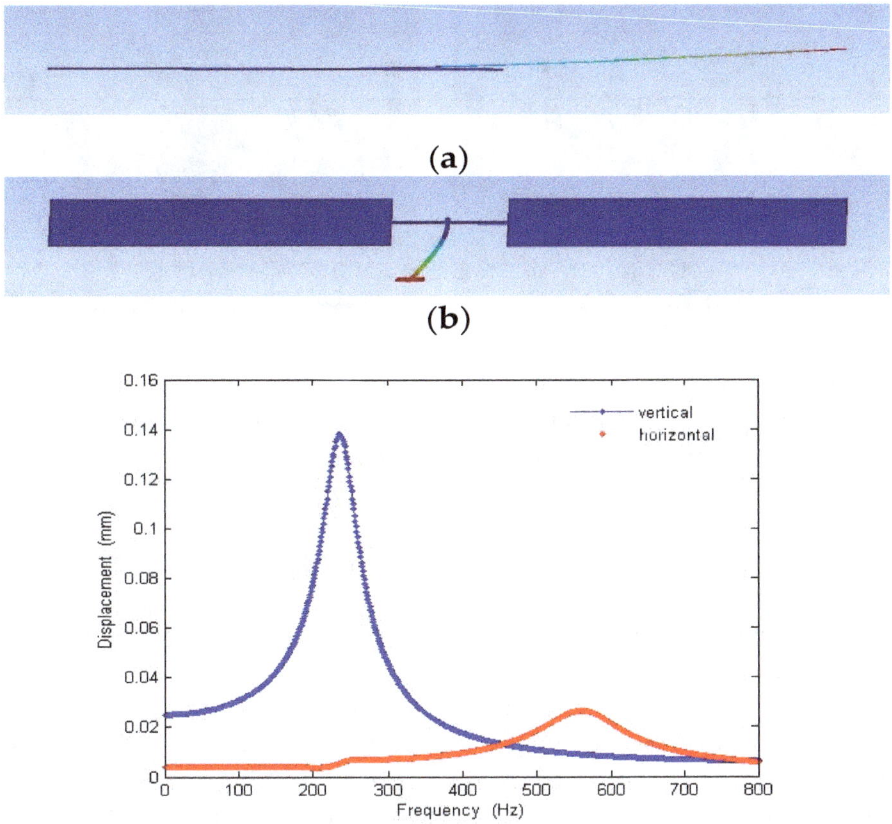

(c)

Figure 25. ANSYS modal analysis of scanner with slab width reduce to 10 microns. The two lowest frequencies 238.32 Hz and 562.68 Hz in the simulation appear closely matching the experiment results. (**a**) Mode shape at 238.32 Hz, (**b**) mode shape at 562.68 Hz. (**c**) Corresponding harmonic responses measured experimentally.

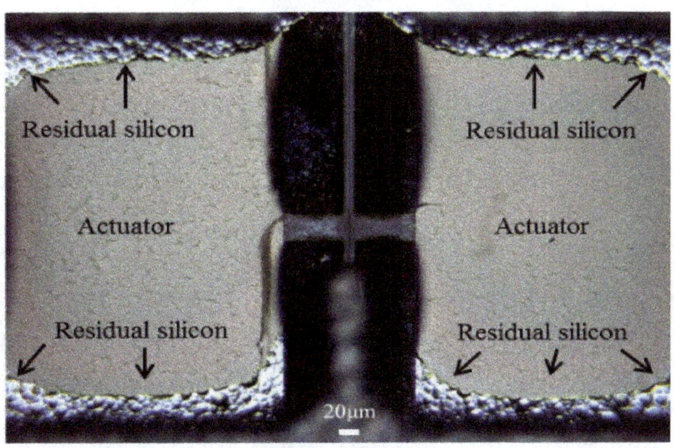

Figure 26. Arrows in the microscopic picture show the residual silicon around corners of the actuators after DRIE. Picture taken from the backside of the actuators.

A 2D scanning motion is successfully demonstrated in the non-resonating configuration with 201 Hz in vertical direction and 20 Hz in horizontal direction (Figure 27). The 34 μm horizontal and 130 μm vertical displacement or 0.019 to 0.072 radians in field of view were obtained. Here the non-resonating mode was performed in the horizontal direction instead of vertical direction as described in the earlier non-resonating simulation because the experiment shows a much improve overall dynamic performance (a larger vertical and horizontal mechanical vibration or FOV) (Figure 21) [22].

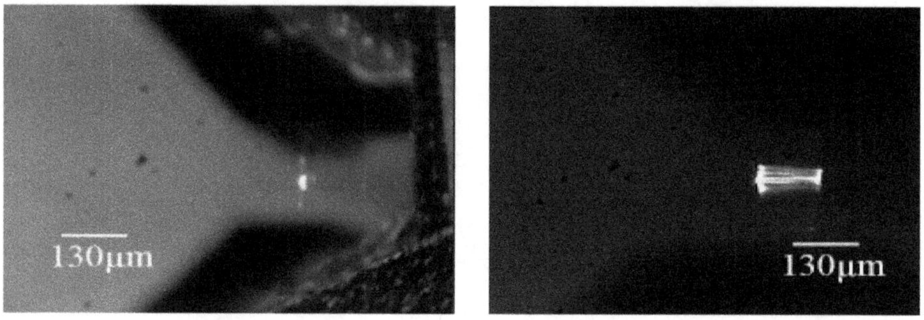

(a) (b)

Figure 27. Microscopic images show the vertical displacement driving at (**a**) 0 Hz, (**b**) non-resonating 2D scanning at 201 Hz in vertical and 20 Hz in horizontal direction. (Pictures are taken directly above the scanner so vertical and horizontal directions are switched).

5. Conclusions

In this paper, we presented a novel, fully integrated MEMS-based 2D mechanical scanning system using 1D push–pull actuators. Detail design, fabrication and tests were performed. The results from the preliminary tests prove the push-pull actuator concept works and two-directional displacements is possible using this new 1D actuator design.

The scanner's mechanical and optical parameters were analyzed and optimized to determine the best line resolution and FOV. Based on the simulation, the dominant factors affecting scanner resolution are the cross-section and length of the waveguide. Higher resolutions can be achieved with a vertically thin or horizontally wide T cross section on a longer waveguide. The best optical single mode operation can be achieved by rib waveguide configuration.

The horizontal resonance of 532 Hz and vertical resonance of 201 Hz were found from the mechanical test. Discrepancy to the simulation results as mentioned in the discussion are mainly due to the dimension reduction in the proof mass and waveguide slab width and thickness. As shown in Figure 25, reduction in proof mass (5×) increases the vertical vibration resonant frequencies (4×) and smaller slab width (2.2×) decreases the horizontal resonant frequencies (2×). It is worth noting that it is extremely difficult to model this scanner design due to the fact that both optical and mechanical structure must both be optimized at the same time. It is also a challenge to correctly model the residual stress and damping and other factors that can only be found experimentally. Other factor contribute to the deviation could be result of fabrication errors. With 10% deviation in the width and/or thickness, the resonant frequencies can vary by more than 10%. The under-etched silicon remained in the backside of the SU-8 waveguide can add additional mass or stiffness to the system and further vary the resonant frequencies.

Initial coupling tests showed a 10% coupling efficiency between the optical fiber and the MEMS waveguide. The measured value is relatively low compared to the optical simulation results. The relatively large cross section (4 μm in height and 20 μm in width) of the double-layer SU-8 rib waveguide design is expected to provide a coupling efficiency of ~94% with a Gaussian beam profile input and broad band single mode operation (λ = 0.4 to 0.65 μm) with a minimal transmission loss (3% output transmission loss–model not including absorption and scattering loss). The coupling efficiency decrease is likely to be caused by imperfections in the fabrication process used during the process and the micron-range precision needed to align the optical fiber with the waveguide coupler for optimal coupling. As shown in simulation, slight offset in input position in either the vertical or horizontal direction creates tremendous coupling loss (e.g., a 1 micron offset from the original x = 0 μm and y = 2 μm input position results in an observed 17% light reduction).

For the FOV and line resolution test, the largest FOV is found to be 0.015 rad at 532 Hz in horizontal and 0.072 rad at 201 Hz in vertical direction (Figure 21) and the largest line resolution is calculated to be about 90 dots per line. The scanner system can definitely be improved. More revisions to the actuator and coupling system are needed to achieve a better FOV and line resolution.

A 2D scanning motion is successfully demonstrated in the non-resonating configuration with 201 Hz in vertical direction and 20 Hz in horizontal direction. A 34 μm horizontal and 130 μm vertical displacement or 0.019 to 0.072 radians in field of view were obtained.

In this paper, we have successfully demonstrated a 2D optical scanner using pairs of 1D electrostatic parallel plate push-pull actuators. Results show tip displacement changing linearly as a function of input actuator voltage. The light beams are well guided and confined within the core of the rib waveguide structure. The optical package with GRIN lens also focuses the output diverging beam as intended. A 2D scanning motion operating at non-resonating configuration is also successfully demonstrated.

Author Contributions: Conceptualization, W.-C.W.; data curation, K.G. and C.T.; formal analysis, W.-C.W., K.G. and C.T.; funding acquisition, W.-C.W.; investigation, W.-C.W., K.G. and C.T.; methodology, W.-C.W.; project administration, W.-C.W.; resources, W.-C.W.; software, W.-C.W. and C.T.; supervision, W.-C.W.; validation, K.G.; visualization, K.G. and C.T.; writing—original draft, W.-C.W.; writing—review and editing, W.-C.W. and C.T.

References

1. Murakami, K.; Murata, A.; Suga, T.; Kitagawa, H.; Kamiya, Y.; Kubo, M.; Katashiro, M. A miniature confocal optical microscope with MEMS gimbal scanner. In Proceedings of the TRANSDUCERS '03. 12th International Conference on Solid-State Sensors, Actuators and Microsystems. Digest of Technical Papers (Cat. No.03TH8664), Boston, MA, USA, 8–12 June 2003.
2. Ra, H.; Piyawattanametha, W.; Taguchi, Y.; Lee, D.; Mandella, M.J.; Solgaard, O. Two-dimensional MEMS scanner for dual-axes confocal microscopy. *J. Microelectromech. Syst.* **2007**, *16*, 969–976. [CrossRef]
3. Miyajima, H.; Asaoka, N.; Isokawa, T.; Ogata, M.; Aoki, Y.; Imai, M.; Matsumoto, K. A MEMS electromagnetic optical scanner for a commercial confocal laser scanning microscope. *J. Microelectromech. Syst.* **2003**, *12*, 243–251. [CrossRef]
4. Shin, H.J.; Pierce, M.C.; Lee, D.; Ra, H.; Solgaard, O.; Richards-Kortum, R. Fiber-optic confocal microscopeusing a MEMS scanner and miniature objective lens. *Opt. Express* **2007**, *15*, 9113–9122. [CrossRef] [PubMed]
5. Hwang, Y.; Park, J.; Kim, Y.; Kim, J. Large-scale full color laser projection display. In Proceedings of the 18th International Display Research Conference ASIA Display'98, Seoul, Korea, 28 September–1 October 1998.
6. Yamada, K.; Kuriyama, T. A novel asymmetric silicon micro-mirror for optical beam scanning display. In Proceedings of the 11th Annual International Workshop on Micro Electro Mechanical Systems, Heidelberg, Germany, 25–29 January 1998.
7. Solgaard, O.; Sandejas, F.S.A.; Bloom, D.M. Deformable grating optical modulator. *Opt. Lett.* **1992**, *17*, 688–690. [CrossRef] [PubMed]
8. Amm, D.T.; Corrigan, R.W. 5.2: Grating Light Valve™ Technology: Update and Novel Applications. *SID* **1998**, *29*, 29–32. [CrossRef]
9. Francis, D.A.; Kiang, M.-H.; Solgaard, O.; Lau, K.Y.; Muller, R.S.; Chang-Hasnain, C.J. Compact 2D Laser Beam Scanner with Fan Laser Array and Si Micro-machined Microscanner. *Electron. Lett.* **1997**, *33*, 1143–1145. [CrossRef]
10. Urey, H.; Wine, D.W.; Osborn, T.D. Optical performance requirements for MEMS-scanner-based microdisplays. *Proc. SPIE* **2000**, *4178*, 176–185.
11. Wine, D.W.; Helsel, M.P.; Jenkins, L.; Urey, H.; Osborn, T.D. Performance of a biaxial MEMS-based scanner for microdisplay applications. *Proc. SPIE* **2000**, *4178*, 186–196.
12. Helmchen, F.; Fee, M.S.; Tank, D.W.; Denk, W. A miniature head-mounted two-photon microscope. *Neuron* **2001**, *31*, 903–912. [CrossRef]
13. Muller, R.S.; Lau, K.Y. Surface-Micromachined Microoptical Elements and Systems. *Proc. IEEE* **1998**, *86*, 1705–1720. [CrossRef]

14. Davis, W.O.; Sprague, R.; Miller, J. MEMS-based pico projector display. In Proceedings of the 2008 IEEE/LEOS Internationall Conference on Optical MEMs and Nanophotonics, Freiburg, Germany, 11–14 August 2008.
15. Wang, W.C.; Fauver, M.; Ho, J.N.; Seibel, E.J.; Reinhall, P. Micromachined optical waveguide cantilever as a resonant optical scanner. *Sens. Actuators, A* **2002**, *102*, 165–175. [CrossRef]
16. Takahshi, C.; Wang, H.J.; Hua, W.S.; Reinhall, P.; Wang, W.C. Polymeric waveguide design of 2D display system. In Proceedings of the SPIE Health Monitoring and Smart Nondestructive Evaluation of Structural and Biological Systems V, San Diego, CA, USA, 26 February–2 March 2006.
17. Panergo, R.; Huang, C.S.; Liu, C.S.; Reinhall, P.; Wang, W.C. Resonant polymeric optical waveguide cantilever integrated for image acquisition. *J. Lightwave Technol.* **2007**, *25*, 850–860. [CrossRef]
18. Wang, W.C.; Reinhall, P. Scanning polymeric waveguide design of a 2D display system. *OSA J. Disp. Technol.* **2008**, *4*, 28–38. [CrossRef]
19. Wang, W.C.; Tsui, C.L. Two-dimensional mechanically resonating fiber optic scanning display system. *Opt. Eng.* **2010**, *49*, 097401.
20. Hua, W.S.; Wang, W.C.; Wu, W.J.; Tsui, C.L.; Cui, W.; Shih, W.P. Development of 2D Microdisplay Using an Integrated Microresonating Waveguide Scanning System. *J. Intell. Mater. Syst. Struct.* **2011**, *22*, 1613–1622. [CrossRef] [PubMed]
21. Gu, K.; Lee, C.C.; Cui, W.; Wu, M.; Wang, W.C. Design and fabrication of mechanical resonance based scanning endoscope. In Proceedings of the 16th International Conference on Solid-State Sensors, Actuators and Microsystems (TRANSDUCERS'11), Beijing, China, 5–10 June 2011.
22. Gu, K.; Lin, K.; Wang, W.C. 2D MEMS electrostatic cantilever waveguide scanner for potential image display application. In Proceedings of the 2015 International Symposium of Optomechatronics Technology (ISOT 2015), Neuchantel, Switzerland, 14–16 October 2015.
23. Acar, C. Robust Micromachined Vibratory Gyroscopes. Ph.D. Thesis, University of California, Irvine, CA, USA, 2004.
24. Rao, S.S. *Mechanical Vibrations*, 3rd ed.; Addison-Wesley Publishing Company: Boston, MA, USA, 1995.
25. Wang, W.; Reinhall, P.; Yee, S. Fluid viscosity measurement using forward light scattering. *Meas. Sci. Technol.* **1999**, *10*, 316–322. [CrossRef]
26. Soref, R.A.; Schmidtchen, J.; Petermann, K. Large single-mode rib waveguides in Ge-Si and Si-on-SiO. *IEEE J. Quantum Electron.* **1991**, *27*, 1971–1974. [CrossRef]
27. Available online: http://microchem.com/Appl-IIIVs-Waveguides.htm (accessed on 2 July 2019).

14

Recent Progress on Photoacoustic Imaging Enhanced with Microelectromechanical Systems (MEMS) Technologies

Changho Lee [1,†], Jin Young Kim [2,†] and Chulhong Kim [2,3,*]

1 Department of Nuclear Medicine, Chonnam National University Medical School & Hwasun Hospital, Hwasun 58128, Korea; ch31037@jnu.ac.kr
2 Departments of Mechanical Engineering, Pohang University of Science and Technology (POSTECH), Pohang 37673, Korea; ronsan@postech.ac.kr
3 Departments of Creative IT Engineering and Electrical Engineering, Pohang University of Science and Technology (POSTECH), Pohang 37673, Korea
* Correspondence: chulhong@postech.edu
† These authors have equally contributed to this work.

Abstract: Photoacoustic imaging (PAI) is a new biomedical imaging technology currently in the spotlight providing a hybrid contrast mechanism and excellent spatial resolution in the biological tissues. It has been extensively studied for preclinical and clinical applications taking advantage of its ability to provide anatomical and functional information of live bodies noninvasively. Recently, microelectromechanical systems (MEMS) technologies, particularly actuators and sensors, have contributed to improving the PAI system performance, further expanding the research fields. This review introduces cutting-edge MEMS technologies for PAI and summarizes the recent advances of scanning mirrors and detectors in MEMS.

Keywords: photoacoustic imaging; microelectromechanical systems (MEMS); MEMS scanning mirror; micromachined US transducer; microring resonator; acoustic delay line

---

1. Introduction

Photoacoustic imaging (PAI) is a new rapidly growing biomedical imaging tool that is based on the photoacoustic (PA) effect using the configuration of light excitation and the ultrasound (US) capture. It has opto-ultrasound contrast mechanisms and multi-scale imaging ability. Thanks to the characteristics of PA wave generation, PAI enables visualization of relatively deep biological tissues (i.e., from a few millimeters to a few centimeters) as compared to typical pure optical imaging techniques (i.e., up to 1 mm), while maintaining high spatial resolution [1–11]. Also, due to excellent intrinsic optical absorbers in bodies, such as hemoglobin, collagen, melanoma, lipids, etc., PAI provides both anatomical and physiological features. Anatomical features include blood vessels, tendon, melanin, and lipid distributions, and physiological features include hemoglobin concentration, oxygen saturation, blood flow rate, metabolism rates, etc. [12–14]. Furthermore, using exogenous contrast agents, PAI can also delineate transparent biological organs, such as lymphatic systems, bladder, intestines, etc. and monitor theranostic process [3,15–24]. These benefits contribute significantly to basic life sciences and expedite clinical translation in dermatology, oncology, ophthalmology, neurology, etc. [14,25–28].

PAI systems generally fall into two categories: photoacoustic microscopy (PAM) and photoacoustic computed tomography (PACT), depending on systems performance and hardware configuration [29]. The PAM generates superior spatial resolution using laser or US focusing approach [30,31]. When a small focused laser beam is used to achieve a spatial resolution of the system, the technique is called optical-resolution PAM (OR-PAM). It enables the visualization of microvasculatures in small animals and humans with a resolution of about several micrometers [32–34]. Unfortunately, the imaging depth of the OR-PAM cannot be deeper than 1.2 mm due to optical diffusion [13]. When a focused US transducer is utilized to create a high spatial resolution, the technique is called acoustic-resolution PAM (AR-PAM). Even though the US focusing configuration in AR-PAM cannot achieve better spatial resolution than OR-PAM, AR-PAM still provides an enhanced depth penetration of few millimeters. The PACT relies on three-dimensional (3D) reconstruction methods to generate cross-sectional and volumetric PA images. Various types of US transducer arrays are used with improved image acquisition speed for real-time PAI, thus reducing the need for mechanical scanning [35]. Each temporal PA signal of the PA source provides time-resolved and spatially resolved one-dimensional radial data through ultrasonic detection. By combining the temporal and spatial PA data, it is possible to reconstruct a three-dimensional PA image of the source. There are several approaches for determining an optimal reconstruction algorithm that is based on the configuration of US transducer aperture and detection geometry (e.g., planar, cylindrical, or spherical) and are described in [36,37].

These PAI systems with high spatial resolution and multi-scale capabilities are well suited for preclinical applications but they have bottlenecks for clinical translation. In the case of PAM, the rate of image acquisition typically depends on the speed of the scanner. Previous approaches, such as mechanical translation stages and optical galvanometer scanners, have either limited scan speed or low signal sensitivity [13,38,39]. In particular, optical galvanometer scanner can provide high scanning speed in the reflection mode, but it is only valid for unfocused ultrasonic detection configuration because normal optical scanners cannot operate on acoustically coupled media (i.e., water and gel). In the case of the transmission mode, although the optical galvanometer scanner can achieve high sensitivity with the increased speed, the instrumental configuration is not appropriate for clinical use [40]. On the other hand, PACT has limitations in comprehensively visualizing biological organs and tissues, due to several transducer limitations, including limited frequency bandwidth and low sensitivity [41]. For high-frequency transducers, the production process needs thin crystals that are fragile and need complex fabricating process [42]. If a multi-element transducer is used, then a large number of expensive data acquisition (DAQ) are required [43]. For example, a 128 elements transducer array requires 128 DAQs, which is a significant part of the system price. The fabrication of small noise-free transducers for endoscopic and handheld probes is difficult, and they suffer from the shallow field of view (FOV) [44,45].

Microelectromechanical system (MEMS) technology can be a good solution to address these existing PAI challenges. The MEMS-based on micromachining technology has been widely used in industrial and scientific research for more than 30 years [46]. It has several advantages, including size, low weight, low cost with mass production, and excellent performance [47]. Generally, MEMS technology has helped to fabricate functional micro-devices such as sensors, switches, and filters using silicon materials with integrated circuit (IC) fabrication. MEMS technology has also revolutionized several biomedical tools for fabricating miniaturized diagnostic modalities and screening assays, such as micro-sensors, actuators, micro-channels, micro-optics, etc. [48]. These micro-devices based on MEMS technology provide good opportunities to create a new generation of micro-endoscopic and handheld probing systems with the capability of high-resolution in vivo real-time imaging [49–54].

In this review, we summarize the current progress of MEMS technologies for PAI and its applications. In Sections 2 and 3, we briefly introduce the progress made in general silicon MEMS scanning mirrors and the 1- & 2-axis water immersible MEMS scanning mirrors and their applications for PAI systems. In Section 4, we introduce diverse PAI detectors, such as micromachined US transducers (MUTs), microring resonators (MRRs), and micromachined silicon acoustic delay lines and multiplexer.

2. Conventional Silicon MEMS Scanning Mirror for PAI

2.1. First Generation PAI System Based on MEMS Scanning Mirror

MEMS scanning mirrors have been a major part of current MEMS research [55]. MEMS scanning mirror has a small micro-scale form factor and it has superior scanning characteristics, such as fast and large scanning angle along two axes. Thanks to these advantages, it has been widely used in optical imaging systems, such as optical coherence tomography [56], multiphoton microscopy [57], confocal microscopy [58], head-up display [59], and digital micromirror device (DMD) [60]. In the last decade, MEMS scanning mirrors have been similarly adopted in PAI system to develop small imaging probes for portable applications.

The first MEMS scanning-mirror based PAI system was reported in 2010 [61]. The custom two-dimensional (2D) MEMS scanning mirror developed in this system is shown in Figure 1(ai). A mirror plate was actuated by four electrothermal bimorph-based actuators. As shown in Figure 1(aii), the fabricated MEMS mirror scans unfocused light through the hollow center of the US transducer. Measured lateral and axial resolutions were 0.7 mm and 0.5 mm, respectively. Imaging depths of up to 2.5 mm and an image area of 9×9 mm^2 was achieved. The PAI of pencil lead in chicken tissue and blood vessels in a human hand (Figure 1(aiii)) was demonstrated. Although the MEMS mirror has a scanning speed of up to 500 Hz, the imaging time was slow (i.e., 250 s) because of the slow repetition rate of the laser (i.e., 10 Hz). This MEMS PAI probe was also adopted in intraoperative applications by the same research group [62]. The MEMS imaging probe was updated with high-frequency US transducer for improved spatial resolution and signal to noise ratio (SNR). Using this system, they acquired volumetric PA images of tumor implanted in a live mouse before (Figure 1(bi)) and after (Figure 1(bii)) surgery. Using the obtained PA images, they confirmed the complete resection of tumor post procedure. The size of the tumor matched within 8.5% error margin with the hematoxylin and eosin (H & E) stained sections (Figure 1(biii)). Thanks to the compact design and the performance of the developed MEMS PA probe, it has the potential to be used for image-guided surgery. The MEMS scanning mirror and the PAI system can be integrated with various other optical imaging systems as well. For example, a dual-modality MEMS imaging probe, which integrates PAI with diffuse optical tomography (DOT), was demonstrated in [63]. The MEMS scanning mirror scanned both the pulse laser for PAI and continuous laser for DOT. A ring transducer at the center of probe detects PA signals and optical fibers at the outside of the probe collects diffused light in DOT (Figure 1(ci)). Since the DOT has a lower resolution than PAI (i.e., 3~4 mm), it can be utilized to confirm the position and approximate volume of the tumor (Figure 1(cii)). The PAI with much better resolution (i.e., 0.2~0.7 mm) can be used to display tumor margins accurately (Figure 1(ciii)).

Around the same time, another research group also demonstrated the PAI probe based on a MEMS scanning mirror [64,65]. In their system, they used a commercially available MEMS scanning mirror (TM-2520, Sercalo Microtechnology Ltd., Neuchâtel, Switzerland) to reflect the laser and microring resonator to detect PA signal. These results will be discussed further in a later section.

2.2. Recent Advances in PAI System Based on MEMS Scanning Mirror

While the MEMS scanning mirror based PAI probes showed promise, several optimizations were still needed for practical clinical applications, such as (i) increasing imaging speed, (ii) improving spatial resolution and SNR, and (iii) minimizing the probe size for endoscopic applications. Unlike conventional PAI system with external bulky mechanical scanning devices, the MEMS scanning mirror based PAI probes are smaller and faster, while maintaining high-resolution.

L. Xi group first reported a high-resolution PA endomicroscopy probe using a commercial MEMS scanning mirror (WM-S3.1, WiOTEK, Wuxi, China, commercialized product of Section 2.1) as shown in Figure 2(ai) [66]. This PA endomicroscopy used a 0.7 mm Gradient-index (GRIN) lens to increase the lateral resolution to 10.6 μm. The fast MEMS scanning mirror (i.e., 500 Hz) fully utilized pulse laser's high repetition rate of 20 kHz. For detecting the PA signals, an unfocused customized US transducer with the axial resolution of ~105 μm was used. Phantom and animal experiments were demonstrated (Figure 2(aii)) while using this system. Since the diameter of the probe is almost half the size of the previous studies (i.e., 6 mm), it can potentially be used in the endoscopic channel for imaging gastrointestinal tract. Most recently, a MEMS scanning mirror based OR-PAM probe for human lip imaging was developed by the same research group [67,68]. Although the size of the OR-PAM probe is slightly bigger than endomicroscopy, it has better performance with respect to spatial resolution and FOV. The 20 grams weight and $22 \times 30 \times 13$ mm^3 size of the probe is suitable for imaging the human lip. High lateral resolution of 3.8 μm and FOV of 2×2 mm^2 can provide a PA microvasculature image. This probe was used to image internal organs vasculatures in the rat (Figure 2(bii)) and oral cavity in human (Figure 2(biii)).

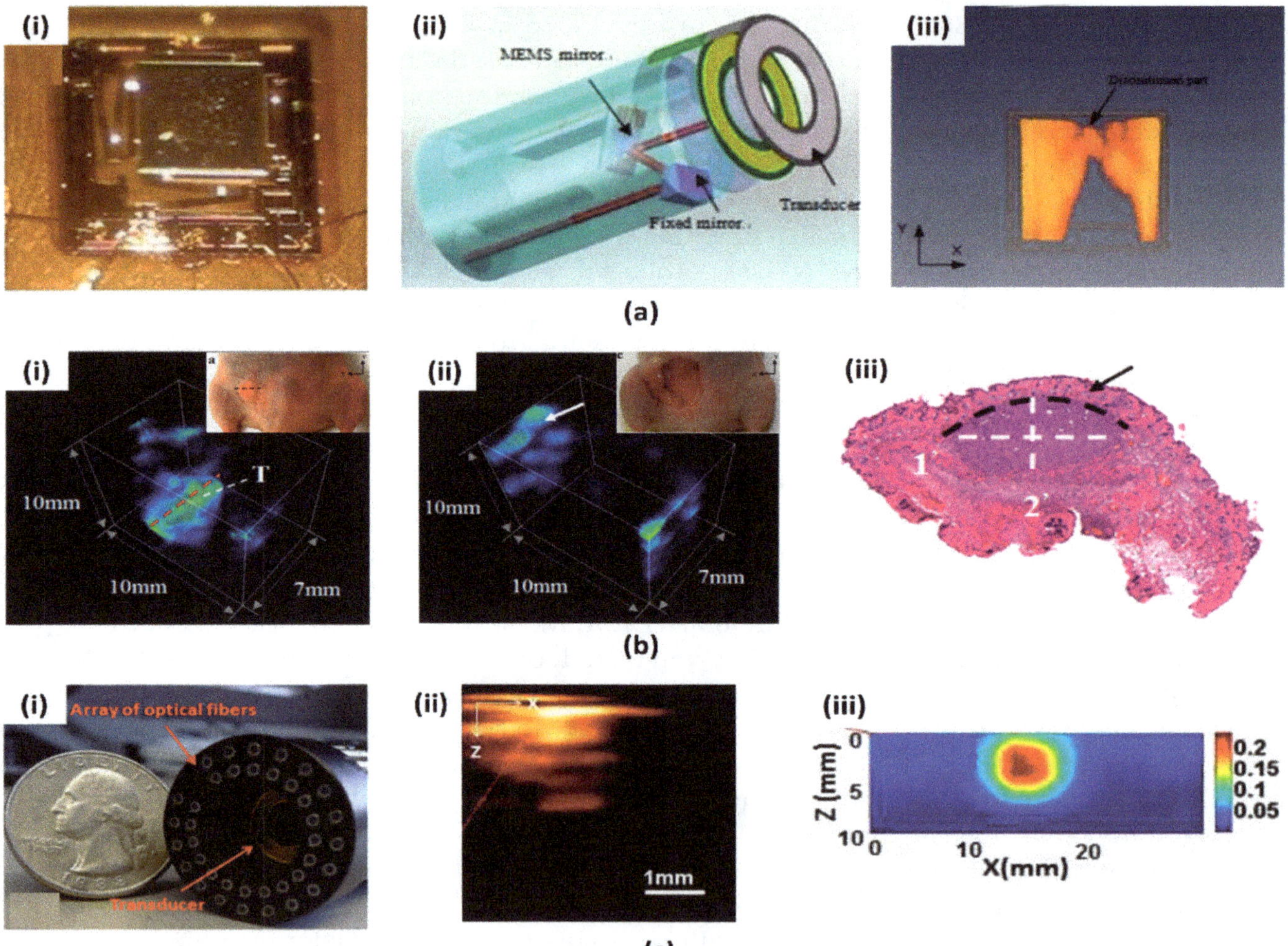

Figure 1. (**a**) Photoacoustic imaging (PAI) probe based on microelectromechanical system (MEMS) scanning mirror (**ai**) Photograph of the MEMS mirror (**aii**) Schematic PAI probe (**aiii**) 3D rendering of the recovered blood vessels of the human hand [61]. Reproduced with permission from Xi, Lei, et al., photoacoustic imaging based on MEMS mirror scanning; published by OSA, 2010. (**b**) In vivo volumetric photoacoustic (PA) image of (**bi**) Tumor before the surgery and (**bii**) the tumor cavity after surgery. (**biii**) H & E stained section along the red dashed line in (**bi**) [62]. Reproduced with permission from Xi, Lei, et al., evaluation of breast tumor margins in vivo with intraoperative photoacoustic imaging; published by OSA, 2012. (**c**): (**ci**) integrated optic fibers and ultrasound transducer probe. (**cii**) Cross-sectional PA image and (**ciii**) optical tomography (DOT) image of the tumor [63]. Reproduced with permission from Yang, Hao, et al., handheld miniature probe integrating diffuse optical tomography with photoacoustic imaging through a MEMS scanning mirror.

The DMD (Discovery 4100, Texas Instruments, Dallas, TX, USA), which consists of several hundred thousand micro mirrors, is another important application of the optical MEMS device. The DMD was also applied in several PAI systems using the spatial and spectral encoding ability of the light [69,70]. Recently, J. Yang et al. reported a motionless volumetric PAM with DMD (Figure 2(ci)) [71]. They used propagation-invariant sinusoidal fringes, by exploiting the field modulation ability of the DMD, for motionless volumetric imaging. The lateral resolution of 1.89 μm that was achieved in this system was 1.5 times higher, and the resolution-invariant axial range of 1800 μm is 30 times higher than the conventional PAM. As shown in Figure 2(cii), they successfully obtained a PA image of zebrafish larva with superior resolution in depth.

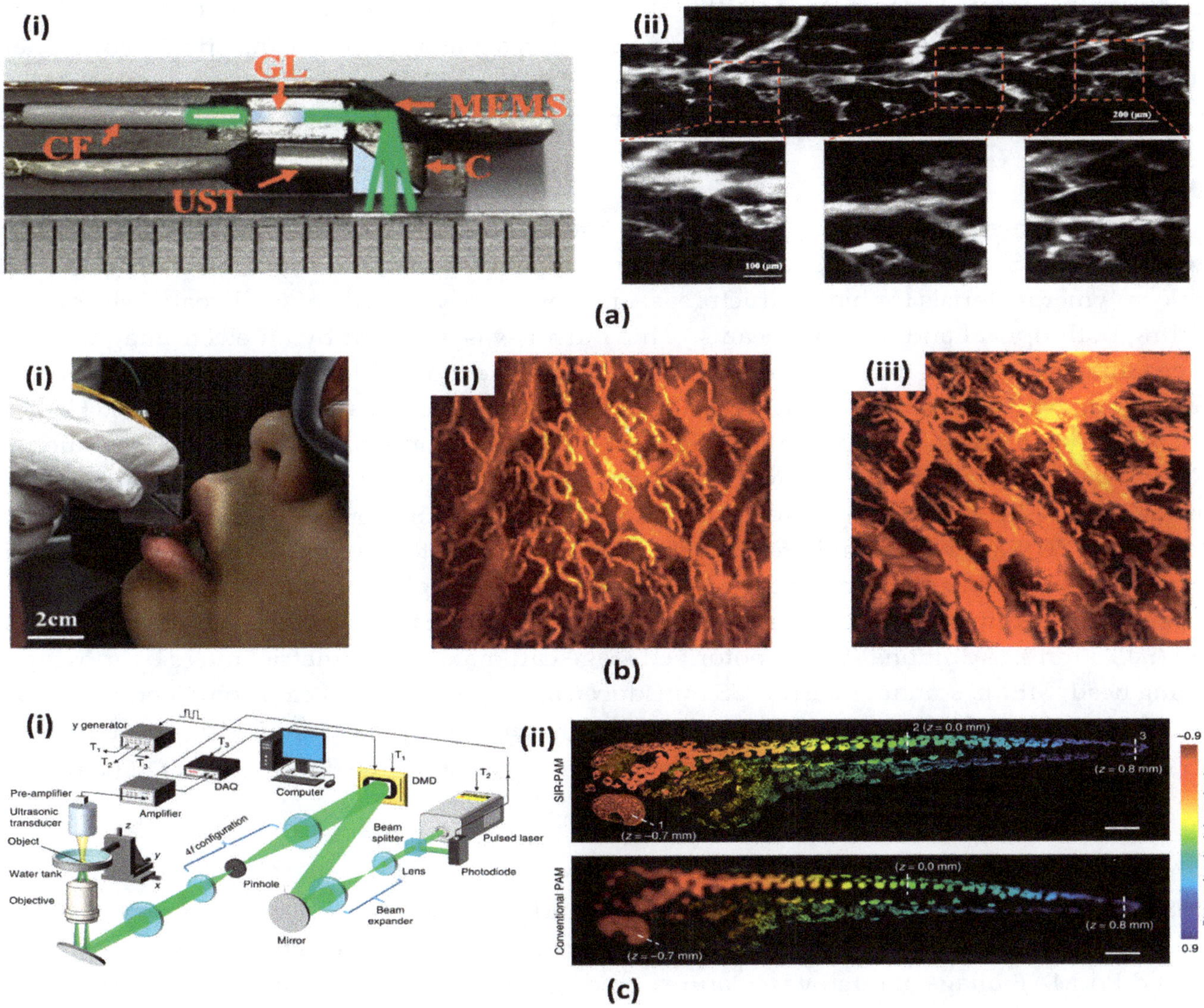

Figure 2. (**a**) MEMS scanning mirror based PA endomicroscopy probe. (**ai**) Photograph of the imaging probe. CF, ceramic ferrule; GL, Gradient-index lens; UST, ultrasound transducer; C, cube. (**aii**) PA image of a mouse colon and sub-images [66]. Reproduced with permission from Guo, Heng, et al., photoacoustic endomicroscopy based on a MEMS scanning mirror; published by OSA, 2017. (**b**) In vivo human oral imaging. (**bi**) Photograph of the PAI probe and a volunteer participating. (**bii**) PA image of the lower lip and (**biii**) back surface of the tongue [67]. Reproduced with permission from Chen, Qian, et al., ultracompact high-resolution photoacoustic microscopy; published by OSA, 2018. (**c**) Digital micromirror device (DMD) based spatially invariant resolution photoacoustic microscopy (PAM) (**ci**) Schematic diagram (**cii**) Depth encoded whole body images of a zebrafish larva. [71].

3. Water Immersible MEMS Scanning Mirror for PAI

3.1. 1-Axis Water Immersible MEMS Scanning Mirror

Although the conventional silicon-based MEMS scanning mirror has many advantages in various optical imaging systems, it has one severe drawback for PAI systems. It is that the MEMS fabrication process is generally based on a silicon wafer, which has brittle and delicate mirror supporting structures. Thus, the previous MEMS scanning mirrors are not appropriate to operate in acoustic coupling medium (e.g., water). The PAI systems, as discussed in Section 2, mainly utilized optical beam scanning with unfocused US transducers, which resulted in low detection sensitivity. However, focused detection of PA signals is essential to have high SNR [72] for diagnostic PA images. Conventional PAM makes one dimensional confocal aligning of focused optical and acoustic beams using special components, such as an opto-acoustic beam combiner [13] or ring transducer [73]. For acquiring volumetric images, motor based linear scanning stages are used to move the heavy components, which results in low imaging speed.

To resolve these above-stated problems, J. Yao et al. [74] developed a special 1-axis water immersible MEMS mirror based OR-PAM. The water immersible MEMS mirror used high-strength flexible polymer materials for hinge structures. A mirror plate was made of gold-coated silicon wafer reflecting both optical and acoustic beams. This mirror was actuated by an electromagnetic force between inductor coil and two permanent magnets under the mirror plate. This polymer based hinge structures and high electromagnetic actuation schemes enabled the fast scanning of up to 400 Hz under water. This system greatly enhanced the imaging speed while maintaining high lateral resolution and SNR. Similar to conventional OR-PAM, this system also can utilize the opto-acoustic beam combiner ensuring high SNR. The main difference in this system is that the confocally aligned optical beam and resultant PA wave were simultaneously scanned in water with the fixed beam combiner position (Figure 3(ai)). With fast scanning of the scanning mirror and high repetition rate of the pulse laser, the speed of two-dimensional cross-sectional imaging (i.e., B-scan) was 400 Hz at a wide scanning range (i.e., 3 mm). Additionally, the motorized stage can make a volumetric image by moving the scanning head, MEMS scanning mirror, US transducer, and opto-acoustic beam combiner. Figure 3(aii) shows the PA maximum amplitude projection (MAP) image of the vasculature in a mouse ear over $2 \times 5\ mm^2$ area. The fast-volumetric imaging rate of 0.8 Hz can show the flow dynamics of hemoglobin in the blood vessels.

A preclinical research study for mouse brain was demonstrated using the high-speed MEMS scanner [75]. Two pulse lasers (i.e., pico- and nano-second pulse), both with a 532 nm single-wavelength, were used to display blood oxygenation with high-resolution. Figure 3(bi) shows the fused PA MAP image of microvasculature and oxygen saturation level in the same mouse brain. The acquisition time for the wide-FOV-mosaic image was about 40 s, which is several hundred times faster than conventional OR-PAM. Figure 3(bii) shows the hemodynamic responses to electrical stimulations in real time. The PA amplitude of right hemisphere was increased in response to electrical stimulation on the left hind limb. The 1-axis water immersible MEMS mirror can also be used in therapy. Y. He et al. demonstrated a PA flow cystography integrated with a laser therapy of melanoma [76]. Similar to the previous results, they first imaged the microvasculature in a mouse ear with a 532 nm wavelength laser. The flow of circulating melanoma cells was acquired while using a 1064 nm wavelength laser. The circulating melanoma cells were immediately killed by another therapy laser, which was self-triggered by the PA signal of the melanoma cells.

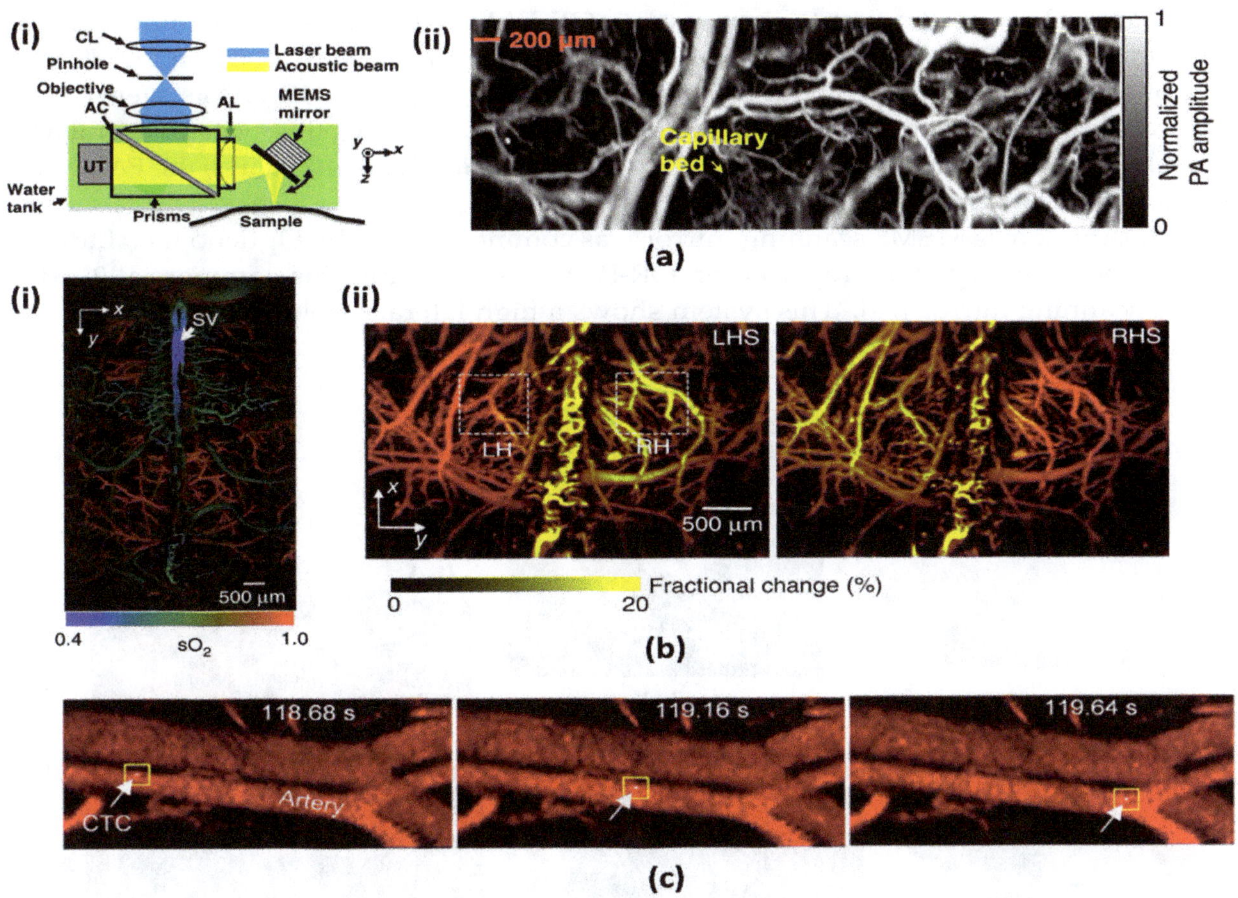

Figure 3. (**a**) A water immersible MEMS mirror based optical-resolution PAM (OR-PAM). (**ai**) Schematic diagram. (**aii**) PA maximum amplitude projection (MAP) image of microvasculature in a mouse ear [74]. Reproduced with permission from Yao, Junjie, et al., wide-field fast-scanning photoacoustic microscopy based on a water-immersible MEMS scanning mirror; published by SPIE, 2012. (**b**) High-speed functional OR-PAM based on MEMS scanning mirror (**bi**) Microvasculatures and oxygen saturation level in a mouse brain. (**bii**) Fractional PA signal changes in response to hindlimb stimulation [75]. Reproduced with permission from Yao, Junjie, et al., high-speed label-free functional photoacoustic microscopy of mouse brain in action; published by Nature, 2015. (**c**) PA snapshots are showing single circulating tumor cells (CTCs) traveling in the vasculature [76].

3.2. 2-Axis Water Immersible MEMS Scanning Mirror

As described in the above section, the 1-axis water immersible MEMS scanning mirror can greatly increase the B-scan imaging speed of OR-PAM. However, it still has limitations such as bulky system size due to the additional motorized stage for volumetric imaging. For clinical translation, such as endoscopy, laparoscopy, or handheld systems, it is essential to have both (i) high imaging speed and (ii) small system size. To overcome these limitations, two kinds of 2-axis water immersible MEMS scanning mirror were developed, as shown in Figure 4(ai,aii) [72,77]. Similar to the 1-axis water immersible MEMS scanning mirror, they are also made of flexible polymer instead of brittle silicon. One was fabricated by a laser cutting of biaxially-oriented polyethylene terephthalate (BOPET) film, and the other was made by soft lithography of polydimethylsiloxane (PDMS). They are commonly adapted to a gimbal structure, which can steer the optical and acoustic beam simultaneously along the two axes on one scanner. Aluminum coated silicon mirror enhanced the reflectivity of optical and acoustic beams. Strong electromagnetic actuation along two axes was used to overcome the water resistance.

J. Y. Kim et al. were the first to demonstrate OR-PAM with 2-axis water immersible MEMS scanning mirror [78]. The fabricated 2 axis MEMS scanning mirror that is based on PDMS stamping has a size of 15 × 15 × 15 mm^3. Without using any motorized stage, this OR-PAM system can achieve a high B-scan rate of 50 Hz and volumetric imaging rate of 0.25 Hz. For this system, lateral and axial resolutions were 3.6 μm and 27.7 μm, respectively. As shown in Figure 4(aiii,aiv), the PA MAP image of a live mouse ear was successfully obtained (Figure 4(aiv)).

Recently, this 2-axis MEMS scanning mirror was commercialized by Opticho Inc., Ltd. in South Korea. M. Moothanchery et al. reported an OR-PAM system using this commercial 2-axis water immersible scanning mirror [79]. This system shows a high lateral resolution of 3.5 μm in spite of using multimode fiber.

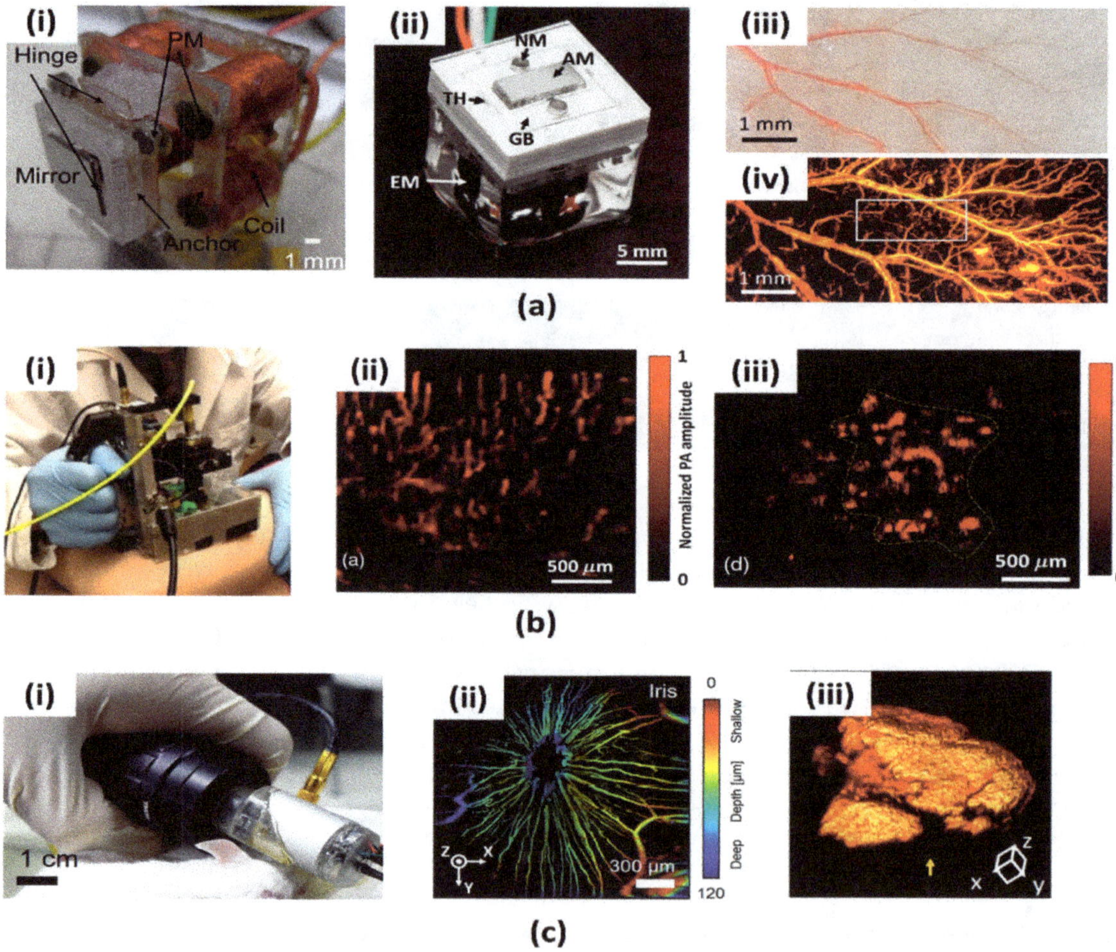

Figure 4. (**a**) 2-axis water immersible MEMS scanning mirror made of (**ai**) biaxially-oriented polyethylene terephthalate (BOPET) film and (**aii**) polydimethylsiloxane (PDMS). (**aiii**) Photograph of a mouse ear and blood micro-vessels in it. (**aiv**) PA MAP image of (**aiii**) [72,77,78]. Reproduced with permission from Huang, Chih-Hsien, et al., a water-immersible 2-axis scanning mirror microsystem for ultrasound andha photoacoustic microscopic imaging applications; published by Springer, 2012. Reproduced with permission from Kim, Jin Young, et al., a PDMS-based 2-axis waterproof scanner for photoacoustic microscopy; published by MDPI, 2015. Fast optical-resolution photoacoustic microscopy using a 2-axis water-proofing MEMS scanner; published by Nature, 2015. (**b**): (**bi**) Photograph of the handheld PAM based on 2-axis water immersible MEMS scanner mirror. (**bii**) PA image of capillaries in a human cuticle. (**biii**) PA image of the red mole on a human leg [80]. Reproduced with permission from Lin, Li, et al., handheld optical-resolution photoacoustic microscopy; published by SPIE, 2016. (**c**): (**ci**) Photograph of the PAM probe. (**cii**) Depth encoded PA image of the microvasculature in a mouse iris. (**ciii**) Volumetric PA image of a mole on a human finger [81].

L. Lin et al. demonstrated a handheld PAM system based on 2-axis water immersible MEMS scanning mirror, as shown in Figure 4(bi) [80]. This handheld OR-PAM system has a dimension of $80 \times 115 \times 150$ mm^3 and is more flexible than conventional benchtop systems. The lateral resolution of the handheld system was 5 μm. The 3D volumetric imaging rate over a region of $2.5 \times 2.0 \times 0.5$ mm^3 was 2 Hz. To verify the usage of the handheld PAM in clinical applications, they acquired PA images of human cuticle (Figure 4(bii)) and a mole on a volunteer's leg (Figure 4(biii)). K. Park et al. reported a much smaller handheld OR-PAM probe, as shown in Figure 4(ci) [81]. They modified the water immersible MEMS scanning mirror to a round shape to reduce the system size. All of the parts, including 2-axis MEMS scanning mirror, were integrated into this small probe (diameter: 17 mm). The lateral resolution was 16 μm, and the B-scan rate was 35 Hz. Thanks to the small size and fast imaging speed, this handheld probe is suitable for both small animal and human imaging. Figure 4(cii) shows the in vivo depth encoded microvasculature image of the mouse iris and Figure 4(ciii) shows the 3D image of a mole on a volunteer's finger. In Table 1, we summarize and present the specifications of all MEMS scanning mirrors compared to conventional scanning methods (i.e., mechanical stage and optical galvanometer scanner).

Table 1. Comparison of the PAI system based on MEMS scanning mirror.

Scanning Methods	System Size	Imaging Speed (B-Scan Rate)	FOV	SNR	Ref.
Mechanical Scanning	Bulky (>300 mm)	1 Hz	>10 mm	+++	[12]
Optical Scanning	Bulky (>200 mm)	100 Hz	<8 mm	+	[39]
Silicon MEMS Mirror	Small (<30 mm)	500 Hz	<3 mm	++	[67]
Water immersible MEMS Mirror	Medium (<100 mm)	1 axis: 400 Hz 2 axis: 50 Hz	<3 mm <9 mm	+++	[75,78]
Handheld PAI Probe	Small (<30 mm)	35 Hz	<2 mm	+++	[81]

4. Micromachined US Detector for PAI

4.1. Micromachined US Transducers (MUTs)

Transducers arrays made of polyvinylidene fluoride (PVDF) have been widely used in clinical PAI systems [82,83]. However, due to the relatively low sensitivity and limited frequency bandwidth of small PVDF, there are limits to using mini-sized probes for endoscopic and vascular applications. MUTs can be an excellent alternative to overcome these issues with broad frequency bandwidth and miniaturized size. MUTs are divided into two types: capacitive MUT (CMUT) and piezoelectric MUT (PMUT).

CMUT utilizes capacitance variation that is related to energy transduction between a silicon substrate and a thin membrane layer to detect the US signal. It has several unique advantages, such as (i) convenient interfacing with front-end electronic circuits and (ii) can be easily manufactured to have diverse array sizes with individually linked electronics [84–87]. This technology has already been applied in compact two & three-dimensional US and PA handheld and endomicroscopic probes. As shown in Figure 5(ai), A. Nikoozadeh et al. reported a ring-type CMUT array that comprised of four concentric rings fabricated with a polysilicon sacrificial release process [88]. All concentric rings were located in the main probe body with different diameters (i.e., 6.0, 7.2, 8.5, and 9.7 mm). Same 128 transducer elements were used at each concentric ring with different center frequencies (i.e., 16, 12, 8, and 6.5 MHz). The probe has an inner diameter of 5.0 mm and the outer diameter of 10.1 mm. The miniaturization provides a good opportunity to use them in endoscopic PAI systems.

To reduce general loss and improve SNR, the ring CMUT arrays were installed into a handcrafted IC in a pin-grid-array (PGA) and was fully connected to commercial PAI systems (Figure 5(aii)). A 128-channel US imaging platform (Verasonics, Inc., Redmond, USA) was used to receive PA waves. In Figure 5(aiii), the volumetric image of the metal spring was obtained by 360 degrees rotation of the B-mode plane along the vertical axis and accumulating the MAP. J. Chen et al. developed an infrared-transparent silicon CMUT array that provides a compact probe size and uniform laser excitation configurations [89].

A multi-band CMUT was also fabricated by J. Zhang et al. to visualize the more comprehensive structure of biological tissues [90]. Figure 5(bi,bii) show the photographs and the magnified optical microscopic image of the multi-band CMUT array comprising of low-frequency (~4 MHz central frequency, 10 μm radius) and high-frequency (~10 MHz central frequency, 15 μm radius) arrays. To fabricate the CMUT array, four-inch silicon wafer consisting of the substrate and a lower electrode was prepared. The CMUT and channels were fabricated through a reactive-ion etching (RIE) process with the polysilicon layer and deposition of the Si_3N_4 layer. Finally, a thin film aluminum of 300 nm was deposited to fabricate an electrode, a connection portion, and a bonding pad. Figure 5b(iii,iv) show the in vivo PA images of zebrafish that were obtained with the multiband CMUT.

PMUT is also an emerging US detector based on flexural vibration induced by a thin-film piezoelectric membrane. The PMUT provides different benefits compared to CMUT including (i) relatively higher capacitance as compared to CMUT, (ii) does not require high polarization voltage, and (iii) has a compatible matching impedance with sample [91–93]. Several types of PMUT-based US transducers are widely used for biomedical applications, such as the catheter type, dome-shape array, and concave array type [94–96]. W. Liao et al. first reported the two-dimensional PMUT array with 144 elements for the PAI [97] system. They developed a PMUT array by fabricating a thin film PZT membranes with a radius of 25 μm and a pitch of 80 μm. The membrane consists of a PZT layer of 0.6 μm, an elastic SiO_2 layer of 1 μm, and covering layer of 5 μm. In the pulse-echo mode, the high resonant frequency of 10 MHz, good spatial gain, and broad capturing angle have been demonstrated.

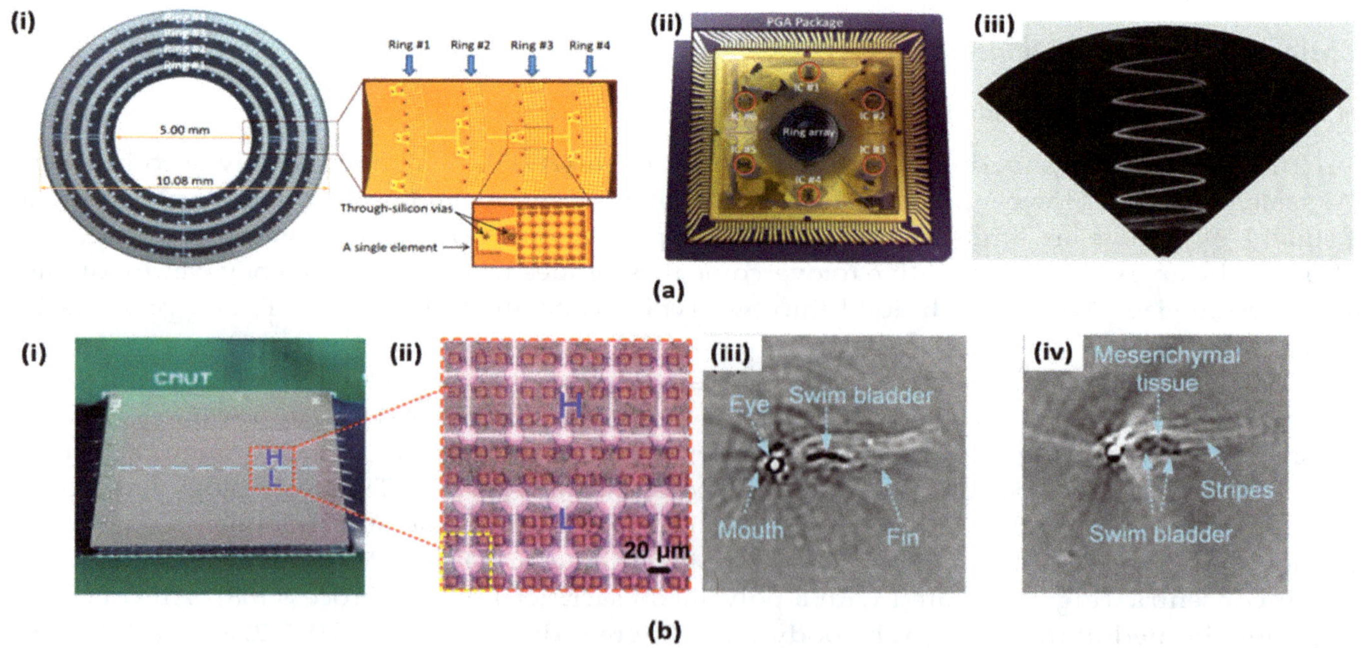

Figure 5. *Cont.*

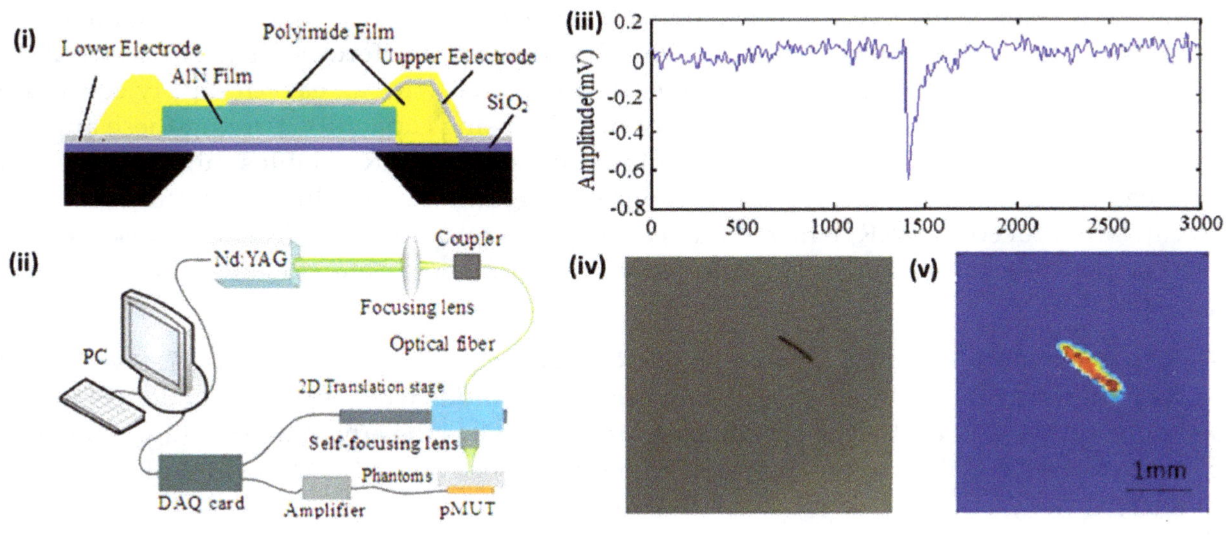

(c)

Figure 5. (**a**) A ring-type capacitive micromachined US transducers (CMUT) array for PAI. (**ai**) Schematic and an optical microscopic view of the 512-element four-ring CMUT array. (**aii**) A ring CMUT array installed into handmade electronics. (**aiii**) Volumetric US image of a metal spring with the ring CMUT array [88]. Reproduced with permission from Nikoozadeh, Amin, et al., an integrated Ring CMUT array for endoscopic ultrasound and photoacoustic imaging; published by IEEE, 2013. (**b**) Multi-band CMUT array for PAI (**bi**) The photograph of multi-band CMUT array. (**bii**) Magnified optical microscopic view of multi-band CMUT array. (**biii,biv**) In vivo PA images of a zebrafish measured by the low- and high-frequency CMUT arrays, respectively [90]. Reproduced with permission from Zhang, Jian, et al., development of a multi-band photoacoustic tomography imaging system based on a capacitive micromachined ultrasonic transducer array; published by OSA, 2017. (**c**) A PMUT based on AlN and acquired PA image (**ci**) Structure of PMUT based on AlN. (**cii**) Experimental setup of photoacoustic imaging with PMUT. (**ciii**) Acquired PA signal of the hair (**civ**) Photography of human hair embedded in the phantom. (**cv**) Reconstructed PA image [98].

B. Chen et al. proposed a new PMUT based on an aluminum nitride (AlN) for PAI applications [98]. As shown in Figure 5(ci), the proposed PMUT has micro-layers comprising of SiO_2, lower/top electrodes, AlN, and polyimide (PI) films. The piezoelectric layer based on AlN was generated from metallic Al samples at room temperature via intermediate frequency magnetron reactive sputtering. The AlN based PMUT shows the enhanced SNR due to AlN's relatively low piezoelectric coefficient. Additionally, its manufacturing process has the benefit of being compatible with the standard ICs. Figure 5(cii) shows the schematic of the PAI experimental setup. A nano-second pulsed laser with 532 nm (Brilliant, QUANTEL) wavelength and was coupled to a mulimodal fiber was excited inside this phantom. The generated PA signal was identified by the PMUT array that was located at the bottom of the phantom. Figure 5(ciii,civ,cv) show one-dimensional PA signal, sample photographs, and reconstructed PA image of human hair within the phantom, respectively. The measured lateral resolution was 240 μm.

4.2. Microring Resonators (MRRs)

Typically, a conventional piezoelectric US transducer works in the resonant frequency band, which is determined by the thickness of the piezoelectric crystal. When a thin piezoelectric crystal film is used to produce a high-frequency transducer, this thin film is fragile and it causes manufacturing complexity and ruggedness issues [42]. Also, these transducers have a low axial resolution because of limited bandwidth and have small FOV because of limited capturing angle. They are also difficult to integrate with high-resolution optical microscopy, which has short working distance (i.e., below 1 mm) [90,99]. To address these drawbacks, diverse optical based ultrasonic detection methods, such as Fabry-Perot polymer film [100], Michelson interferometer [101], Mach Zehnder interferometer [102], and MRR [52,103–105] have been reported with an easy-to-apply configuration for endoscopic and microscopic systems and superior US sensing capability. Among these approaches, MRR has additional strengths. (i) A sub-millimeter sized MRR enables high US sensitivity, which reduces the optical interference in probing configuration. (ii) Broadband ultrasonic wave detection can be achieved in MRR, which enhances the axial resolution in PAI and ultrasonic imaging (USI). (iii) The MRR detector allows for a relatively high ultrasonic detection angle, which improves the FOV.

C.-Y. Chao et al. first reported a polymer MRR detector as a US transducer [52]. It was designed in such a way that the ring and the straight-line bus waveguides were interconnected (Figure 6(ai)). They used polystyrene (PS) as the waveguide material, which has the advantages of high sensitivity for acoustic pressure and low absorption for visible to near IR spectrum light. The width of the waveguide is 2.4 μm and the height is 1.85 μm.

Nanoimprint process was applied to fabricate waveguides with high sensitivity. First, a mold with an inverted pattern was produced using electron beam lithography and RIE. Subsequently, a spin-coated polymer was imprinted onto the substrate by using the fabricated mold at an appropriately increased temperature and pressure. By applying pulse-echo signals, the MRR response was acquired, as shown in Figure 6a(ii). The bandwidth increased by 10 dB from 15 MHz to 58 MHz and decreased approximately from 60 MHz onwards.

The active imaging area was investigated with two-dimensional US emission on the surface of MRR. The measured signal has the full width at half maximum (FWHM) of approximately 130 μm (Figure 6(aiii)). C. Zhang et al. upgraded the polymer bandwidth from dc to 350 MHz, which presented the outstanding axial resolution of 3 μm [106].

The concept of miniaturized PAI and all optical customized PAI were successfully demonstrated based on MRR's advantages [64,103,107]. For instance, S.-L. Chen et al. reported the miniaturized PAM probe with MRR detector and MEMS optical scanning mirror. Figure 6(bi) shows the system configuration. A high speed diode-pumped solid-state Nd:YAG laser at 532 nm was directly inserted into an optical fiber and was transferred to a 2-axis MEMS scanning mirror.

The MRR detector was located 3.7 mm below the sample surface. System performance was demonstrated by visualizing the microvessels in a mouse bladder with lateral and axial resolutions of 17.5 μm and 20 μm, respectively. Even though these MRRs were investigated on silicon plates, they are not optically transparent. Therefore, only permeable PAI system configurations that are not suitable for scanning thin layered samples were possible. H. Li et al. fabricated an optically transparent US detector that was composed of the MRR on a fine coverslip [108]. Figure 6(ci) shows the customized MRR US detector.

The two tapered optical fibers combined with the input and output stages of the ring and bus waveguide simplify the packaging process and improve the coupling efficiency. Due to the optical transparency of the MRR detector, a highly focused laser beam was irradiated on the thin samples via the MRR detector located on the adjustable holder. When compared to the transmission PAI configuration, US deformation was eliminated. The developed MRR US detector has an ultra-wideband frequency range (approx. 140 MHz) and provides an excellent axial resolution of 5.3 μm. A thin film sample was used to obtain a PA image with improved axial resolution and is shown in Figure 6(ciii)).

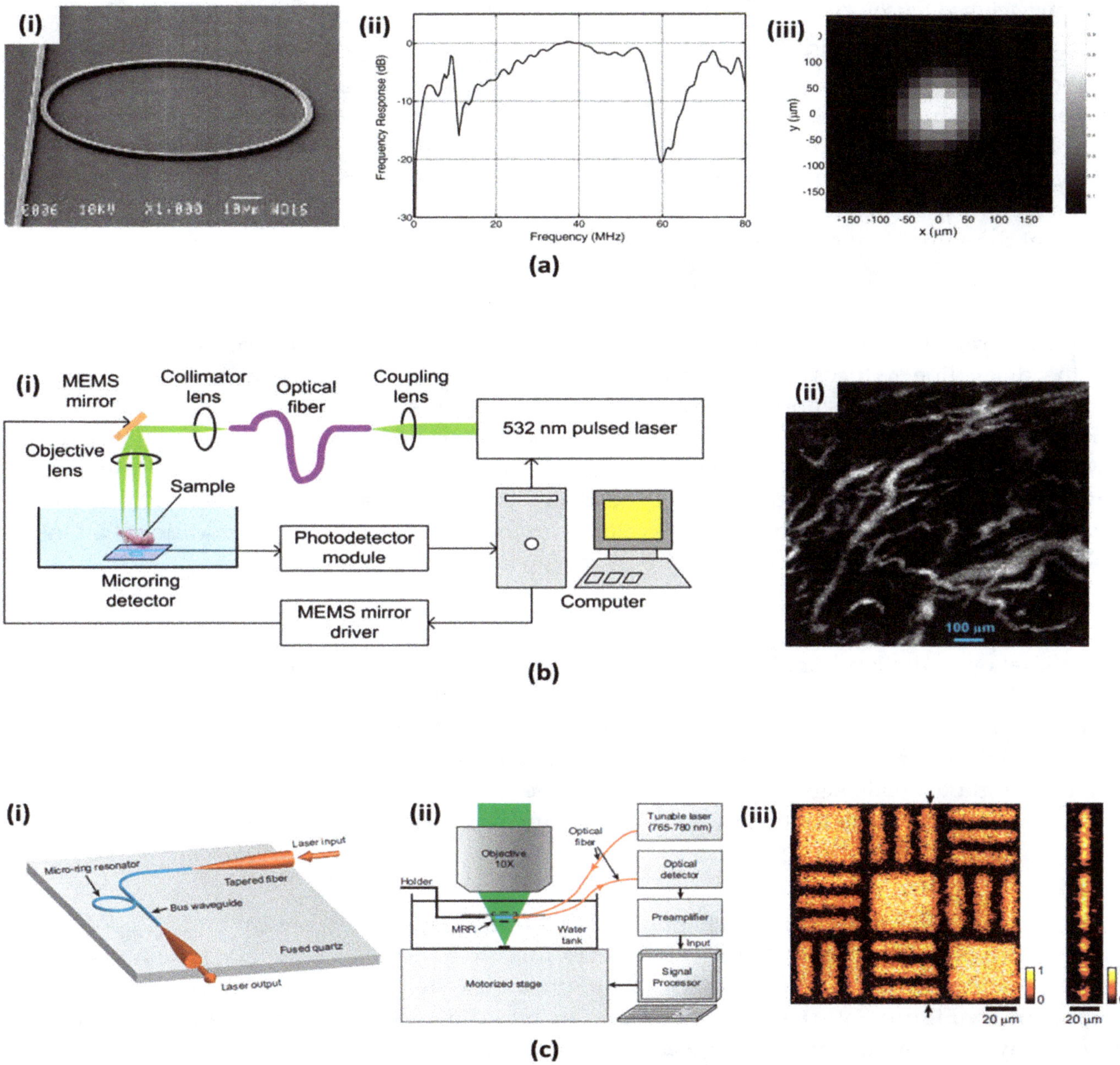

Figure 6. (**a**) Geometry of micro-ring resonator (MRR) US detector and measured properties (**ai**) Scanning electron micrograph of MRR. (**aii**) The frequency response of MRR to a US pulse. (**aiii**) Two-dimensional US pulse response of MRR [52] Reproduced with permission from Chao, Chung-Yen, et al., high-frequency ultrasound sensors using polymer microring resonators; published by IEEE, 2007. (**b**) Miniaturized OR-PAM using MRR (**bi**) Schematic of optical-resolution PAM system using the MRR. (**bii**) MAP image of the microvasculature in the mouse bladder [64]. Reproduced with permission from Chen, Sung-Liang, et al., miniaturized all-optical photoacoustic microscopy based on microelectromechanical systems mirror scanning; published by OSA, 2012. (**c**) Transparent broadband MRR US detector for OR-PAM. (**ci**) Schematic of MRR US detector with tapered optical fibers. (**cii**) Experimental setup for OR-PAM with transparent MRR. (**ciii**) The MAP image of a carbon-black thin film sample along an x-y plate and a two-dimensional PA image of the target at the location indicated by the arrows [108].

4.3. Micromachined Silicon Acoustic Delay Lines and Multiplexer

Typical array-type US transducers used in clinical USI and PAI require multiple complex multi-channel DAQ devices to simultaneously receive large amounts of acoustic data from each transducer element [109]. This increases the overall PAI complexity and cost of the system. Recently, the concepts of acoustic time delay were reported by M. K. Yapici et al. [110] to reduce complexity. The parallel connected acoustic delay line receivers were utilized instead of the transducer elements. Each delay line detected the acoustic signal and generated an appropriate delay time so that the signal arrived at a different time on the other side.

A single transducer was connected on the opposite side for sensing the time delay signal in series. Thus, the delay line reduces the requirements for multi-element transducer elements and multi-channel DAQ devices. This approach would be more cost effective than conventional US detecting systems. The handheld optical fiber based delay line was investigated as a promising method to take several advantages, such as less acoustic loss, microscale size, flexible property, and low cost [111]. However, in order to generate enough time delay in the optical fiber, a considerable length of optical fiber is required due to the high US velocity in the medium. Moreover, additional attenuation and signal distortion could also occur due to the covered jacket layer.

Optimal optical alignment is also necessary to obtain a proper signal and manual assembly. Y. Cho et al. introduced a micromachined silicon acoustic delay line [112]. Thanks to the material property of single crystalline silicon, this method has better transmission efficiency, small size, and more productivity when compared to the optical fiber-based delay lines. Each acoustic channel delivers a single acoustic signal with a specific travel path and delay. To generate sufficient delay length and maintain a compact size, each acoustic channel consists of several U-turns.

As shown in Figure 7(ai,aii), 16-channel parallel lines were fabricated by an RIE process using the aluminum pattern mask. All fabricated delay lines were located on the acrylic housing. Since the ultrasonic pulses propagate different lengths from the delay line, they reached the outputs at different times. Figure 7a(iii) shows the acquired two-dimensional PA image from the proposed parallel delay lines. A similar concept was adopted by the same group to micromachined acoustic multiplexer [113]. Only one transmit and/or receive US transducer was required to resolve multichannel signals in this system. Unlike the acoustic delay line, acoustic multiplexer can selectively transmit the acoustic signal via the movement of mercury droplet in microfluidic channel (Figure 7(bi)).

The assembled multiplexer is shown in Figure 7(bii). The silicon delay line and multiplexer structure were fabricated by the RIE process. Two PDMS sealing pads were used to form a microchannel with the silicon structure, and the PI microtubing was connected to inlet and outlet of the channel. Mercury droplet was driven by a syringe pump. The PA image of the phantom using this system is shown in Figure 7(biii). A pulse laser illuminated a $5 \times 5\,mm^2$ area and the PA signal generated was successfully detected by a single transducer. To collect eight channel signal, illumination and acquisition were repeated eight times.

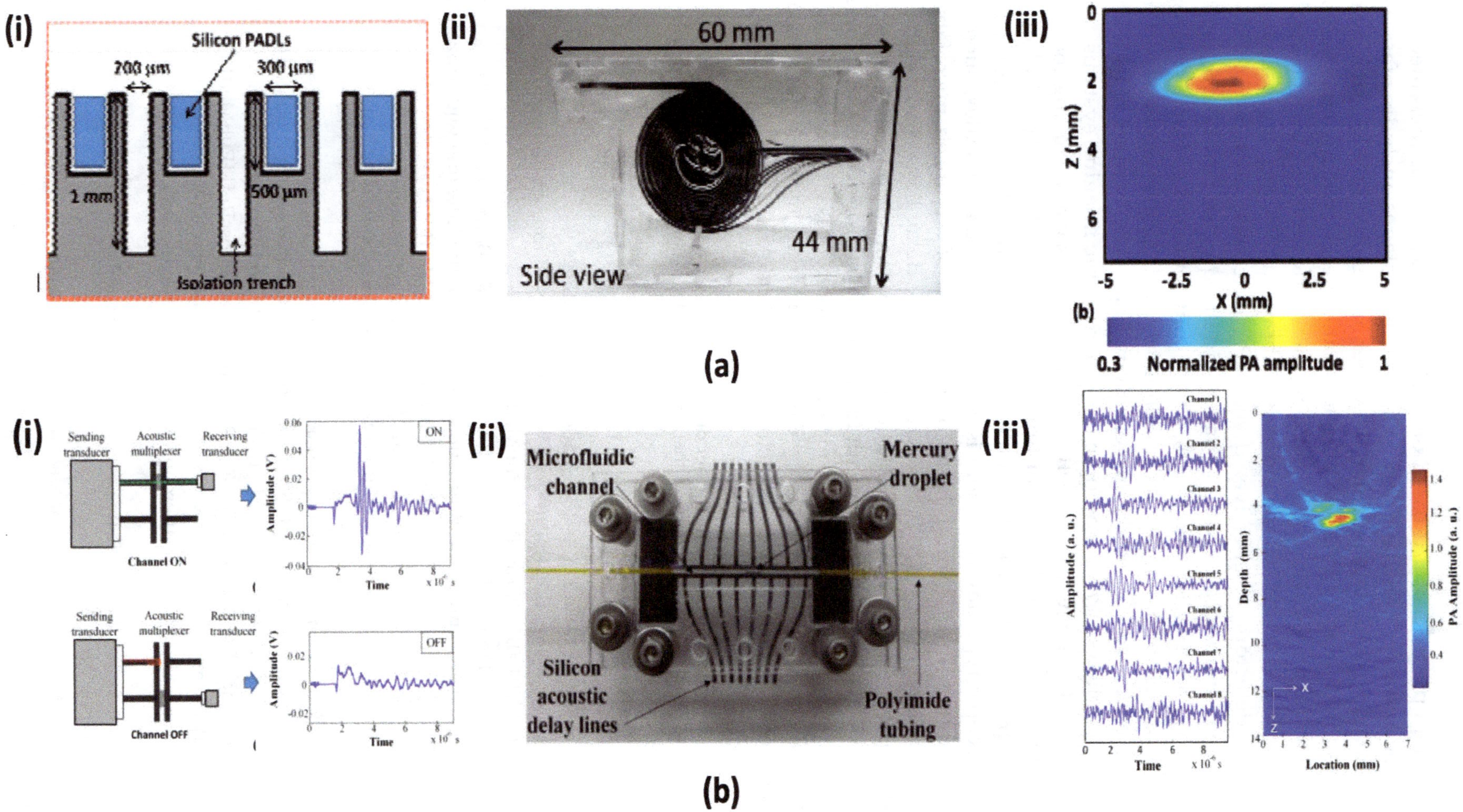

Figure 7. (**a**) Micromachined parallel silicon delay lines. (**ai**) An enlarged view of spacers with detail dimension. (**aii**) Fabricated 16 channels parallel delay lines and assembled on an acrylic housing. (**aiii**) Reconstructed two-dimensional PA image of the absorber in the phantom with 16-channel parallel delay lines [112]. Reproduced with permission from Cho, Young, et al., a micromachined silicon parallel acoustic delay line (PADL) array for real-time photoacoustic tomography (PAT); published by SPIE, 2015. (**b**) Micromachined acoustic multiplexer (**bi**) Acoustic ON/OFF characterization. (**bii**) An assembled acoustic multiplexer (**biii**) Photoacoustic signal and reconstructed image [113].

5. Conclusions

In this review, the current progress of PAI based on MEMS technology was presented. From the MEMS scanning mirrors perspective, they have shown several advantages, including fast scanning abilities, compact sizes, and high SNRs. In particular, the water immersible MEMS scanning mirrors broke through the intrinsic limitation of PAM techniques that were caused by acoustic coupling medium (i.e., water). New advances also contributed to the fabrication of the well-established preclinical PA handheld probes and PA endoscopic systems for brain studies, angiogenesis, and cancer studies. From the MEMS detectors perspective, diverse PA detectors, such as MUTs, MRRs, and acoustic delay lines were introduced. MUTs enable wide frequency bandwidth, small size, and conventional integrating process with electronics. These contribute to develop a multispectral clinical PA system with endoscopic or handheld probes. Similarly, MRRs have excellent performance in the wide frequency band, enhanced FOV, and high sensitivity. Especially, because of its micro-scale resolution, this can also be applied to PA endoscopic and microscopic imaging systems. Acoustic delay lines show the potential for a new cost-effective acoustic delivery and mixing tool. In spite of these advances in MEMS technology, further optimizations are needed for clinical use. First, the currently developed water immersible MEMS scanning mirrors are not yet micro size, which limits their application for endoscopic type device. There is also a need to reduce scales, such as t that of silicon-based MEMS scanning mirror through the development of advanced microfabrication. In addition to the MEMS scanning mirror, MUTs, MRR, and acoustic delay liens, also require special and expensive fabrication process, such as e-beam lithography and anisotropic etching with high aspect ratio. These fabrication processes make it difficult to achieve mass production and stable system performance. Thus, there is a need to develop simple microfabrication process to reduce cost as well as to increase reliability. If these challenges are resolved, we expect the MEMS technologies to contribute greatly to the development of high-performance and clinically useful PAI systems.

Author Contributions: C.L. contributed to writing introduction, Section 4, and conclusions; J.Y.K. contributed to writing Sections 2 and 3; C.K. organized the structure of the review article; all authors participated in writing the paper.

References

1. Bell, A.G. The Photophone. *Science* **1880**, *1*, 130–134. [CrossRef] [PubMed]
2. Cai, X.; Kim, C.; Pramanik, M.; Wang, L.V. Photoacoustic tomography of foreign bodies in soft biological tissue. *J. Biomed. Opt.* **2011**, *16*, 046017. [CrossRef] [PubMed]
3. Zhang, Y.; Jeon, M.; Rich, L.J.; Hong, H.; Geng, J.; Zhang, Y.; Shi, S.; Barnhart, T.E.; Alexandridis, P.; Huizinga, J.D.; et al. Non-invasive multimodal functional imaging of the intestine with frozen micellar naphthalocyanines. *Nat. Nanotechnol.* **2014**, *9*, 631–638. [CrossRef] [PubMed]
4. Lee, C.; Han, S.; Kim, S.; Jeon, M.; Jeon, M.Y.; Kim, C.; Kim, J. Combined photoacoustic and optical coherence tomography using a single near-infrared supercontinuum laser source. *Appl. Opt.* **2013**, *52*, 1824–1828. [CrossRef] [PubMed]
5. Kim, J.Y.; Lee, C.; Park, K.; Han, S.; Kim, C. High-speed and high-SNR photoacoustic microscopy based on a galvanometer mirror in non-conducting liquid. *Sci. Rep.* **2016**, *6*, 34803. [CrossRef] [PubMed]
6. Lee, D.; Lee, C.; Kim, S.; Zhou, Q.; Kim, J.; Kim, C. In Vivo Near Infrared Virtual Intraoperative Surgical Photoacoustic Optical Coherence Tomography. *Sci. Rep.* **2016**, *6*, 35176. [CrossRef] [PubMed]
7. Lee, C.; Jeon, M.; Jeon, M.Y.; Kim, J.; Kim, C. In vitro photoacoustic measurement of hemoglobin oxygen saturation using a single pulsed broadband supercontinuum laser source. *Appl. Opt.* **2014**, *53*, 3884–3889. [CrossRef] [PubMed]
8. Kim, J.; Lee, D.; Jung, U.; Kim, C. Photoacoustic imaging platforms for multimodal imaging. *Ultrasonography* **2015**, *34*, 88–97. [CrossRef] [PubMed]
9. Choi, W.; Park, E.-Y.; Jeon, S.; Kim, C. Clinical photoacoustic imaging platforms. *Biomed. Eng. Lett.* **2018**, *8*, 139–155. [CrossRef]

10. Park, S.; Jung, U.; Lee, S.; Lee, D.; Kim, C. Contrast-enhanced dual mode imaging: Photoacoustic imaging plus more. *Biomed. Eng. Lett.* **2017**, *7*, 121–133. [CrossRef]
11. Lee, S.; Kwon, O.; Jeon, M.; Song, J.; Shin, S.; Kim, H.; Jo, M.; Rim, T.; Doh, J.; Kim, S.; et al. Super-resolution visible photoactivated atomic force microscopy. *Light Sci. Appl.* **2017**, *6*, e17080. [CrossRef] [PubMed]
12. Hu, S.; Maslov, K.; Wang, L.V. Second-generation optical-resolution photoacoustic microscopy with improved sensitivity and speed. *Opt. Lett.* **2011**, *36*, 1134–1136. [CrossRef] [PubMed]
13. Wang, Y.; Maslov, K.; Zhang, Y.; Hu, S.; Yang, L.; Xia, Y.; Liu, J.; Wang, L.V. Fiber-laser-based photoacoustic microscopy and melanoma cell detection. *J. Biomed. Opt.* **2011**, *16*, 011014. [CrossRef] [PubMed]
14. Yao, J.; Maslov, K.I.; Zhang, Y.; Xia, Y.; Wang, L.V. Label-free oxygen-metabolic photoacoustic microscopy in vivo. *J. Biomed. Opt.* **2011**, *16*, 076003. [CrossRef] [PubMed]
15. Lee, C.; Kwon, W.; Beack, S.; Lee, D.; Park, Y.; Kim, H.; Hahn, S.K.; Rhee, S.-W.; Kim, C. Biodegradable nitrogen-doped carbon nanodots for non-invasive photoacoustic imaging and photothermal therapy. *Theranostics* **2016**, *6*, 2196–2208. [CrossRef] [PubMed]
16. Lovell, J.F.; Jin, C.S.; Huynh, E.; Jin, H.; Kim, C.; Rubinstein, J.L.; Chan, W.C.W.; Cao, W.; Wang, L.V.; Zheng, G. Porphysome nanovesicles generated by porphyrin bilayers for use as multimodal biophotonic contrast agents. *Nat. Mater.* **2011**, *10*, 324. [CrossRef] [PubMed]
17. Chen, J.; Yang, M.; Zhang, Q.; Cho, E.C.; Cobley, C.M.; Kim, C.; Glaus, C.; Wang, L.V.; Welch, M.J.; Xia, Y. Gold nanocages: A novel class of multifunctional nanomaterials for theranostic applications. *Adv. Funct. Mater.* **2010**, *20*, 3684–3694. [CrossRef]
18. Lee, M.Y.; Lee, C.; Jung, H.S.; Jeon, M.; Kim, K.S.; Yun, S.H.; Kim, C.; Hahn, S.K. Biodegradable photonic melanoidin for theranostic applications. *ACS Nano* **2016**, *10*, 822–831. [CrossRef] [PubMed]
19. Kim, C.; Jeon, M.; Wang, L.V. Nonionizing photoacoustic cystography in vivo. *Opt. Lett.* **2011**, *36*, 3599–3601. [CrossRef] [PubMed]
20. Lee, C.; Kim, J.; Zhang, Y.; Jeon, M.; Liu, C.; Song, L.; Lovell, J.F.; Kim, C. Dual-color photoacoustic lymph node imaging using nanoformulated naphthalocyanines. *Biomaterials* **2015**, *73*, 142–148. [CrossRef] [PubMed]
21. Lee, D.; Beack, S.; Yoo, J.; Kim, S.-K.; Lee, C.; Kwon, W.; Hahn, S.K.; Kim, C. In vivo photoacoustic imaging of livers using biodegradable hyaluronic acid-conjugated silica nanoparticles. *Adv. Funct. Mater.* **2018**, *28*, 1800941. [CrossRef]
22. Roy, I.; Shetty, D.; Hota, R.; Baek, K.; Kim, J.; Kim, C.; Kappert, S.; Kim, K. A Multifunctional subphthalocyanine nanosphere for targeting, labeling, and killing of antibiotic-resistant bacteria. *Angew. Chem. Int. Ed.* **2015**, *54*, 15152–15155. [CrossRef] [PubMed]
23. Yoo, S.W.; Jung, D.; Min, J.-J.; Kim, H.; Lee, C. Biodegradable contrast agents for photoacoustic imaging. *Appl. Sci.* **2018**, *8*, 1567. [CrossRef]
24. Xia, J.; Kim, C.; Lovell, J.F. Opportunities for photoacoustic-guided drug delivery. *Curr. Drug Targets* **2015**, *16*, 571–581. [CrossRef] [PubMed]
25. Zhou, Y.; Xing, W.; Maslov, K.I.; Cornelius, L.A.; Wang, L.V. Handheld photoacoustic microscopy to detect melanoma depth in vivo. *Opt. Lett.* **2014**, *39*, 4731–4734. [CrossRef] [PubMed]
26. Zhang, C.; Wang, L.V.; Cheng, Y.J.; Chen, J.; Wickline, A.S. Label-free photoacoustic microscopy of myocardial sheet architecture. *J. Biomed. Opt.* **2012**, *17*, 060506. [CrossRef] [PubMed]
27. Hu, S.; Wang, L.V. Neurovascular photoacoustic tomography. *Front. Neuroenergetics* **2010**, *2*, 10. [CrossRef] [PubMed]
28. Jiao, S.; Jiang, M.; Hu, J.; Fawzi, A.; Zhou, Q.; Shung, K.K.; Puliafito, C.A.; Zhang, H.F. Photoacoustic ophthalmoscopy for in vivo retinal imaging. *Opt. Express* **2010**, *18*, 3967–3972. [CrossRef] [PubMed]
29. Zhang, Y.; Hong, H.; Cai, W. Photoacoustic imaging. *Cold Spring Harb. Protoc.* **2011**, *2011*. [CrossRef] [PubMed]
30. Beard, P. Biomedical photoacoustic imaging. *Interface Focus* **2011**, *1*, 602–631. [CrossRef] [PubMed]
31. Park, S.; Lee, C.; Kim, J.; Kim, C. Acoustic resolution photoacoustic microscopy. *Biomed. Eng. Lett.* **2014**, *4*, 213–222. [CrossRef]
32. Lan, B.; Liu, W.; Wang, Y.C.; Shi, J.; Li, Y.; Xu, S.; Sheng, H.; Zhou, Q.; Zou, J.; Hoffmann, U.; et al. High-speed widefield photoacoustic microscopy of small-animal hemodynamics. *Biomed. Opt. Express* **2018**, *9*, 4689–4701. [CrossRef] [PubMed]

33. Lin, L.; Yao, J.; Zhang, R.; Chen, C.C.; Huang, C.H.; Li, Y.; Wang, L.; Chapman, W.; Zou, J.; Wang, L.V. High-speed photoacoustic microscopy of mouse cortical microhemodynamics. *J. Biophotonics* **2016**, *10*, 792–798. [CrossRef] [PubMed]
34. Park, J.; Jeon, S.; Meng, J.; Song, L.; Lee, J.S.; Kim, C. Delay-multiply-and-sum-based synthetic aperture focusing in photoacoustic microscopy. *J. Biomed. Opt.* **2016**, *21*, 036010. [CrossRef] [PubMed]
35. Su, J.L.; Wang, B.; Wilson, K.E.; Bayer, C.L.; Chen, Y.S.; Kim, S.; Homan, K.A.; Emelianov, S.Y. Advances in clinical and biomedical applications of photoacoustic imaging. *Expert Opin. Med. Diagn.* **2010**, *4*, 497–510. [CrossRef] [PubMed]
36. Xu, M.; Wang, L.V. Photoacoustic imaging in biomedicine. *Rev. Sci. Instrum.* **2006**, *77*, 041101. [CrossRef]
37. Xia, J.; Yao, J.; Wang, L.V. Photoacoustic tomography: Principles and advances. *Prog. Electromagn. Res.* **2014**, *147*, 1–22. [CrossRef]
38. Maslov, K.; Zhang, H.F.; Hu, S.; Wang, L.V. Optical-resolution photoacoustic microscopy for in vivo imaging of single capillaries. *Opt. Lett.* **2008**, *33*, 929–931. [CrossRef] [PubMed]
39. Xie, Z.; Jiao, S.; Zhang, H.F.; Puliafito, C.A. Laser-scanning optical-resolution photoacoustic microscopy. *Opt. Lett.* **2009**, *34*, 1771–1773. [CrossRef] [PubMed]
40. Hajireza, P.; Forbrich, A.; Zemp, R. In-vivo functional optical-resolution photoacoustic microscopy with stimulated Raman scattering fiber-laser source. *Biomed. Opt. Express* **2014**, *5*, 539–546. [CrossRef] [PubMed]
41. Chee, R.K.W.; Zhang, P.; Maadi, M.; Zemp, R.J. Multifrequency interlaced CMUTs for photoacoustic imaging. *IEEE Trans. Ultrason. Ferroelectr. Freq. Control* **2017**, *64*, 391–401. [CrossRef] [PubMed]
42. Oraevsky, A.A.; Karabutov, A.A. Ultimate sensitivity of time-resolved optoacoustic detection. In Proceedings of the International Symposium on Biomedical Optics, San Jose, CA, USA, 19 May 2000.
43. Kim, C.; Erpelding, T.N.; Jankovic, L.; Pashley, M.D.; Wang, L.V. Deeply penetrating in vivo photoacoustic imaging using a clinical ultrasound array system. *Biomed. Opt. Express* **2010**, *1*, 278–284. [CrossRef] [PubMed]
44. Qiu, Y.; Gigliotti, J.; Wallace, M.; Griggio, F.; Demore, C.; Cochran, S.; Trolier-McKinstry, S. Piezoelectric micromachined ultrasound transducer (PMUT) arrays for integrated sensing, actuation and imaging. *Sensors* **2015**, *15*, 8020–8041. [CrossRef] [PubMed]
45. Chee, R.K.W.; Sampaleanu, A.; Rishi, D.; Zemp, R.J. Top orthogonal to bottom electrode (TOBE) 2-D CMUT arrays for 3-D photoacoustic imaging. *IEEE Trans. Ultrason. Ferroelectr. Freq. Control* **2014**, *61*, 1393–1395. [CrossRef] [PubMed]
46. Voldman, J.; Gray, M.L.; Schmidt, M.A. microfabrication in biology and medicine. *Annu. Rev. Biomed. Eng.* **1999**, *1*, 401–425. [CrossRef] [PubMed]
47. Khoshnoud, F.; De Silva, C.W. Recent advances in MEMS sensor technology–biomedical applications. *IEEE Instrum. Meas. Mag.* **2012**, *15*, 8–14. [CrossRef]
48. Sant, S.; Tao, S.L.; Fisher, O.Z.; Xu, Q.; Peppas, N.A.; Khademhosseini, A. Microfabrication technologies for oral drug delivery. *Adv. Drug Deliv. Rev.* **2012**, *64*, 496–507. [CrossRef] [PubMed]
49. Yang, J.-M.; Favazza, C.; Chen, R.; Yao, J.; Cai, X.; Maslov, K.; Zhou, Q.; Shung, K.K.; Wang, L.V. Simultaneous functional photoacoustic and ultrasonic endoscopy of internal organs in vivo. *Nat. Med.* **2012**, *18*, 1297. [CrossRef] [PubMed]
50. Elahi, S.F.; Wang, T.D. Future and advances in endoscopy. *J. Biophotonics* **2011**, *4*, 471–481. [CrossRef] [PubMed]
51. Fu, L.; Gu, M. Fibre-optic nonlinear optical microscopy and endoscopy. *J. Microsc.* **2007**, *226*, 195–206. [CrossRef] [PubMed]
52. Chao, C.; Ashkenazi, S.; Huang, S.W.; Donnell, M.O.; Guo, L.J. High-frequency ultrasound sensors using polymer microring resonators. *IEEE Trans. Ultrason. Ferroelectr. Freq. Control* **2007**, *54*, 957–965. [CrossRef]
53. Tearney, G.J.; Brezinski, M.E.; Bouma, B.E.; Boppart, S.A.; Pitris, C.; Southern, J.F.; Fujimoto, J.G. In vivo endoscopic optical biopsy with optical coherence tomography. *Science* **1997**, *276*, 2037–2039. [CrossRef] [PubMed]
54. Denk, W.; Strickler, J.H.; Webb, W.W. Two-photon laser scanning fluorescence microscopy. *Science* **1990**, *248*, 73–76. [CrossRef] [PubMed]
55. Holmström, S.T.S.; Baran, U.; Urey, H. MEMS laser scanners: A review. *J. Microelectromech. Syst.* **2014**, *23*, 259–275. [CrossRef]

56. Pan, Y.; Xie, H.; Fedder, G.K. Endoscopic optical coherence tomography based on a microelectromechanical mirror. *Opt. Lett.* **2001**, *26*, 1966–1968. [CrossRef] [PubMed]
57. Jung, W.; Tang, S.; McCormic, D.T.; Xie, T.; Ahn, Y.C.; Su, J.; Tomov, I.V.; Krasieva, T.B.; Tromberg, B.J.; Chen, Z. Miniaturized probe based on a microelectromechanical system mirror for multiphoton microscopy. *Opt. Lett.* **2008**, *33*, 1324–1326. [CrossRef] [PubMed]
58. Dickensheets, D.L.; Kino, G.S. Silicon-micromachined scanning confocal optical microscope. *J. Microelectromech. Syst.* **1998**, *7*, 38–47. [CrossRef]
59. Hedili, M.K.; Freeman, M.O.; Urey, H. Microstructured head-up display screen for automotive applications. In Proceedings of the SPIE Photonics Europe, Brussels, Belgium, 8 May 2012; p. 84280.
60. Hornbeck, L.J. The DMD™ projection display chip: A MEMS-based technology. *MRS Bull.* **2001**, *26*, 325–327. [CrossRef]
61. Xi, L.; Sun, J.; Zhu, Y.; Wu, L.; Xie, H.; Jiang, H. Photoacoustic imaging based on MEMS mirror scanning. *Biomed. Opt. Express* **2010**, *1*, 1278–1283. [CrossRef] [PubMed]
62. Xi, L.; Grobmyer, S.R.; Wu, L.; Chen, R.; Zhou, G.; Gutwein, L.G.; Sun, J.; Liao, W.; Zhou, Q.; Xie, H.; et al. Evaluation of breast tumor margins in vivo with intraoperative photoacoustic imaging. *Opt. Express* **2012**, *20*, 8726–8731. [CrossRef] [PubMed]
63. Yang, H.; Xi, L.; Samuelson, S.; Xie, H.; Yang, L.; Jiang, H. Handheld miniature probe integrating diffuse optical tomography with photoacoustic imaging through a MEMS scanning mirror. *Biomed. Opt. Express* **2013**, *4*, 427–432. [CrossRef] [PubMed]
64. Chen, S.-L.; Xie, Z.; Ling, T.; Guo, L.J.; Wei, X.; Wang, X. Miniaturized all-optical photoacoustic microscopy based on microelectromechanical systems mirror scanning. *Opt. Lett.* **2012**, *37*, 4263–4265. [CrossRef] [PubMed]
65. Chen, S.L.; Xie, Z.; Guo, L.J.; Wang, X. A fiber-optic system for dual-modality photoacoustic microscopy and confocal fluorescence microscopy using miniature components. *Photoacoustics* **2013**, *1*, 30–35. [CrossRef] [PubMed]
66. Guo, H.; Song, C.; Xie, H.; Xi, L. Photoacoustic endomicroscopy based on a MEMS scanning mirror. *Opt. Lett.* **2017**, *42*, 4615–4618. [CrossRef] [PubMed]
67. Chen, Q.; Guo, H.; Jin, T.; Qi, W.; Xie, H.; Xi, L. Ultracompact high-resolution photoacoustic microscopy. *Opt. Lett.* **2018**, *43*, 1615–1618. [CrossRef] [PubMed]
68. Qi, W.; Chen, Q.; Guo, H.; Xie, H.; Xi, L. Miniaturized optical resolution photoacoustic microscope based on a microelectromechanical systems scanning mirror. *Micromachines* **2018**, *9*, 288. [CrossRef]
69. Liang, J.; Gao, L.; Li, C.; Wang, L.; Wang, L.V. Spatially fourier-encoded photoacoustic microscopy using a digital micromirror device. *Opt. Lett.* **2014**, *39*, 430–433. [CrossRef] [PubMed]
70. Wang, Y.; Maslov, K.; Wang, L.V. Spectrally encoded photoacoustic microscopy using a digital mirror device. *J. Biomed. Opt.* **2012**, *17*, 066020. [CrossRef] [PubMed]
71. Yang, J.; Gong, L.; Xu, X.; Hai, P.; Shen, Y.; Suzuki, Y.; Wang, L.V. Motionless volumetric photoacoustic microscopy with spatially invariant resolution. *Nat. Commun.* **2017**, *8*, 1–7. [CrossRef] [PubMed]
72. Kim, J.Y.; Lee, C.; Park, K.; Lim, G.; Kim, C. A PDMS-based 2-axis waterproof scanner for photoacoustic microscopy. *Sensors* **2015**, *15*, 9815–9826. [CrossRef] [PubMed]
73. Li, L.; Yeh, C.; Hu, S.; Wang, L.; Soetikno, B.T.; Chen, R.; Zhou, Q.; Shung, K.K.; Maslov, K.I.; Wang, L.V. Fully motorized optical-resolution photoacoustic microscopy. *Opt. Lett.* **2014**, *39*, 2117–2120. [CrossRef] [PubMed]
74. Yao, J.; Huang, C.H.; Wang, L.; Yang, J.M.; Gao, L.; Maslov, K.I.; Zou, J.; Wang, L.V. Wide-field fast-scanning photoacoustic microscopy based on a water-immersible MEMS scanning mirror. *J. Biomed. Opt.* **2012**, *17*, 080505. [CrossRef] [PubMed]
75. Yao, J.; Wang, L.; Yang, J.M.; Maslov, K.I.; Wong, T.T.W.; Li, L.; Huang, C.H.; Zou, J.; Wang, L.V. High-speed label-free functional photoacoustic microscopy of mouse brain in action. *Nat. Methods* **2015**, *12*, 407–410. [CrossRef] [PubMed]
76. He, Y.; Wang, L.; Shi, J.; Yao, J.; Li, L.; Zhang, R.; Huang, C.H.; Zou, J.; Wang, L.V. In vivo label-free photoacoustic flow cytography and on-the-spot laser killing of single circulating melanoma cells. *Sci. Rep.* **2016**, *6*, 6–13. [CrossRef] [PubMed]
77. Huang, C.H.; Yao, J.; Wang, L.V.; Zou, J. A water-immersible 2-axis scanning mirror microsystem for ultrasound andha photoacoustic microscopic imaging applications. *Microsyst. Technol.* **2013**, *19*, 577–582. [CrossRef]

78. Kim, J.Y.; Lee, C.; Park, K.; Lim, G.; Kim, C. Fast optical-resolution photoacoustic microscopy using a 2-axis water-proofing MEMS scanner. *Sci. Rep.* **2015**, *5*, 7932. [CrossRef] [PubMed]
79. Moothanchery, M.; Bi, R.; Kim, J.Y.; Jeon, S.; Kim, C.; Olivo, M. Optical resolution photoacoustic microscopy based on multimode fibers. *Biomed. Opt. Express* **2018**, *9*, 1190–1197. [CrossRef] [PubMed]
80. Lin, L.; Zhang, P.; Xu, S.; Shi, J.; Li, L.; Yao, J.; Wang, L.; Zou, J.; Wang, L.V. Handheld optical-resolution photoacoustic microscopy. *J. Biomed. Opt.* **2016**, *22*, 041002. [CrossRef] [PubMed]
81. Park, K.; Kim, J.Y.; Lee, C.; Jeon, S.; Lim, G.; Kim, C. Handheld Photoacoustic Microscopy Probe. *Sci. Rep.* **2017**, *7*, 13359. [CrossRef] [PubMed]
82. Aguirre, A.; Guo, P.; Gamelin, J.K.; Yan, S.; Sanders, M.M.; Brewer, M.A.; Zhu, Q. Coregistered three-dimensional ultrasound and photoacoustic imaging system for ovarian tissue characterization. *J. Biomed. Opt.* **2009**, *14*, 054014. [CrossRef] [PubMed]
83. Ermilov, S.A.; Khamapirad, T.; Conjusteau, A.; Leonard, M.H.; Lacewell, R.; Mehta, K.; Miller, T.; Oraevsky, A.A. Laser optoacoustic imaging system for detection of breast cancer. *J. Biomed. Opt.* **2009**, *14*, 024007. [CrossRef] [PubMed]
84. Daft, C.; Calmes, S.; Da Graca, D.; Patel, K.; Wagner, P.; Ladabaum, I. Microfabricated ultrasonic transducers monolithically integrated with high voltage electronics. In Proceedings of the 2004 IEEE International Symposium on Circuits and Systems, Montreal, QC, Canada, 23–27 August 2004; pp. 493–496.
85. Eccardt, P.C.; Niederer, K. Micromachined ultrasound transducers with improved coupling factors from a CMOS compatible process. *Ultrasonics* **2000**, *38*, 774–780. [CrossRef]
86. Erguri, A.S.; Yongli, H.; Xuefeng, Z.; Oralkan, O.; Yarahoglu, G.G.; Khuri-Yakub, B.T. Capacitive micromachined ultrasonic transducers: Fabrication technology. *IEEE Trans. Ultrason. Ferroelectr. Freq. Control* **2005**, *52*, 2242–2258. [CrossRef]
87. Ladabaum, I.; Jin, X.; Soh, H.T.; Atalar, A.; Khuri-Yakub, B.T. Surface micromachined capacitive ultrasonic transducers. *IEEE Trans. Ultrason. Ferroelectr. Freq. Control* **1998**, *45*, 678–690. [CrossRef] [PubMed]
88. Nikoozadeh, A.; Chienliu, C.; Choe, J.W.; Bhuyan, A.; Byung Chul, L.; Moini, A.; Khuri-Yakub, P.T. An integrated Ring CMUT array for endoscopic ultrasound and photoacoustic imaging. In Proceedings of the 2013 IEEE International Ultrasonics Symposium (IUS), Prague, Czech Republic, 21–25 July 2013; pp. 1178–1181.
89. Chen, J.; Wang, M.; Cheng, J.C.; Wang, Y.H.; Li, P.C.; Cheng, X. A photoacoustic imager with light illumination through an infrared-transparent silicon CMUT array. *IEEE Trans. Ultrason. Ferroelectr. Freq. Control* **2012**, *59*, 766–775. [CrossRef] [PubMed]
90. Zhang, J.; Pun, S.H.; Yu, Y.; Gao, D.; Wang, J.; Mak, P.U.; Lei, K.F.; Cheng, C.H.; Yuan, Z. Development of a multi-band photoacoustic tomography imaging system based on a capacitive micromachined ultrasonic transducer array. *Appl. Opt.* **2017**, *56*, 4012–4018. [CrossRef] [PubMed]
91. Lu, Y.; Horsley, D.A. Modeling, Fabrication, and Characterization of Piezoelectric Micromachined Ultrasonic Transducer Arrays Based on Cavity SOI Wafers. *J. Microelectromech. Syst.* **2015**, *24*, 1142–1149. [CrossRef]
92. Lu, Y.; Rozen, O.; Tang, H.Y.; Smith, G.L.; Fung, S.; Boser, B.E.; Polcawich, R.G.; Horsley, D.A. Broadband piezoelectric micromachined ultrasonic transducers based on dual resonance modes. In Proceedings of the 2015 28th IEEE International Conference on Micro Electro Mechanical Systems (MEMS), Estoril, Portugal, 18–22 January 2015; pp. 146–149.
93. Lu, Y.; Tang, H.Y.; Fung, S.; Boser, B.E.; Horsley, D.A. Short-range and high-resolution ultrasound imaging using an 8 MHz aluminum nitride PMUT array. In Proceedings of the 2015 28th IEEE International Conference on Micro Electro Mechanical Systems (MEMS), Estoril, Portugal, 18–22 January 2015; pp. 140–143.
94. Akhbari, S.; Sammoura, F.; Shelton, S.; Yang, C.; Horsley, D.; Lin, L. Highly responsive curved aluminum nitride pMUT. In Proceedings of the 2014 IEEE 27th International Conference on Micro Electro Mechanical Systems (MEMS), San Francisco, CA, USA, 26–30 January 2014; pp. 124–127.
95. Dausch, D.E.; Gilchrist, K.H.; Carlson, J.B.; Hall, S.D.; Castellucci, J.B.; Von Ramm, O.T. In vivo real-time 3-D intracardiac echo using PMUT arrays. *IEEE Trans. Ultrason. Ferroelectr. Freq. Control* **2014**, *61*, 1754–1764. [CrossRef] [PubMed]
96. Hajati, A.; Latev, D.; Gardner, D.; Hajati, A.; Imai, D.; Torrey, M.; Schoeppler, M. Three-dimensional micro electromechanical system piezoelectric ultrasound transducer. *Appl. Phys. Lett.* **2012**, *101*, 253101. [CrossRef]

97. Liao, W.; Liu, W.; Rogers, J.E.; Usmani, F.; Tang, Y.; Wang, B.; Jiang, H.; Xie, H. Piezoelectric micromachined ultrasound tranducer array for photoacoustic imaging. In Proceedings of the 2013 Transducers & Eurosensors XXVII: The 17th International Conference on Solid-State Sensors, Actuators and Microsystems, Barcelona, Spain, 16–20 June 2013; pp. 1831–1834.
98. Chen, B.; Chu, F.; Liu, X.; Li, Y.; Rong, J.; Jiang, H. AlN-based piezoelectric micromachined ultrasonic transducer for photoacoustic imaging. *Appl. Phys. Lett.* **2013**, *103*, 031118. [CrossRef]
99. Shung, K.K.; Cannata, J.M.; Zhou, Q.F. Piezoelectric materials for high frequency medical imaging applications: A review. *J. Electroceram.* **2007**, *19*, 141–147. [CrossRef]
100. Zhang, E.; Laufer, J.; Beard, P. Backward-mode multiwavelength photoacoustic scanner using a planar Fabry-Perot polymer film ultrasound sensor for high-resolution three-dimensional imaging of biological tissues. *Appl. Opt.* **2008**, *47*, 561–577. [CrossRef] [PubMed]
101. Rousseau, G.; Gauthier, B.; Blouin, A.; Monchalin, J.P. Non-contact biomedical photoacoustic and ultrasound imaging. *J. Biomed. Opt.* **2012**, *17*, 061217. [CrossRef] [PubMed]
102. Schneider, F.; Fellner, T.; Wilde, J.; Wallrabe, U. Mechanical properties of silicones for MEMS. *J. Micromech. Microeng.* **2008**, *18*, 065008. [CrossRef]
103. Xie, Z.; Chen, S.L.; Ling, T.; Guo, L.J.; Carson, P.L.; Wang, X. Pure optical photoacoustic microscopy. *Opt. Express* **2011**, *19*, 9027–9034. [CrossRef] [PubMed]
104. Ling, T.; Chen, S.-L.; Guo, L.J. High-sensitivity and wide-directivity ultrasound detection using high Q polymer microring resonators. *Appl. Phys. Lett.* **2011**, *98*, 204103. [CrossRef] [PubMed]
105. Peng, X.; Huang, J.; Deng, H.; Xiong, C.; Fang, J. A multi-sphere indentation method to determine Young's modulus of soft polymeric materials based on the Johnson–Kendall–Roberts contact model. *Meas. Sci. Technol.* **2011**, *22*, 027003. [CrossRef]
106. Zhang, C.; Ling, T.; Chen, S.L.; Guo, L.J. Ultrabroad bandwidth and highly sensitive optical ultrasonic detector for photoacoustic imaging. *ACS Photonics* **2014**, *1*, 1093–1098. [CrossRef]
107. Hsieh, B.Y.; Chen, S.L.; Ling, T.; Guo, L.J.; Li, P.C. All-optical scanhead for ultrasound and photoacoustic dual-modality imaging. *Opt. Express* **2012**, *20*, 1588–1596. [CrossRef] [PubMed]
108. Li, H.; Dong, B.; Zhang, Z.; Zhang, H.F.; Sun, C. A transparent broadband ultrasonic detector based on an optical micro-ring resonator for photoacoustic microscopy. *Sci. Rep.* **2014**, *4*, 4496. [CrossRef] [PubMed]
109. Song, L.; Kim, C.; Maslov, K.; Shung, K.K.; Wang, L.V. High-speed dynamic 3D photoacoustic imaging of sentinel lymph node in a murine model using an ultrasound array. *Med. Phys.* **2009**, *36*, 3724–3729. [CrossRef] [PubMed]
110. Yapici, M.K.; Kim, C.; Chang, C.C.; Jeon, M.; Guo, Z.; Cai, X.; Zou, J.; Wang, L.V. Parallel acoustic delay lines for photoacoustic tomography. *J. Biomed. Opt.* **2012**, *17*, 116019. [CrossRef] [PubMed]
111. Cho, Y.; Chang, C.C.; Yu, J.; Jeon, M.; Kim, C.; Wang, L.V.; Zou, J. Handheld photoacoustic tomography probe built using optical-fiber parallel acoustic delay lines. *J. Biomed. Opt.* **2014**, *19*, 086007. [CrossRef] [PubMed]
112. Cho, Y.; Chang, C.C.; Wang, L.V.; Zou, J. A micromachined silicon parallel acoustic delay line (PADL) array for real-time photoacoustic tomography (PAT). In Proceedings of the SPIE BiOS, San Francisco, CA, USA, 11 March 2015.
113. Chang, C.; Cho, Y.; Zou, J. A micromachined acoustic multiplexer for ultrasound and photoacoustic imaging applications. *J. Microelectromech. Syst.* **2014**, *23*, 514–516. [CrossRef]

15

Three-Dimensional Printed Piezoelectric Array for Improving Acoustic Field and Spatial Resolution in Medical Ultrasonic Imaging

Zeyu Chen [1,2,†], Xuejun Qian [2,†], Xuan Song [3], Qiangguo Jiang [4], Rongji Huang [4], Yang Yang [5], Runze Li [2], Kirk Shung [2], Yong Chen [5,*] and Qifa Zhou [2,6,*]

1 College of Mechanical & Electrical Engineering, Central South University, Changsha 410083, China; zeyuchen@usc.edu
2 Department of Biomedical Engineering, University of Southern California, Los Angeles, CA 90089, USA; xuejunqi@usc.edu (X.Q.); runzeli@usc.edu (R.L.); kkshung@usc.edu (K.S.)
3 Department of Mechanical and Industrial Engineering, The University of Iowa, Iowa City, IA 52242, USA; xuan-song@uiowa.edu (X.S.)
4 School of Electro-Mechanical Engineering, Guangdong University of Technology, Guangzhou 510006, China; qiangguojiang@gdut.edu.cn (Q.J.); rongji.huang@hotmail.com (R.H.)
5 Epstein Department of Industrial and Systems Engineering, University of Southern California, Los Angeles, CA 90089, USA; yang610@usc.edu (Y.Y.)
6 Roski Eye Institute, University of Southern California, Los Angeles, CA 90089, USA
* Correspondence: yongchen@usc.edu (Y.C.), qifazhou@usc.edu (Q.Z.)
† These authors contributed equally.

Abstract: Piezoelectric arrays are widely used in non-destructive detecting, medical imaging and therapy. However, limited by traditional manufacturing methods, the array's element is usually designed in simple geometry such as a cube or rectangle, restricting potential applications of the array. This work demonstrates an annular piezoelectric array consisting of different concentric elements printed by Mask-Image-Projection-based Stereolithography (MIP-SL) technology. The printed array displays stable piezoelectric and dielectric properties. Compared to a traditional single element transducer, the ultrasonic transducer with printed array successfully modifies the acoustic beam and significantly improves spatial resolution.

Keywords: 3D Printing; piezoelectric array; ultrasonic transducer; ultrasonic imaging

---

1. Introduction

With exceptional piezoelectric, dielectric, and electronics properties, piezoelectric materials have been the focus of significant interest in the botch industry and academic fields. The wide applications ranging from signal sensor and energy harvesting devices to electromechanical actuator [1–3]. Among this material, piezoelectric ceramic with high piezoelectric constant and electromechanical coupling coefficient can effectively convert electrical signals into mechanical vibrations and vise versa, which results in obvious advantages in drug delivery, particle manipulation, ultrasonic imaging, and therapy [4–7]. The corresponding ceramic array with complex geometry has great potential to improve the performance of piezoelectric devices. For example, a piezoelectric array incorporating a hexagonal shape element demonstrated the evenly distributed sidelobe compared with rectangular shape element for nondestructive testing [8]. However, a piezoelectric array with complex geometry is challenging using traditional manufacturing methods such as dicing and etching [9,10]. In this regard, digital, additive, and automatic printing technologies offer a promising approach.

Additive manufacturing, or more commonly, 3D printing technology, is widely considered a revolutionary manufacturing technology. During past decades, direct inkjet based printing, extrusion-based direct write technique, and light exposure based Stereolithography Apparatus (SLA) have been used in ceramic component fabrication [11–20]. SLA involving the light exposure on photocurable polymer allows for the manufacture of complex geometry layer-by-layer with small resolution (X-Y resolution < 25 μm). It is compatible with multilaterals and composites printing, offering a distinct advantage for integrating functional materials in 3D objects [21–23]. Therefore, SLA has significant promise in a broad range of fields including mechanical and biomedical engineering. In previous work, Xuan et al. reported composite fabrication using Mask-Image-Projection-based stereolithograhpy integrated with tape-casting (MIP-SL) [24]. This method has been used for manufacturing a variety of materials such as resin and alumina ceramic. With MIP-SL method, we fabricated piezoelectric ceramic nanoparticles into 3D objects in previous work [25]. Since the decrease in surface energy due to a reduction in surface area is the main driving force for ceramic sintering, the nanoparticle-based fabrication results in improved piezoelectric property. After a specifically designed post processing, the 3D objects display the abilities on energy focusing and ultrasonic sensing. This method has great potential in applications of piezoelectric devices. The single element focused transducer concentrates an ultrasonic beam at a certain point (focus zone) with constant distance away from the transducer. The focus point has the highest intensity and the smallest lateral resolution. However, the lateral resolution at other positions besides except the focus point is unsatisfactory for ultrasonic imaging. Compared to a single element transducer, an array transducer has the potential to improve the focus zone and lateral resolution [26,27].

In this study, we present here the design, fabrication, and post processing of piezoelectric array with piezoelectric effect and precisely controlled geometry using the MIP-SL system (Figure 1a). The 3D model was produced by Solidworks (Figure 1c,d,e). A Digital Micromirror Device (DMD) controlled the image pattern projected on the slurry (Figure 1b). An annular array with a limited number of elements was assembled in the ultrasonic array transducer that improved the lateral resolution and depth of field (focus zone). The resulting piezoelectric array structures are mechanically robust in the device, with stable dielectric and piezoelectric properties. Overall, the additive manufactured piezoelectric array enables improved performance and differing function of the corresponding device.

2. Materials and Methods

The $BaTiO_3$ Nano powder (solid loading, 100 nm, Sigma-Aldrich St. Louis, MO, USA) was used as the raw materials. To modify the powder surface, an azeotropic mixture and dispersant (Triton x-100, Sigma-Aldrich, Saint Louis, MO, USA 0.5–0.8 wt.% on a dry weight basis of ceramic powders) were mixed with the powder by planetary mill (pulverisette 5, FRITSCH Idar-Oberstein, Germany) with 200 rpm rotation speed for 12 h. The azeotropic mixture consisted of methylethylketone (66 v/v%, 99%, MEK, Sigma-Aldrich, Saint Louis, MO, USA) and ethanol (34 v/v%, 99.5%, Sigma-Aldrich, Saint Louis, MO, USA). The mixture with powder was then dried at 50 °C for 12 h. After the evaporation of the solvent in the dispersion, deagglomerated $BaTiO_3$ powders with dispersant adsorbed on to their surface can be obtained.

The deagglomerated $BaTiO_3$ powder was mixed with a photocurable resin (SI500, EnvisionTec Inc., Ferndale, MI, USA) by ball milling for 1 h. The solid loading was 70 wt.%. MIP-SL system was used to fabricate 3D green part with the slurry. When the slurry was exposed under visible light, the photocurable resin in the slurry produced a cross-linked matrix, forming a strong bond between $BaTiO_3$ powders and polymer network. The 3D model was produced by Solidworks (Figure 1a). A Digital Micromirror Device (DMD) controlled the images pattern projected on the slurry (Figure 1b). After the layer-by-layer process, a 3D green part was fabricated (Figure 2b).

The post-processing steps involved organic binder removal and high-temperature sintering. The 3D green part was debinded in a muffle furnace with Argon under 600 °C for 3 h. After the furnace cooling, the debinded part was put in a regular muffle furnace with air at 1300 °C for 2 h.

The sintered samples and bulk samples were poling under 30 kV/cm at 100 °C for 30 min. Dielectric constant and dielectric loss (tanδ) measured by an impedance analyzer (Agilent 4294A, Santa Clara, CA, USA). Density was measured by ASTM B962-14 standard. Piezoelectric constant was measured by d33 meter (APC International, Ltd., Mackeyville, PA, USA).

The array transducer was fabricated using the annular array. Epoxy (Epo-Tek 301, Billerica, MA, USA) was filled into the kerf between each element. A 150 nm Cr/Au layer was sputtered on the annular array to serve as the electrode Figure 3a. Four electric cables were connected on the elements with conductive epoxy (E-Solder 3022, Von Roll Isola Inc., New Haven, CT, USA) shown in Figure 3b. The housing was an Aluminum Silicate.

Epoxy (Epo-Tek 301) with an acoustic impedance of ~6 MRayl was inserted into the housing to serve as the backing layer (Fgiure 3c). A Cr/Au layer was sputtered on the other side of the annular array with a cable attached on the layer (Figure 3d.) After that, a 10μm-thick parylene was vapor-deposited by Specialty Coating System (SCS, Indianapolis, IN, USA) on the other Au surface to protect the transducer array. The impulse-echo response of each element in the array transducer was measured by an ultrasonic system consisting of PC, gage card, JSR500, function generator, motor and quartz target (Figure 5).

The transducers were driven by JSR500 (Ultrasonics, Imaginant Inc., Pittsford, NY, USA) and triggered by the function generator with a pulse repetition frequency (PRF) of 1kHz. The ultrasonic signals were filtered by an analog band-pass filter. A 12-bit digitizer card (ATS9360, Alazartech, Montreal, QC, Canada) with a 1.8 GHz sampling rate was used to record the signals (Figure 5). To obtain a 2D image, the transducers were mounted on a stepper motor (SGSP33-200, OptoSigma Corporation, Santa Ana, CA, USA) for mechanical scanning with 36 μm increment.

3. Results and Discussion

3.1. Characterization of Sintered-Parts

An annular array (Figure 2a,b,c), self-focused linear array (Figure 2d,e,f), and cylinder array (Figure 2g,h,i) were fabricated using MIP-SL and the post-processing method. Figure 2a,d,g show the green-part involving piezoelectric nanoparticles printed by the MIP-SL system. Figure 2b,e,h display the piezoelectric array after post-processing and Figure 2c,f,I are the optical images of the array under a microscope. The scanning electron microscope images of the debinded part and sintered sample were shown in Figure 2j and k, respectively.

The figures show that after post-processing, the density of printed ceramics increased obviously. Limited by traditional machining technology, the piezoelectric elements of array are usually designed in square or rectangular shape with fixed kerf, while the three types of printed array demonstrates more flexibility of complex geometry. The specific designed annular array can not only focus ultrasound, but also improve the depth of acoustic field (Focus zone). The design and application will be discussed later.

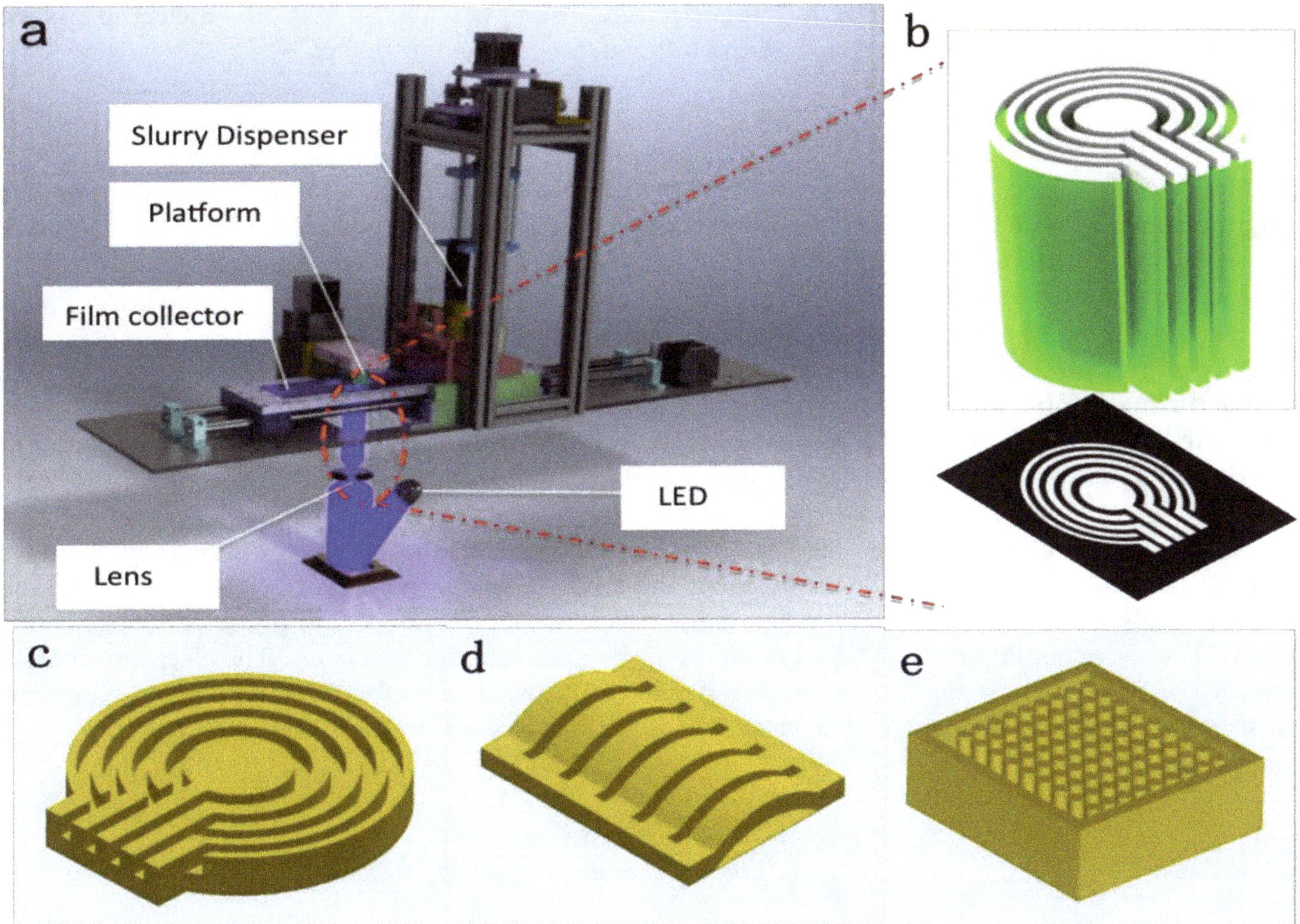

Figure 1. (**a**) sketch of Mask-Image-Projection-based Stereolithography system. (**b**) Green part controlled by image pattern. (**c–e**) 3D model designed by SolidWork.

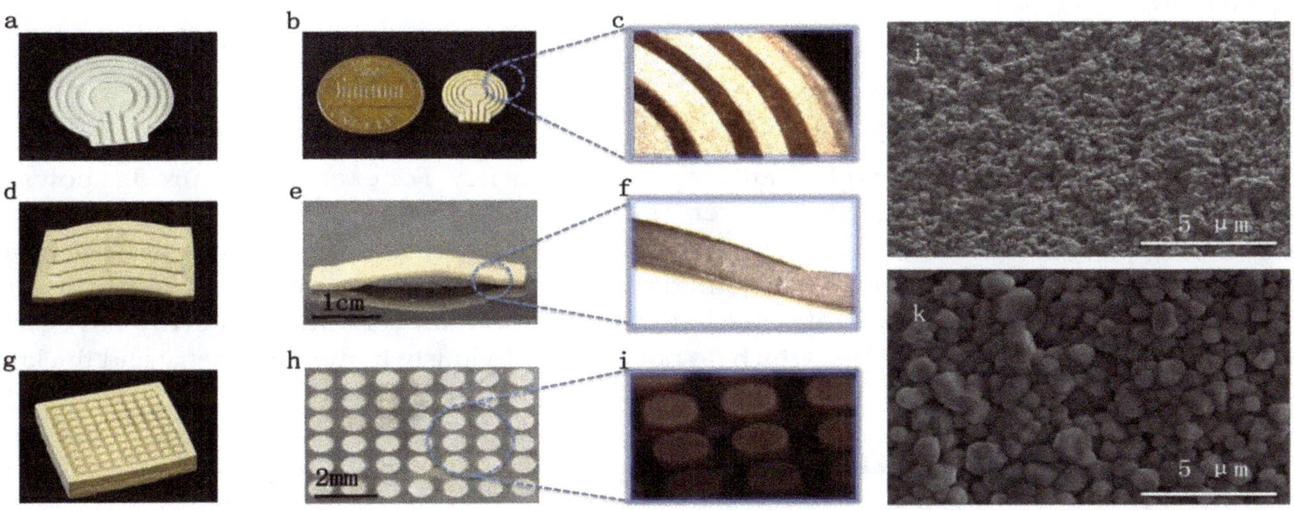

Figure 2. (**a**), (**d**), (**g**) Green-part fabricated by MIP-SL system. (**b**), (**e**), (**h**) Optical images of piezoelectric array after sintering. (**c**), (**f**), (**i**) Details of the array under microscope. (**j**) Scanning electron microscope image of printed sample after debinding process. (**k**) SEM image of printed sample after sintering process.

A set of cylindrical samples with 10mm diameter and different thickness (400 μm, 800 μm, 1.2 mm, 1.6 mm) were fabricated using the same fabrication process. The bulk cylindrical samples and the printed array with complex geometry were used to characterize the printed piezoelectric ceramics. The poling filed was 30 kV/cm at 100°C for 30 min. The dielectric constant was 1300~13,500, the dielectric loss was 0.018~0.02. Density was 5.62~5.64 g/cm^3. Piezoelectric constant was 146~160 pCN^{-1}.

3.2. Annular Array Transducer

Here we designed an annular array and fabricated it with the MIP-SL method. A transducer using the printed annular array with a limited number of elements can provide an improved depth of field and improve lateral resolution over the field, when compared with a single element transducer with the same total aperture and focal length.

The annular array consists of 5 concentric elements and the outermost element can prevent damage during sample transfer. After sintering, the outermost element was removed from the annular array. The thickness of the array was 400 μm. The area and center frequency of 4 working elements were designed as 13.5 mm^2 and 6 MHz.

An ultrasonic transducer was fabricated using the printed annular array (Shown in Figure 3). Figure 3f numbers each element after sintering, the actual area can be found in Table 1. Impedance analyzer (Agilent 4294A) was used to measure the spectrum of impedance and phase. The spectrum of element 1 is shown in Figure 3g. The other elements have the similar spectrum. The electromechanical coupling coefficient of piezoelectric materials is defined as the ratio of the mechanical energy accumulated in response to an electrical input or vice versa, which can be expressed in the following equation:

$$k_t = \sqrt{\frac{\text{Mechanical energy stroed}}{\text{Electrical energy applied}}} \tag{1}$$

$$= \sqrt{\frac{\text{Electrical energy stored}}{\text{Mechanical energy applied}}} \tag{2}$$

k_t can be formulated as [28]:

$$k_t = \sqrt{\frac{\pi f_r}{2f_a} \times \cot\frac{\pi f_r}{2f_a}} \tag{3}$$

where f_r is resonant frequency, and f_a is anti-resonant frequency. For example, Figure 3g shows the spectrum of the element in the array transducer. The f_r and f_a are 5.54 MHz and 6.1 MHz, respectively, and the corresponding k_t is 46.5%. The coupling coefficient of printed bulk ceramics and other array elements were measured with the same method and the values do not have an obvious difference (46.3~46.5%). The results demonstrate that both the printed bulk ceramics and array have stable dielectric and piezoelectric properties, which do not change obviously in their geometry and thickness.

Table 1. The measured pulse and echo characteristics for all elements.

Characteristics	Element 1	Element 2	Element 3	Element 4
Center Frequency (MHz)	5.72	5.86	6.39	6.12
−6 dB Bandwidth (%)	19.6	12.9	19.8	23.6
V_{pp} (mV)	402	793	626	1039
−20 dB Pulse Length (ns)	1940	1621	989	2949
Area (mm^2)	13.7	13.2	13.6	13.5

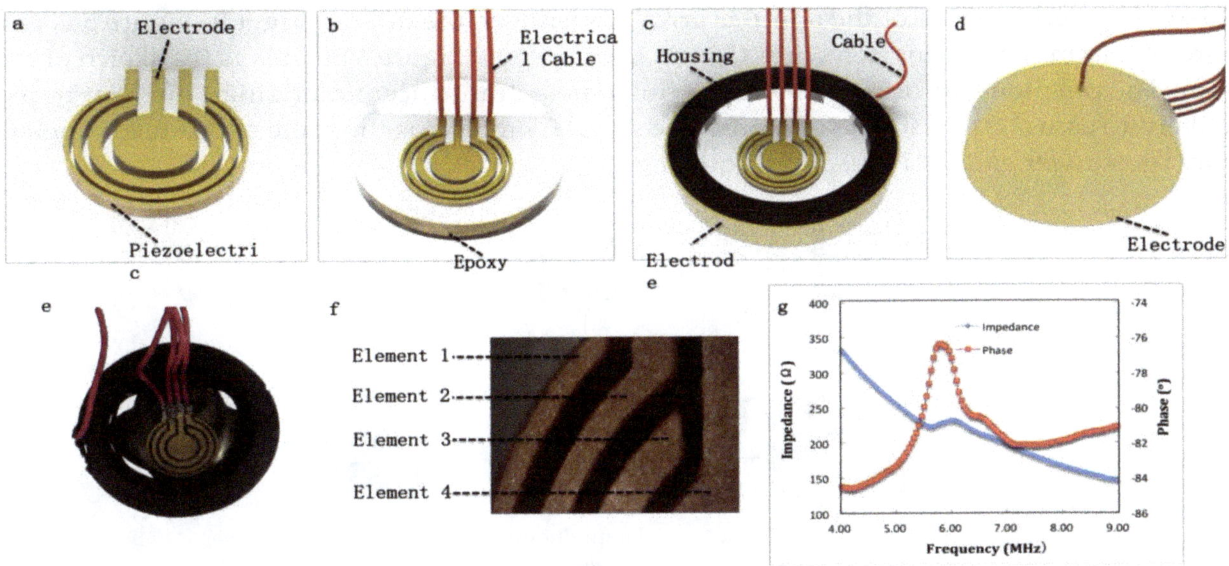

Figure 3. (**a–d**) Structure of annular array transducer. (**e**) Optical image of annular array transducer. (**f**) Four elements of annular array. (**g**) Element's spectrum of impedance and phase.

Each element can transfer electrical impulses to mechanical oscillation and then generates ultrasound. After a target reflects the ultrasound, the elements converted the returned echoes back into electrical impulses, which could be further processed to from an ultrasonic image. The impulse-echo response was measured by an ultrasonic system. Figure 4 represents the pulse-echo waveform (solid line) in time domain and normalized spectrum in frequency domain of each element. Table 1 shows the measured pulse and echo characteristics for all array elements. V_{PP} is peak-to-peak voltage. The variations between four elements may be caused by the debinding and sintering process, which lead to inaccuracy of the geometry.

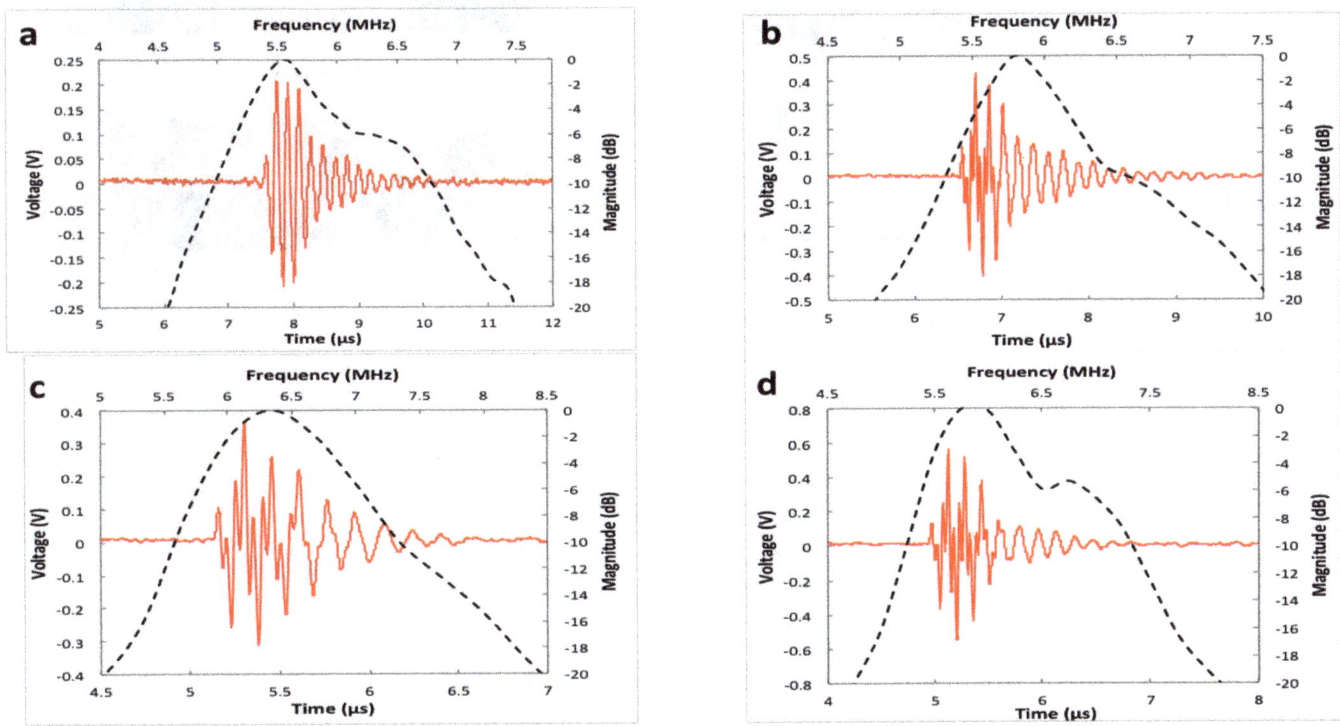

Figure 4. Pulse-echo waveform (solid line) and normalized spectrum of element 1 (**a**), element 2 (**b**), element 3 (**c**) and element 4 (**d**).

To test the performance of the annular array transducer, the quartz target in Figure 5 is replaced by a wire phantom with 3 tungsten wires (50 μm in diameter). Figure 6a displays the sketch of the wire phantom. The phantom was imaged by the annular array transducer and a single element transducer, respectively, to assess the lateral resolutions. The single element has the same aperture (diameter) with the array transducer and 6MHz center frequency.

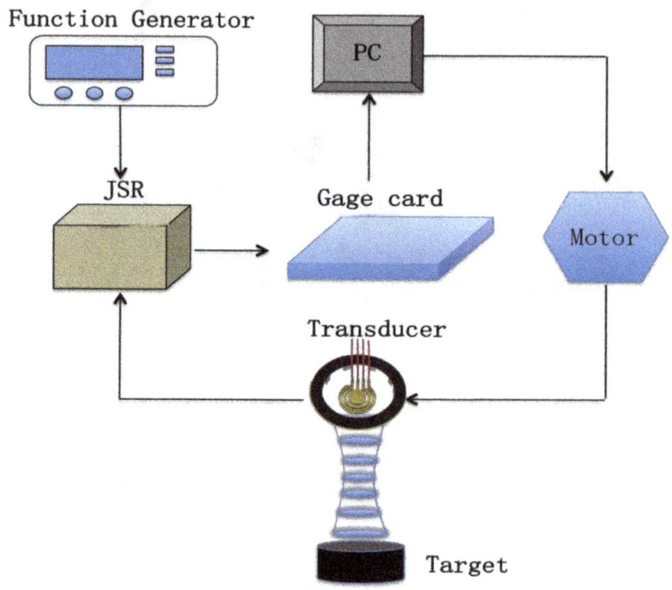

Figure 5. Schematic of the test system setup for pulse-echo detecting and ultrasonic imaging.

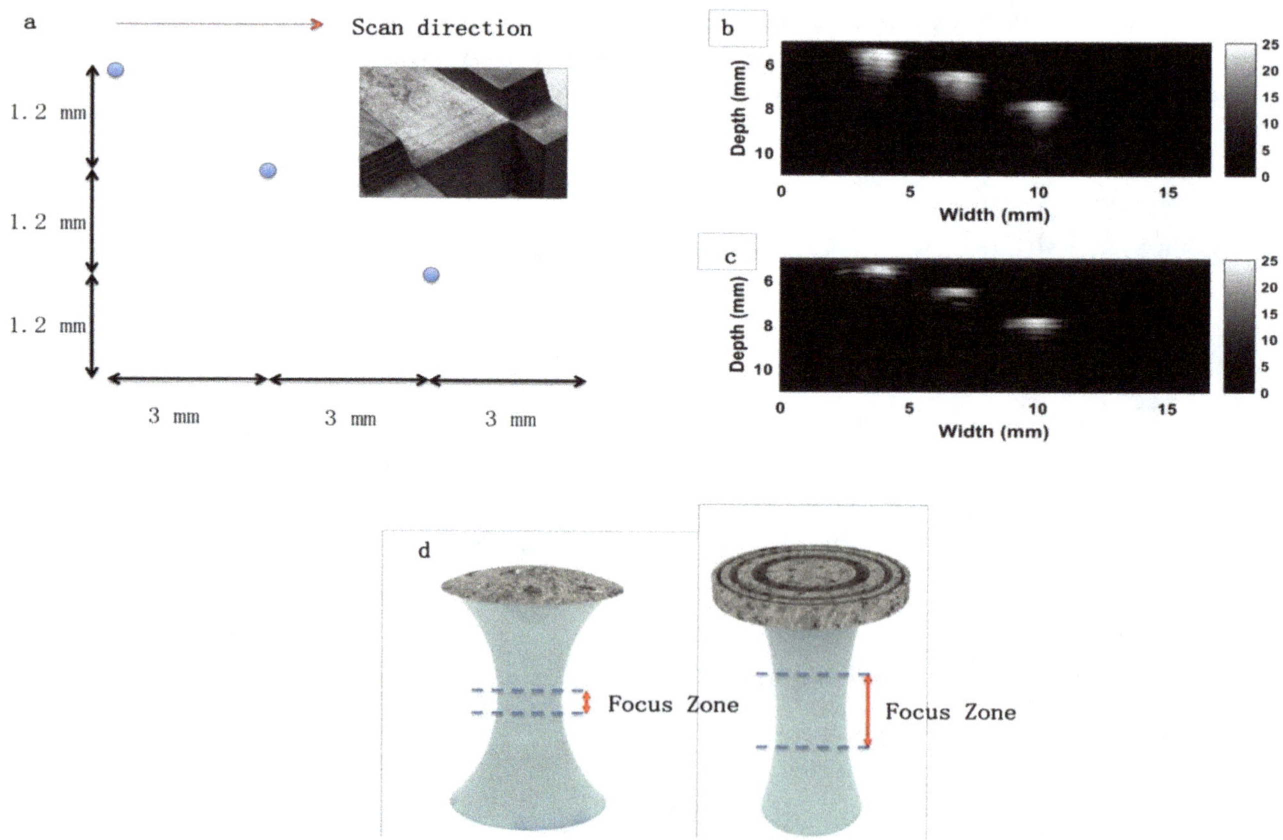

Figure 6. (**a**) Sketch of the wire phantom. The inset is the optical photo of the wires. (**b**) Phantom imaging by single element transducer. (**c**) Phantom imaging by annular array transducer. (**d**) Schematic of the acoustic beam for single element (**left**) and annular array (**right**).

The array transducer is controlled by a stepper motor. The scan direction is labeled as a red arrow shown in Figure 6a. As the transducer changes scanning distance, it detects the wire at different depths. After one element transmits an initial signal, an element receives the echo signal. This process is a transmit-to-receive combination. So in this study, 4 elements have 16 transmit-to-receive combinations ($4 \times 4 = 16$). These transmit-to-receive combinations were processed with a specific beam forming technology reported in reference [29] for the ultrasonic images. Figure 6b,c demonstrates the phantom images of the single element and annular array transducer when the dynamic range was −25 dB. The phantom image of the array transducer (Figure 6c) displays an improved signal to noise ratio compared to the single element transducer (Figure 6b). Figure 7 shows the dB (signal magnitude) versus scanning distance for single element (Figure 7a,b,c) and annular array (Figure 7d,e,f) transducer when the wires were set at different distances away from the transducer. As Figure 7a shows, the lateral resolution is the intercept (read dash line) when dB (magnitude) is the maximum value (black dash line) minus 6 dB. Table 2 shows the lateral resolutions at a different depth of different transducers. Because the ultrasonic beam diverges quickly when the depth is larger than 8.0 mm, we studied the lateral resolution within 8 mm.

Table 2. Resolution of single element and annular array.

Depth (mm)	Resolution (mm)	
	Single Element	Annular Array
5.6	1.4	1
6.8	1.5	1.05
8	1.1	1.1

The results indicate that the focus point of the single element transducer is located at 8 mm away from the transducer, when the lateral resolution is 1.1 mm. But the lateral resolution (beam width) of the single element at another depth is obviously larger than 1.1 mm. For example, the lateral resolution at 5.6 mm depth is 1.4 mm. In contrast, the array transducer provides similar and small lateral resolutions (beam width) less than 1.1 mm from 5.6 mm to 8 mm. A sketch of ultrasonic beams generated by two different transducers is shown in Figure 6d. With the tunable focus zone, medical imaging for the target at a different depth can be achieved. Not only medical imaging, but also particle manipulation and ultrasonic therapy can benefit from the boarder focus zone. There are two downsides to this method. Firstly, the density of printed samples is lower than bulk materials. Secondly, the debinding and sintering process would lead to defects and inaccuracy of the geometry.

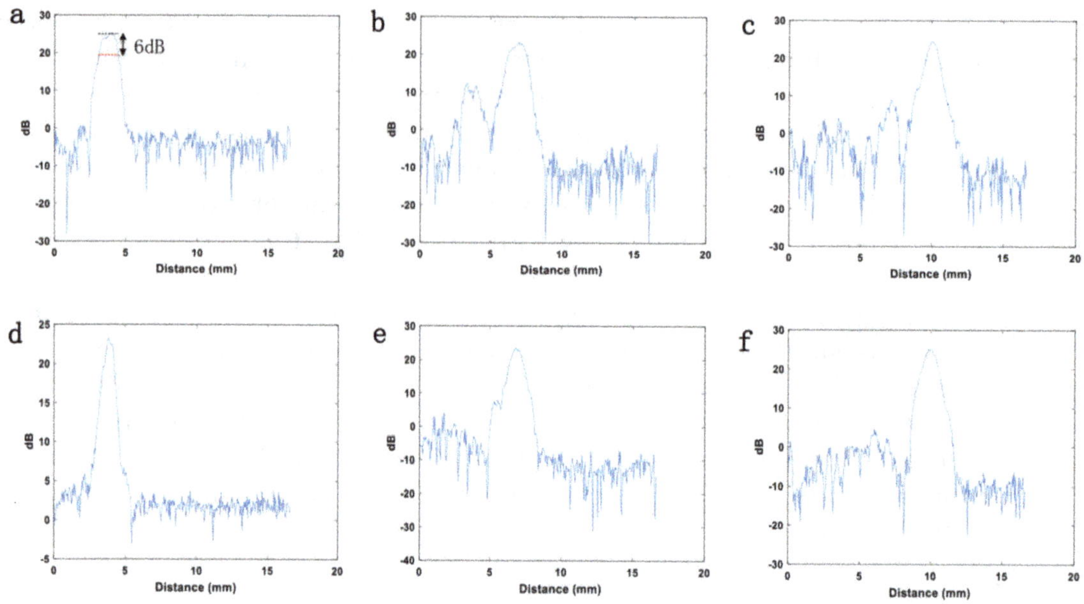

Figure 7. Signal magnitude (dB) versus scanning distance for lateral resolution measurement. The resolution was measured when the depth between wire and single element were 5.6 mm (**a**), 6.8 mm (**b**) and 8 mm (**c**). The resolution was then measured when the depth between wire and annular array were 5.6 mm (**d**), 6.8 mm (**e**) and 8 mm (**f**).

4. Conclusions

Using Mask-Image-Projection-based Stereolithography, photocurable resin and nano ceramic particles can be 3D-printed into arbitrarily shaped arrays. After post-processing, the dense ceramic arrays display stable piezoelectric and dielectric properties. A specifically designed annular array was printed with our method. Each element of this array can convert electric signals to mechanical vibration, and vice versa. With a beam forming, the ultrasonic transducer with printed array improved the acoustic field and signal-to-noise ratio, which resulted in a longer focus zone and the smaller lateral resolution. This array transducer with tunable focus zone and resolution has many benefits in medical imaging, non-destructive detecting and high intensity focused ultrasound. The 3D printing enabled morphology of the piezoelectric array can lend itself to a range of potential applications in the medical transducer, composite design, and wearable and implantable electronics.

Author Contributions: Conceptualization, Z.Q. and C.Y.; Methodology, C.Z.; Software, Q.X.; Validation, S.X., J.Q. and H.R.; Formal Analysis, Y.Y.; Investigation, L.R.; Resources, C.Z.; Data Curation, Q.X.; Writing-Original Draft Preparation, C.Z.; Writing-Review & Editing, Q.X.; Visualization, S.K.; Supervision, S.K.; Project Administration, Z.Q.; Funding Acquisition, Z.Q.

References

1. Dagdeviren, C.; Su, Y.; Joe, P.; Yona, R.; Liu, Y.; Kim, Y.S.; Huang, Y.; Damadoran, A.R.; Xia, J.; Martin, L.W.; et al. Conformable amplified lead zirconate titanate sensors with enhanced piezoelectric response for cutaneous pressure monitoring. *Nat. Commun.* **2014**, *5*, 4496. [CrossRef] [PubMed]
2. Fan, F.R.; Tang, W.; Wang, Z.L. Flexible Nanogenerators for Energy Harvesting and Self-Powered Electronics. *Adv. Mater.* **2016**, *28*, 4283–4305. [CrossRef] [PubMed]
3. Hwang, G.T.; Park, H.; Lee, J.H.; Oh, S.; Park, K.I.; Byun, M.; Park, H.; Ahn, G.; Jeong, C.K.; No, K.; et al. Self-powered cardiac pacemaker enabled by flexible single crystalline PMN-PT piezoelectric energy harvester. *Adv. Mater.* **2014**, *26*, 4880–4887. [CrossRef] [PubMed]

4. Atul, S.T.; Babu, M.L. Characterization of valveless micropump for drug delivery by using piezoelectric effect. In Proceedings of the Advances in Computing, Communications and Informatics (ICACCI), Jaipur, India, 21–24 September 2016; IEEE: Piscataway, NJ, USA, 2016; pp. 2138–2144. [CrossRef]
5. Chen, X.; Lam, K.h.; Chen, R.; Chen, Z.; Yu, P.; Chen, Z.; Shung, K.K.; Zhou, Q. An adjustable multi-scale single beam acoustic tweezer based on ultrahigh frequency ultrasonic transducer. *Biotech. Bioeng.* **2017**. [CrossRef] [PubMed]
6. Hu, H.; Zhu, X.; Wang, C.; Zhang, L.; Li, X.; Lee, S.; Huang, Z.; Chen, R.; Chen, Z.; Wang, C. Stretchable ultrasonic transducer arrays for three-dimensional imaging on complex surfaces. *Sci. Adv.* **2018**, *4*, eaar3979. [CrossRef] [PubMed]
7. Kennedy, J.E. High-intensity focused ultrasound in the treatment of solid tumours. *Nat. Rev. Cancer* **2005**, *5*, 321. [CrossRef] [PubMed]
8. Dziewierz, J.; Ramadas, S.; Gachagan, A.; O'Leary, R.; Hayward, G. A 2D Ultrasonic Array design incorporating Hexagonal-shaped Elements and Triangular-cut Piezocomposite Substructure for NDE applications. In Proceedings of the Ultrasonics Symposium (IUS), Rome, Italy, 20–23 September 2009; IEEE: Piscataway, NJ, USA, 2009; pp. 422–425.
9. Lee, H.J.; Zhang, S.; Bar-Cohen, Y.; Sherrit, S. High temperature, high power piezoelectric composite transducers. *Sensors* **2014**, *14*, 14526–14552. [CrossRef] [PubMed]
10. He, L.; Yang, H.; Zhou, D.; Niu, Y.; Xiang, F.; Wang, H. Improved dielectric and magnetic properties of 1–3-type Ni0. 5Zn0. 5Fe2O4/epoxy composites for high-frequency applications. *J. Phys. D* **2013**, *46*, 125003. [CrossRef]
11. Lee, D.H.; Derby, B. Preparation of PZT suspensions for direct ink jet printing. *J. Eur. Ceram. Soc.* **2004**, *24*, 1069–1072. [CrossRef]
12. Lewis, J.A. Direct ink writing of 3D functional materials. *Adv. Funct. Mater.* **2006**, *16*, 2193–2204. [CrossRef]
13. Özkol, E.; Wätjen, A.M.; Bermejo, R.; Deluca, M.; Ebert, J.; Danzer, R.; Telle, R. Mechanical characterisation of miniaturised direct inkjet printed 3Y-TZP specimens for microelectronic applications. *J. Eur. Ceram. Soc.* **2010**, *30*, 3145–3152. [CrossRef]
14. Smay, J.E.; Cesarano, J.; Lewis, J.A. Colloidal inks for directed assembly of 3-D periodic structures. *Langmuir* **2002**, *18*, 5429–5437. [CrossRef]
15. Franco, J.; Hunger, P.; Launey, M.E.; Tomsia, A.P.; Saiz, E. Direct write assembly of calcium phosphate scaffolds using a water-based hydrogel. *Acta Biomat.* **2010**, *6*, 218–228. [CrossRef] [PubMed]
16. Sun, J.; Ngernchuklin, P.; Vittadello, M.; Akdoğan, E.; Safari, A. Development of 2-2 piezoelectric ceramic/polymer composites by direct-write technique. *J. Electroceram.* **2010**, *24*, 219–225. [CrossRef]
17. Yang, H.; Yang, S.; Chi, X.; Evans, J.R. Fine ceramic lattices prepared by extrusion freeforming. *J. Biomed. Mater. Res. Part B* **2006**, *79*, 116–121. [CrossRef] [PubMed]
18. Griffith, M.L. Stereolithography of ceramics. PhD Thesis, University of Michigan, Ann Arbor, MI, USA, 1995.
19. O'connor, K.F.; Nohns, D.C.; Chattin, W.A. Method of combining metal and ceramic inserts into stereolithography components. U.S. Patent No. 5705117, 1998.
20. Zhang, X.; Jiang, X.; Sun, C. Micro-stereolithography of polymeric and ceramic microstructures. *Sens. Actuators A* **1999**, *77*, 149–156. [CrossRef]
21. Song, X.; Zhang, Z.; Chen, Z.; Chen, Y. Porous Structure Fabrication Using a Stereolithography-Based Sugar Foaming Method. *J Manufact. Sci. Eng.* **2017**, *139*, 031015. [CrossRef]
22. Yang, Y.; Chen, Z.; Song, X.; Zhang, Z.; Zhang, J.; Shung, K.K.; Zhou, Q.; Chen, Y. Biomimetic anisotropic reinforcement architectures by electrically assisted nanocomposite 3D printing. *Adv. Mater.* **2017**, *29*. [CrossRef] [PubMed]
23. Yang, Y.; Chen, Z.; Song, X.; Zhu, B.; Hsiai, T.; Wu, P.-I.; Xiong, R.; Shi, J.; Chen, Y.; Zhou, Q. Three dimensional printing of high dielectric capacitor using projection based stereolithography method. *Nano Energy* **2016**, *22*, 414–421. [CrossRef]
24. Song, X.; Chen, Z.; Lei, L.; Shung, K.; Zhou, Q.; Chen, Y. Piezoelectric component fabrication using projection-based stereolithography of barium titanate ceramic suspensions. *Rapid Prototyping J.* **2017**, *23*, 44–53. [CrossRef]
25. Chen, Z.; Song, X.; Lei, L.; Chen, X.; Fei, C.; Chiu, C.T.; Qian, X.; Ma, T.; Yang, Y.; Shung, K. 3D printing of piezoelectric element for energy focusing and ultrasonic sensing. *Nano Energy* **2016**, *27*, 78–86. [CrossRef]

26. Cannata, J.M.; Ritter, T.A.; Chen, W.-H.; Silverman, R.H.; Shung, K.K. Design of efficient, broadband single-element (20-80 MHz) ultrasonic transducers for medical imaging applications. *IEEE Trans. Ultrason. Ferroelectr. Freq. Control* **2003**, *50*, 1548–1557. [CrossRef] [PubMed]
27. Krause, M.; Mielentz, F.; Milman, B.; Müller, W.; Schmitz, V.; Wiggenhauser, H. Ultrasonic imaging of concrete members using an array system. *NDT E Int.* **2001**, *34*, 403–408. [CrossRef]
28. Kim, T.; Kim, J.; Dalmau, R.; Schlesser, R.; Preble, E.; Jiang, X. High-temperature electromechanical characterization of AlN single crystals. *IEEE Trans. Ultrason. Ferroelectr. Freq. Control* **2015**, *62*, 1880–1887. [CrossRef] [PubMed]
29. Ketterling, J.A.; Filoux, E. Synthetic-focusing strategies for real-time annular-array imaging. *IEEE Trans. Ultrason. Ferroelectr. Freq. Control* **2012**, *59*, 1830–1839. [CrossRef] [PubMed]

16

Adaptive Absolute Ego-Motion Estimation Using Wearable Visual-Inertial Sensors for Indoor Positioning

Ya Tian [1,2,3,*], Zhe Chen [1], Shouyin Lu [1,2,3] and Jindong Tan [4]

1 School of Information and Electrical Engineering, Shandong Jianzhu University, Jinan 250101, China; chenzhe19930517@163.com(Z.C.); lusy@sdjzu.edu.cn(S.L.)
2 Shandong Provincial Key Laboratory of Intelligent Buildings Technology, Jinan 250101, China
3 Shandong Provincial Key Laboratory of Intelligent Technology for New Type Man-Machine Interaction and Robot System, Jinan 250101, China
4 Department of Mechanical, Aerospace, and Biomedical Engineering, The University of Tennessee, Knoxville, TN 37996, USA; tan@utk.edu
* Correspondence: ytian@sdjzu.edu.cn

Abstract: This paper proposes an adaptive absolute ego-motion estimation method using wearable visual-inertial sensors for indoor positioning. We introduce a wearable visual-inertial device to estimate not only the camera ego-motion, but also the 3D motion of the moving object in dynamic environments. Firstly, a novel method dynamic scene segmentation is proposed using two visual geometry constraints with the help of inertial sensors. Moreover, this paper introduces a concept of "virtual camera" to consider the motion area related to each moving object as if a static object were viewed by a "virtual camera". We therefore derive the 3D moving object's motion from the motions for the real and virtual camera because the virtual camera's motion is actually the combined motion of both the real camera and the moving object. In addition, a multi-rate linear Kalman-filter (MR-LKF) as our previous work was selected to solve both the problem of scale ambiguity in monocular camera tracking and the different sampling frequencies of visual and inertial sensors. The performance of the proposed method is evaluated by simulation studies and practical experiments performed in both static and dynamic environments. The results show the method's robustness and effectiveness compared with the results from a Pioneer robot as the ground truth.

Keywords: ego-motion estimation; indoor navigation; monocular camera; scale ambiguity; wearable sensors

---

1. Introduction

Recently, with the increasing number of elderly people in many countries, the age-related problems will become increasingly serious, such as hearing loss, sight loss, memory loss and other increased health problems, which definitely lead to a burning issue for all modern societies around the world [1]. Commonly, most aging people with these age-related problems have difficulties in safety and mobility of daily life, especially within unfamiliar environments, so they usually rely on some aiding devices, like a positioning system, to carry out tasks and activities.

As is known, the Global Positioning System (GPS) has been available for a wide variety of navigation applications over the past 50 years because of its high accuracy. Therefore, it is one of the most important parts for positioning and tracking systems and especially plays a key role in outdoor positioning. However, for indoors, and outdoor environments with tall buildings and trees, GPS-based positioning is not suitable due to the unreliable satellite signals. With recent development of miniature sensor technology, more and more researchers have been attracted to developing various wearable electronic aids for aging people to avoid collision and motion risks. However, these aiding devices still have limited functionality and flexibility so that developing a novel wearable indoor positioning system is desirable to make the aging people's daily life much easier and more convenient.

In this paper, we mainly focus on the integration of ego- and ambient-motion tracking in indoor environments using wearable visual-inertial sensors, where global positioning (GPS-denied) is unavailable or inaccurate. The goal of this work is to obtain not only accurate ego-motion estimation, but also the motion of moving object with a metric scale under dynamic scenes. In our work, a moving visual IMU (Inertial Measurement Unit) system (vIMU) is developed to observe both a 3D static scene as shown in Figure 1a and a 3D dynamic scene as shown in Figure 1b. Rotational and translational motion is estimated individually by visual and inertial sensors. Outliers from visual estimations due to the variety of dynamic indoor environment are rejected via our proposed adaptive orientation method using MARG (Magnetic, Angular Rate and Gravity) sensors [2]. Moreover, a concept of "virtual camera" is presented to consider the motion area of each moving object as if a static object were observed by a "virtual camera", while the motion of the "real camera" is estimated by the extracted features from the static background. In particular, considering of the different sampling rates of visual and inertial sensors and the scale ambiguity in monocular camera tracking, we propose a multi-rate linear Kalman-filter (MR-LKF) to integrate visual and inertial estimations.

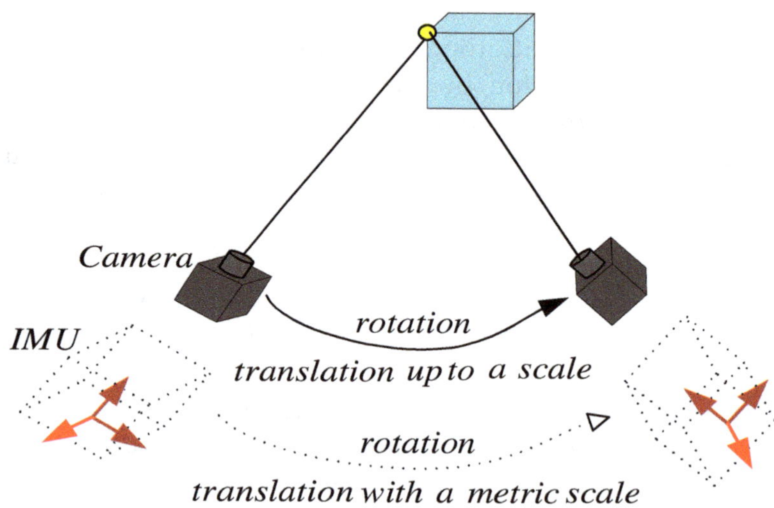

(a)

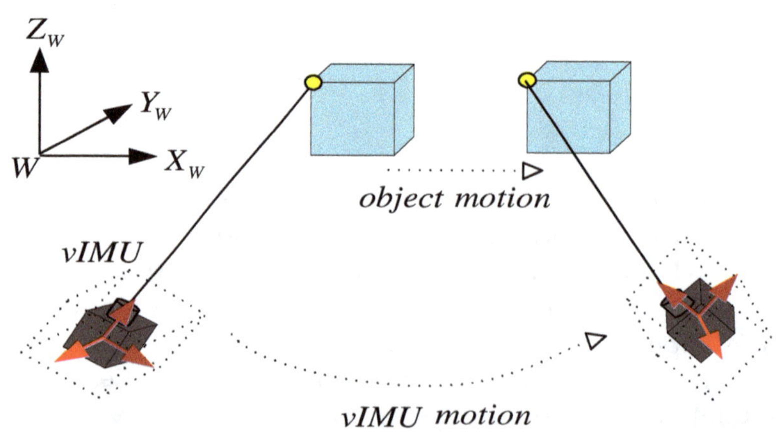

(b)

Figure 1. Static and dynamic scene. (**a**) in a static scene, a camera integrated with an IMU can infer the information of the metric scale; (**b**) in a dynamic scene, the problem is how to accurately infer both the vIMU motion and the object motion.

The main contributions of this paper are summarized as follows: (1) a novel method for dynamic scene segmentation based on AGOF-aided (Adaptive-Gain Orientation Filter) homography recovery constraint and epipolar geometry constraint shown as process (B) in Figure 2; (2) a new concept of "virtual camera" for robust ego- and ambient-estimation in dynamic environments; and (3) an MR-LKF fusion method for solving the problems of two different sampling rates and scale ambiguity.

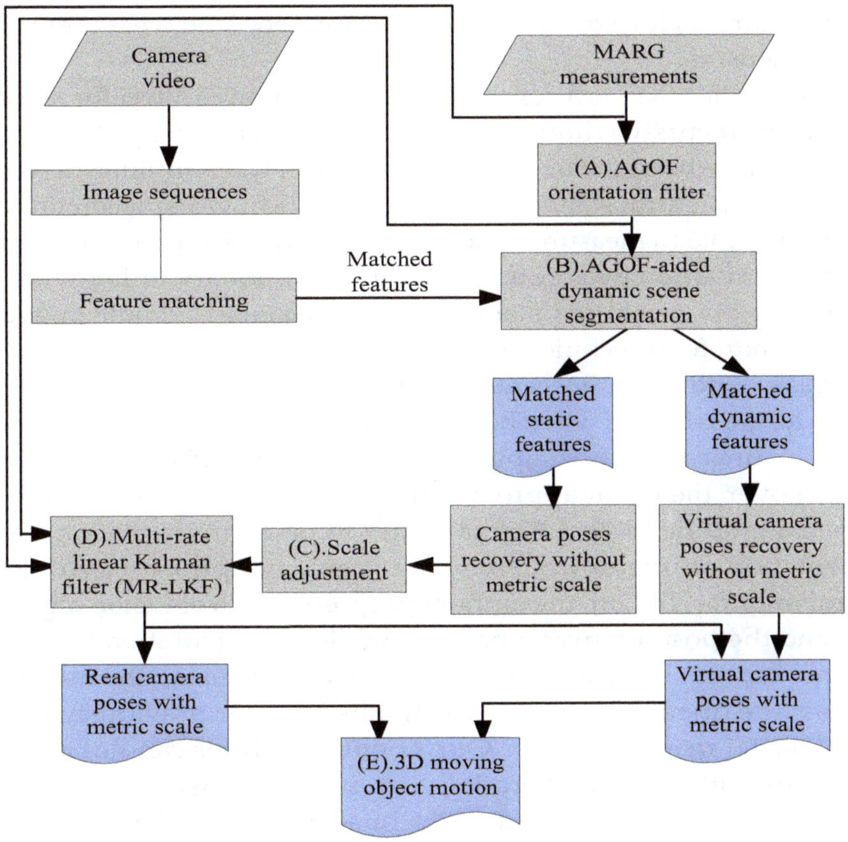

Figure 2. The main framework of the proposed method.

2. Related Work

In recent years, with the development of technology in computer vision, more and more researchers have been attracted to develop monocular visual-based localization algorithms based on the theory of structure from motion (SFM) [3–6]. However, there are two main problems with monocular visual-based localization algorithms. One is the triangulation problem, which can only be enabled in at least two views where the 3D scene is commonly assumed to be static. If there are other objects moving in the 3D scene, which is referred to as the dynamic 3D scene, the rule of triangulation will fail unless some constraints are further applied [7]. The other is the visual scale problem, which is usually lost when projecting a 3D scene on a 2D imaging plane. The most common approach for doing so is stereo vision [8,9]. Although these systems work well in many environments, stereo vision is fundamentally limited by two specific cameras. In addition, the structure of 3D environment and the motion of camera could be recovered from a monocular camera using structure from motion (SFM) techniques [10–14], but they are up to an arbitrary scale. Methods appearing in structure from motion to infer the scale of the 3D structure is to place an artificial reference with a known scale into the scene. However, it limits its applications to place a marker before the 3D reconstruction .

In the past 10 years, the integration of visual and inertial sensors has shown more significant performance than a single sensor system, especially in positioning and tracking systems [8,15–17] due to their complementary properties [18]. Inertial sensors provide good signals with high-rate motions in the short term but suffer from accumulated drift due to the double integration during the estimation of position. On the contrary, visual sensors offer accurate ego-motion estimation with low-rate motion in the long term, but are sensitive to blurred features during unpredicted and fast motions [19]. Therefore, recently, these complementary properties have been utilized by more and more researchers as the basic principle for integrating visual and inertial sensors together. Moreover, the inertial sensors can not only be small in size, light weight and low in cost, but also easily adopt wireless communication technologies, so it is much easier for people to wear them. This is why we call them "wearable" inertial sensors.

In general, the Kalman filter (KF) is a common and popular algorithm for sensor fusion and data fusion, which is an efficient recursive filter and widely used in many applications. In recent years, more and more researchers have been attracted to develop novel Kalman-filter-based algorithms to deal with structural systems. In structural systems, the states including displacements and velocities are difficult or sometimes impossible to measure, so a variety of novel Kalman filters have been developed from Kalman's original formulation by accounting for non-stationary unknown external inputs and theoretical investigation of observability, stability and associated advancements [20–23]. To our knowledge, nonlinear Kalman filter techniques are usually applied to almost all of the inertial-visual fusion algorithms, such as extended KF, unscented KF, etc. [8,17,24–26], because a large state vector and a complex nonlinear model are required when both the orientation and the position are optimized in the same process. However, an unacceptable computational burden would be imposed because of so many recursive formulas. Moreover, the linear approximations of EKF may result in non optimal estimates. Although [27] proposed a modified linear Kalman filter to perform the fusion of inertial and visual data, the accurate orientation estimates were based on the assumption of gyroscope measurements trusted for up to several minutes. In [28], the authors proposed a novel fusion algorithm by separating the orientation fusion and the position fusion process, while the orientation estimation could only be robust for a static or slow movement without magnetic distortions using the method proposed in [29]. In contrast, in this paper, the orientation is firstly estimated by our previously proposed orientation filter in [2] only from inertial measurements. Our orientation filter can not only obtain the robust orientation in real time for both extra acceleration and magnetic distortions, but also eliminate the bias and noise in angular velocity and acceleration. In addition, the sampling rates for visual and inertial sensors are inherently different. As a result, an efficient inertial-visual fusion algorithm, called multi-rate AGOF/Linear Kalman filter (MR-LKF), is proposed to separate the orientation and the position estimation; thus, this results in a small state vector and a linear model. A summary of the related work on inertial-visual integration is presented in Table 1.

Table 1. Related work on inertial-visual fusion (OS, FFT, OFP, OPSP, SE, DFSV, KF, DKF, EKF, UKF, Gyro, Mag and Acc stand for Orientation Source, Fusion Filter Type, Orientation-aided Feature points, Orientation and Position in the Same Process, Scale Estimation, Dimension of Filter's State Vector, Kalman Filter, Decentralized Kalman Filter, Extended Kalman Filter, Unscented Kalman Filter, Gyroscope, Magnetometer and Accelerometer respectively; x—No and √—Yes).

Reference	OS	FFT	OFP	OPSP	SE	DFSV
Chen et al. [24]	vision + Gyro + Acc	EKF	x	x	x	16
. Diel et al. [27]	Gyro	KF	x	x	x	18
Bleser et al. [17]	vision + Gyro + Acc	EKF	x	x	x	16–22
Randeniya et al. [7]	vision + Gyro + Acc	DKF	x	x	x	17
Tardif et al. [8]	vision + Gyro + Acc	EKF	x	x	x	15
Li et al. [25]	vision + Gyro + Acc	EKF	x	x	x	17
Panahandeh et al. [26]	vision + Gyro + Acc	UKF	x	x	x	16
Liu et al. [28]	vision + Gyro + Acc	KF	x	√	x	13
This paper	Mag + Gyro + Acc	MR-LKF	√	√	√	13

Table 2. Definitions of mathematical symbols and variables.

Symbol	Meaning	Symbol	Meaning
t	time	f	focal length
s	sensor frame	$(x, y)^T$	2D image point
c	camera frame	$(X, Y, Z)^T$	3D point
e	earth frame	$(c_x, c_y)^T$	camera principal point
${}^{e}\boldsymbol{g}$	gravity in e	K	camera intrinsic parameter
${}^{s}\boldsymbol{a}$	acceleration in s	$\mathbf{F}$	fundamental matrix
${}^{s}\boldsymbol{\omega}$	angular velocity in s	$\mathbf{E}$	essential matrix
${}^{s}\boldsymbol{m}$	magnetic field in s	$\boldsymbol{b}$	baseline between two consecutive views
${}^{s}_{e}\hat{\boldsymbol{q}}_{f,t}$	final orientation from s to e at t	R_1^2	relative rotation from frame 2 to 1
${}^{c}_{s}\boldsymbol{q}$	relative orientation from c to s	$\boldsymbol{l}$	epipolar line
${}^{c}_{s}\boldsymbol{b}$	relative translation from c to s	$\boldsymbol{e}$	epipole
${}^{s}\boldsymbol{\omega}_{c,t}$	compensated angular velocity in s at t	f_c	sample rate of camera
${}^{s}\boldsymbol{a}_{b,t}$	compensated acceleration in s at t	λ	reciprocal of the scale factor
f_s	sample rate of sensor	$\mathbf{T}$	camera ego-motion in homogeneous representation

3. Sensors

This section introduces some preliminary notations and definitions for the camera and integrated visual-inertial (vIMU) system. For brevity and clarity, Table 2 gives the definitions of mathematical symbols and variables.

3.1. Camera

3.1.1. Camera Model

A camera is a mapping between the 3D world and a 2D image, so the most specialized and simplest camera modle, called the basic pinhole camera model [10], is used here to deduce the mapping between a point in 2D image coordinate system and a point in 3D camera coordinate system. Under this model, a 3D point $\boldsymbol{M}^c = (X, Y, Z)^T$ in the camera coordinate system c is mapped to the 2D point $\boldsymbol{m}^i = (x, y)^T$ in the image coordinate system i, which is located on the image plane ($Z = f$). A line joining the point $\boldsymbol{M}^c$ to the center of projection (called camera centre) meets the image plane illustrated in Figure 3. Based on triangle similarity, the relationship between $\boldsymbol{m}^i$ and $\boldsymbol{M}^c = (X, Y, Z)$ is given in Label (1):

$$\begin{aligned} x &= fX/Z, \\ y &= fY/Z, \end{aligned} \tag{1}$$

where f denotes the focal length. Based on the representation of homogeneous coordinates, Label (1) can be rewritten as a linear mapping using a matrix representation denoted in Label (2):

$$Z * \begin{bmatrix} x \\ y \\ 1 \end{bmatrix} = \begin{bmatrix} f & 0 & 0 & 0 \\ 0 & f & 0 & 0 \\ 0 & 0 & 1 & 0 \end{bmatrix} * \begin{bmatrix} X \\ Y \\ Z \\ 1 \end{bmatrix}. \tag{2}$$

By introducing a non-zero homogenous scaling factor s, Label (2) can be rewritten in Label (3):

$$\begin{bmatrix} x \\ y \\ 1 \end{bmatrix} = s * \begin{bmatrix} f & 0 & 0 & 0 \\ 0 & f & 0 & 0 \\ 0 & 0 & 1 & 0 \end{bmatrix} * \begin{bmatrix} X \\ Y \\ Z \\ 1 \end{bmatrix}. \tag{3}$$

3.1.2. Intrinsic Camera Parameters

Usually, most of the current imaging systems use pixels to measure image coordinates where the origin of the pixel coordinate system is located at the top-left pixel of the image. Therefore, in order to describe a projected point in the pixel coordinate system, the intrinsic camera parameters have to be taken into account. If $\boldsymbol{m}^p = (u, v)^T$ represents the 2D point in the pixel coordinate system p corresponding to the 2D point $\boldsymbol{m}^i = (x, y)^T$ in image coordination system i, the relationship between $\boldsymbol{m}^p = (u, v)^T$ and $\boldsymbol{m}^i = (x, y)^T$ can be rewritten in Label (4):

$$\begin{aligned} u &= k_x x + c_x, \\ v &= k_y y + c_y, \end{aligned} \tag{4}$$

where k_x and k_y, respectively, represent the number of pixels per unit of length in the direction of x and y. Based on Label (4) and the representation of homogeneous coordinates, the correlation of $(\boldsymbol{m}^i = (x, y)^T$ and $\boldsymbol{m}^p = (u, v)^T$ can be easily denoted in Label (5) using a matrix representation:

$$\begin{bmatrix} u \\ v \\ 1 \end{bmatrix} = \begin{bmatrix} k_x & 0 & c_x \\ 0 & k_y & c_y \\ 0 & 0 & 1 \end{bmatrix} * \begin{bmatrix} x \\ y \\ 1 \end{bmatrix}. \tag{5}$$

Depending on Labels (3) and (5), we can easily express the mapping between a 3D point $\boldsymbol{M}^c = (X, Y, Z)$ in the camera frame and its corresponding 2D point $\boldsymbol{m}^p = (u, v)^T$ in the pixel frame using the camera intrinsic calibration matrix K as shown in the following equation:

$$\begin{aligned} \begin{bmatrix} u \\ v \\ 1 \end{bmatrix} &= \begin{bmatrix} k_x & 0 & c_x \\ 0 & k_y & c_y \\ 0 & 0 & 1 \end{bmatrix} * \begin{bmatrix} x \\ y \\ 1 \end{bmatrix} \\ &= s * \begin{bmatrix} f_x & 0 & c_x & 0 \\ 0 & f_y & c_y & 0 \\ 0 & 0 & 1 & 0 \end{bmatrix} * \begin{bmatrix} X \\ Y \\ Z \\ 1 \end{bmatrix} = s * K * \begin{bmatrix} X \\ Y \\ Z \\ 1 \end{bmatrix}, \end{aligned} \tag{6}$$

where f_x and f_y, called focal distances, can be respectively obtained by using k_x and k_y multiplied by the focal length f.

3.1.3. Extrinsic Camera Parameters

Generally, 3D points are not expressed in the moving camera coordinate system c but in a fixed reference frame, called the world coordinate system w. The relationship between those coordinate systems can be given by a rigid transformation consisting of a rotation ${}^c_w R$ and a translation ${}^c_w \boldsymbol{t}$ called the extrinsic camera parameters or the camera pose. This is illustrated on the right side of Figure 3. The mapping of a point $\boldsymbol{M}^w$ expressed in the world frame to a point $\boldsymbol{M}^c$ expressed in the camera frame can be denoted as follows:

$$\boldsymbol{M}^c = {}^c_w R(\boldsymbol{M}^w - \boldsymbol{C}^w), \tag{7}$$

where $\boldsymbol{C}^w$ is the position of the camera center in the world frame. Label (7) can be rewritten in another commonly used form as illustrated in Lable (8):

$$\boldsymbol{M}^c = {}^c_w R \boldsymbol{M}^w + {}^c_w \boldsymbol{t}, \tag{8}$$

where the rotation ${}^{c}_{w}R$ is pre-estimated only from inertial sensors and then used for calculating the translation ${}^{c}_{w}\boldsymbol{t}$ denoted as ${}^{c}_{w}\boldsymbol{t} = -{}^{c}_{w}RC^{w}$. By introducing homogeneous coordinates, Label (8) can be expressed as a linear operation shown in Label (9):

$$\begin{bmatrix} X^c \\ Y^c \\ Z^c \\ 1 \end{bmatrix} = \begin{bmatrix} {}^{c}_{w}R & {}^{c}_{w}\boldsymbol{t} \\ \mathbf{0}_3^T & 1 \end{bmatrix} * \begin{bmatrix} X^w \\ Y^w \\ Z^w \\ 1 \end{bmatrix}, \tag{9}$$

where ${}^{c}_{w}R$ and ${}^{c}_{w}\boldsymbol{t}$ are the camera's extrinsic parameters.

3.1.4. From World to Pixel Coordinates

By combining the forward transformations given in Label (6) and Label (9), the expected pixel location $\boldsymbol{m}^p$ can be computed from each point $\boldsymbol{M}^w$ using Label (10):

$$\begin{bmatrix} u \\ v \\ 1 \end{bmatrix} = s * K * \begin{bmatrix} X^c \\ Y^c \\ Z^c \\ 1 \end{bmatrix} = s * K * \begin{bmatrix} {}^{c}_{w}R & {}^{c}_{w}\boldsymbol{t} \\ \mathbf{0}_3^T & 1 \end{bmatrix} * \begin{bmatrix} X^w \\ Y^w \\ Z^w \\ 1 \end{bmatrix}, \tag{10}$$

so the mapping can be simply expressed as $\boldsymbol{m}^p \sim \mathrm{P}\boldsymbol{M}^w$, where the matrix $\mathrm{P} = K[{}^{c}_{w}R \mid {}^{c}_{w}\boldsymbol{t}]$ is called the camera projection matrix, and $\sim$ means equivalence up to a scale factor.

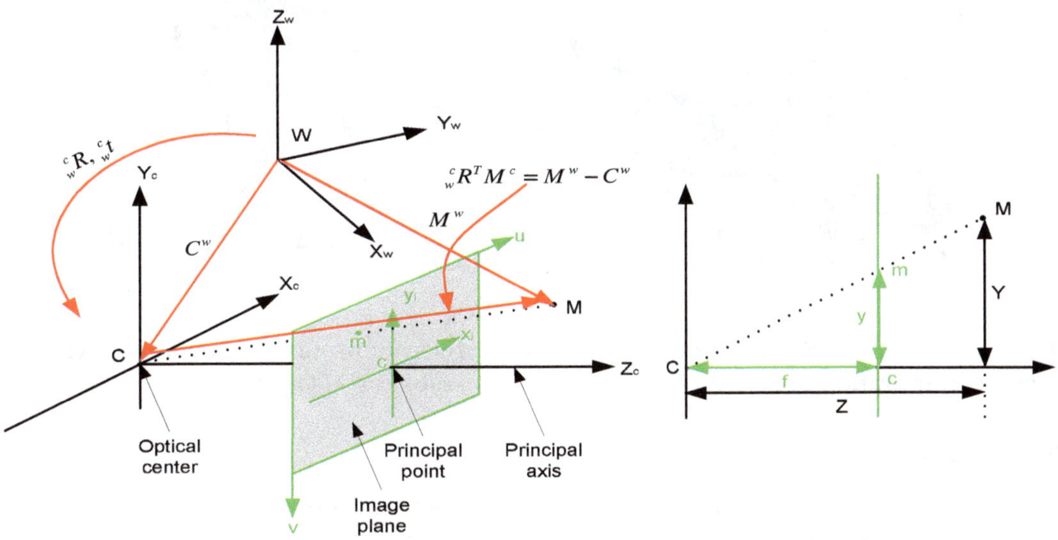

Figure 3. left: the relationship between the camera and image coordinates and between the camera and world coordinates; **right**: side view of the left figure is used to derive the relationship between the camera and image coordinates based on the principle of similarity.

3.2. Visual IMU System

A wearable visual IMU (vIMU) system is shown in Figure 4c. It integrates a camera and a newly developed MARG sensor together on a sunglass, so it is convenient for people to wear. The camera has a feature of 170 degree wide-angle, HD (High Definition) camera lens with 5.0 Mage 720P. Figure 4a shows the prototype of MARG sensor, which contains a tri-axis accelerometer (LIS3LV02D), a tri-axis gyroscope (ITG3200) and a tri-axis magnetometer (HMC5843) in a small sensor package. All signals are transmitted through Bluetooth. Moreover, an processor (TI MSP430F2618) is embedded in the small chip for convenient computation. The hardware configurations of the MARG sensor is shown in Figure 4b.

In order to integrate the measurements from different sensors, their measurements have to be timely and spatially synchronized due to each physical sensor providing measurements in its own time and spatial reference. The proposed vIMU system provides timely synchronized image sequences and inertial readings. The sample rate of MARG sensor is 60 Hz and the sample rate of camera can be lower due to the accurate baseline from epipolar geometry constraint. The related coordinate systems connected to the camera and the MARG sensor have already been presented in our previous work [2,30].

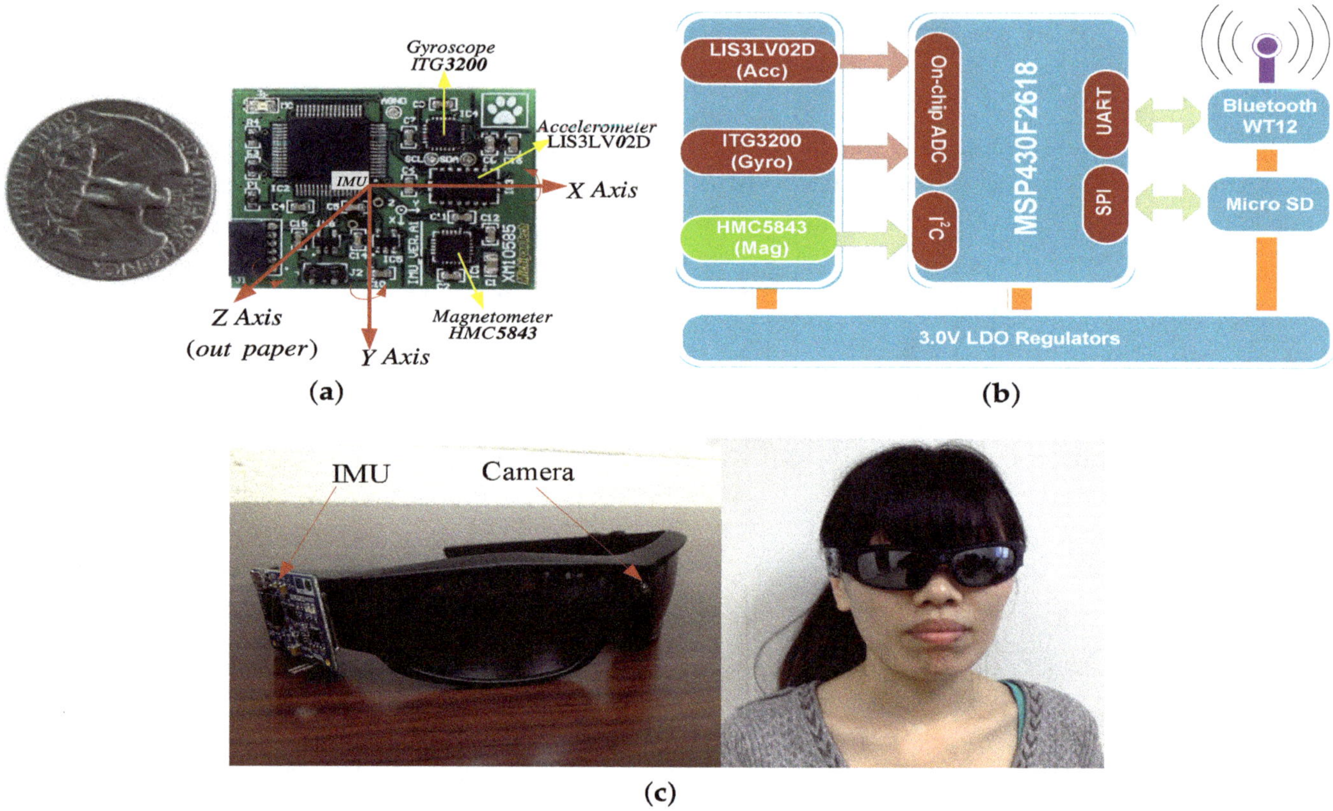

Figure 4. Prototype of MARG sensor and wearable vIMU system. (**a**) the developed MARG sensor; (**b**) hardware configuration of MARG sensor; (**c**) the wearable vIMU system.

4. Motion Estimation

In this section, an adaptive method is presented to estimate motion from visual measurements with the help of inertial measurements. Inertial motion estimation outputs the real-time orientation using an adaptive-gain orientation filter (AGOF) from our previous work [2], which aids visual motion estimation to not only segment dynamic scenes, but also compute the camera transformation from corresponding features between consecutive images.

4.1. AGOF-Aided Dynamic Scene Segmentation

The SIFT (Scale-Invariant Feature Transform) algorithm is selected to generate a SIFT descriptor corresponding to each key-point [31] and then all 2D matched feature points are obtained. The goal of our work is to propose a robout algorithm to classify these matched feature points. As a result, different groups of matched featuer points are used to recover the corresponding motions. In this subsection, we present the sorted method for matched feature points: AGOF-aided homography recovery constraint and epipolar geometry constraint.

4.1.1. Homography Recovery

When the camera undergoes a pure translation, a general motion of camera can be transformed to a special motion with the help of the preestimated robust orientation from our AGOF filter. Usually, there are two special cases: one is parallel to the image plane and the other is perpendicular to the image plane.

As shown in Figure 5, the homography H can recover rotation between two consecutive images because it directly connects the corresponding 2D points of a 3D point. If the camera intrinsic parameter K and the rotation R are known, the homography H can be directly obtained using Label (11):

$$\begin{aligned} \boldsymbol{m}_{k+1}^T &= H\boldsymbol{m}_k, \\ H &= KRK^{-1}, \end{aligned} \tag{11}$$

where $\boldsymbol{m}_k = (u_k, v_k)$ and $\boldsymbol{m}_{k+1} = (u_{k+1}, v_{k+1})$ are corresponding 2D points in two consecutive frames k and $k+1$ of a 3D point $\boldsymbol{M}$. As we mentioned previously, the rotation R can be preestimated, so a bunch of motion lines, which connect the corresponding 2D matched feature points of a 3D point, are obtained. These lines can be sorted by computing the slope of them or checking if they can intersect at the same point called "epipole". The slope of motion line ρ can be expressed in Label (12) according to $\boldsymbol{m}_k$ and $\boldsymbol{m}_{k+1}$:

$$\rho = \frac{u_{k+1} - u_k}{v_{k+1} - v_k}, \text{ if } \|v_{k+1} - v_k\| \neq 0. \tag{12}$$

If $\|v_{k+1} - v_k\|$ equals 0, then the real camera moves along x-axis of the camera coordinate system.

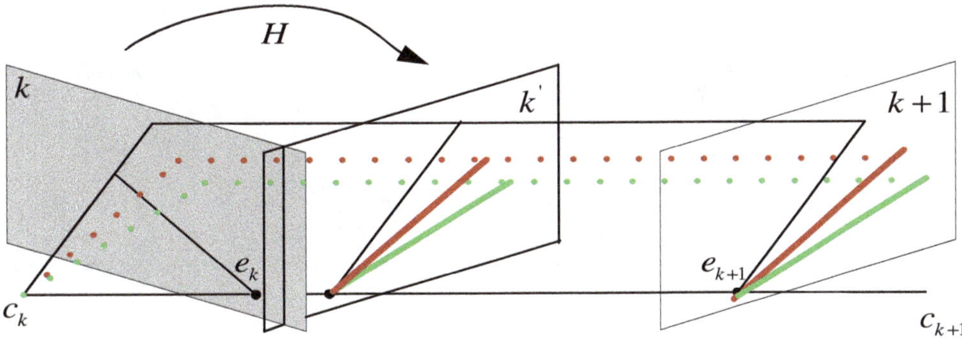

Figure 5. Homography recovery under a general motion of camera.

4.1.2. Epipolar Geometry

According to the definition in reference [10], two epipolar lines can be obtained in Label (13) based on the optical flows:

$$\begin{aligned} \boldsymbol{l}_k &= \boldsymbol{e}_k \times \boldsymbol{m}_k &&= [\boldsymbol{e}_k]_\times \boldsymbol{m}_k, \\ \boldsymbol{l}_{k+1} &= \boldsymbol{e}_{k+1} \times \boldsymbol{m}_{k+1} &&= [\boldsymbol{e}_{k+1}]_\times \boldsymbol{m}_{k+1}, \end{aligned} \tag{13}$$

where $\boldsymbol{e}_k$ and $\boldsymbol{e}_{k+1}$ are the epipoles; $[\boldsymbol{e}_k]_\times$ and $[\boldsymbol{e}_{k+1}]_\times$ are 3×3 skew-symmetric matrixes; $\boldsymbol{l}_k$ and $\boldsymbol{l}_{k+1}$ respectively denote lines connecting $\boldsymbol{e}$ and $\boldsymbol{m}$ in frame k and frame $k+1$ respectively as shown in Figure 6. Moreover, based on the constraint of epipolar geometry as depicted in Label (14), two epipolar lines $\boldsymbol{l}_k'$ and $\boldsymbol{l}_{k+1}'$ could be inferred from the fundamental matrix F as shown in Label (15):

$$\boldsymbol{m}_{k+1}^T \mathrm{F} \boldsymbol{m}_k = 0, \tag{14}$$

$$\boldsymbol{l}_k' = \mathrm{F}^T \boldsymbol{m}_{k+1}, \quad \boldsymbol{l}_{k+1}' = \mathrm{F} \boldsymbol{m}_k. \tag{15}$$

Based on two constraints of optical flow and epipolar geometry for static points, we can obtain $\boldsymbol{l}_k \cong \boldsymbol{l}'_k$ and $\boldsymbol{l}_{k+1} \cong \boldsymbol{l}'_{k+1}$, where $\cong$ means up to a scale factor. Nevertheless, the constrain of epipolar geometry will be not satisfied if the points belong to moving objectgs. Therefore, for feature points from moving objects in the scene, the distance from the 2D point to the corresponding epipolar line is chosen to evaluate how discrepant this epipolar line is, and it can be derived in Label (16) from the constraint of epipolar geometry:

$$\begin{aligned} d_k &= \frac{\boldsymbol{m}_k^T(\mathrm{F}^T\boldsymbol{m}_{k+1})}{\parallel \mathrm{F}^T\boldsymbol{m}_{k+1} \parallel^2}, \\ d_{k+1} &= \frac{\boldsymbol{m}_{k+1}^T(\mathrm{F}\boldsymbol{m}_k)}{\parallel \mathrm{F}\boldsymbol{m}_k \parallel^2}. \end{aligned} \tag{16}$$

In general, the distance for a static point is non-zero due to image noises and estimation errors of epipolar geometry. Actually, the larger the distance, the more confidently the 3D point is considered to be part of a moving object.

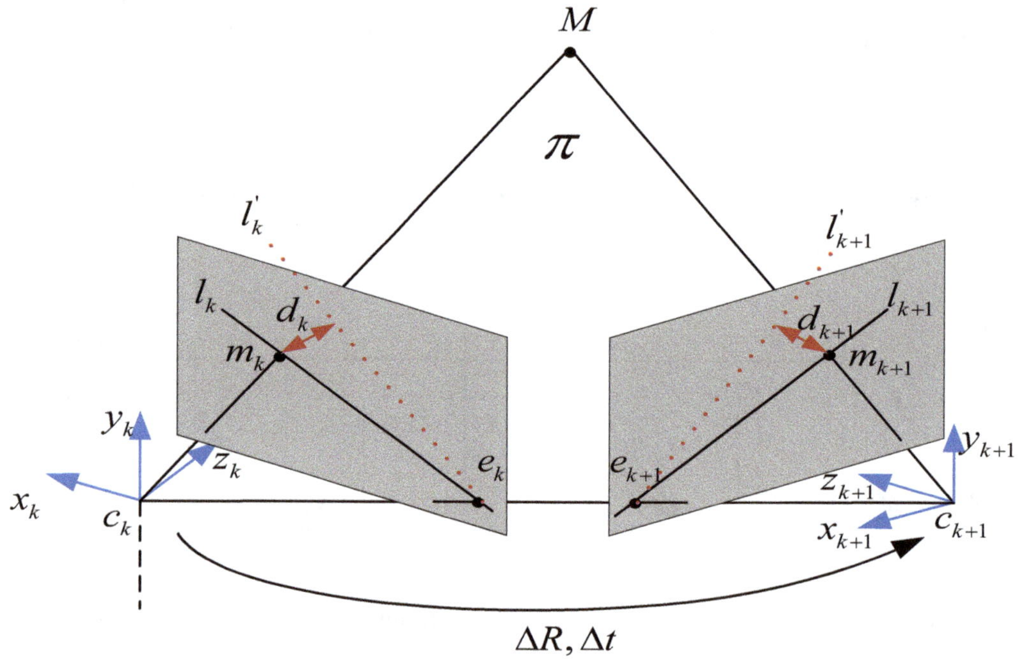

Figure 6. Epipolar geometry.

4.2. Real and Virtual Camera Motion Recovery

Based on the matched 2D feature points from a moving object viewed by a moving camera, the recovered poses actually reflect the combined motion of the moving object and the moving camera. For better understanding, a novel concept of a "virtual" camera is proposed to consider as if the object were static observed by a "virtual" moving camera in comparison with the "real" camera as depicted in Figure 7. This section will emphasize how to recover the motion of real and virtual camera.

4.2.1. Relative Motion Recovery for Real Camera

After dividing 2D matched feature points based on two pre-presented constraints, the essential matrix E can be derived from the fundamental matrix F and the camera's intrinsic parameter matrix K using Labels (14) and (17):

$$\mathrm{E} = K^T \mathrm{F} K. \tag{17}$$

As we know, the relative translation $\Delta \boldsymbol{t}$ and rotation ΔR of camera can be obtained from the essential matrix E, so $\Delta \boldsymbol{t}$ and ΔR could differentiate the relative motion of camera from the absolute motion of camera. Authors in [10] retrieved the camera matrices from the essential matrix E using $\mathrm{E} = [\boldsymbol{t}]_{\times} R$, so the relative rotation ΔR and the relative translation $\Delta \boldsymbol{t}$, as shown in Figure 6, can be recovered from E by using Labels (18) and (19) based on the method proposed in [32]:

$$\begin{aligned} \Delta \boldsymbol{t}\, \Delta \boldsymbol{t}^T &= \frac{1}{2} Trace(\mathrm{E}\mathrm{E}^T)\mathrm{I} - \mathrm{E}\mathrm{E}^T, \\ (\Delta \boldsymbol{t} \cdot \Delta \boldsymbol{t})\Delta R &= \mathrm{E}^{*T} - \Delta \boldsymbol{t} \times \mathrm{E}, \end{aligned} \tag{18}$$

where E^* is E's cofactor and I is a 3×3 identity matrix. As a result, two solutions $\Delta \boldsymbol{t}_1$ and $\Delta \boldsymbol{t}_2$ could be obtained for $\Delta \boldsymbol{t}$ by finding the largest row of matrix $\mathbb{T} = \Delta \boldsymbol{t}\, \Delta \boldsymbol{t}^T$ as shown in Label (19):

$$\Delta \boldsymbol{t} = \pm \mathbb{T}(i,:)^T / \sqrt{\mathbb{T}(i,i)}, \tag{19}$$

where $\mathbb{T}(i,i)$ is the largest element of diagonal of matrix $\mathbb{T}$ ($i = 1,2,3$). Therefore, the camera matrix has only two different solutions: $\mathrm{P}_1 = [\Delta R \mid \Delta \boldsymbol{t}_1]$ and $\mathrm{P}_2 = [\Delta R \mid \Delta \boldsymbol{t}_2]$ due to pre-estimated accurate ΔR in [2]. Here, we use the rule that a reconstructed 3D point should be in front of the camera between two consecutive views to check which one of these two solutions is satisfied.

Finally, a refining process called "Bundle Adjustment" is used to optimize the parameters of the relative motion $\Delta \boldsymbol{t}$ and the optical characteristics of the camera K, according to a nonlinear least square solution to minimize the total reprojection errors of all points in two consecutive images at k and $k+1$ as shown in Label (20):

$$\begin{aligned} \epsilon &= [\epsilon_k, \epsilon_{k+1}]^T, \\ \epsilon_k &= \textstyle\sum_i \|{}^i\boldsymbol{m}_k - K[eye(3)|\boldsymbol{0}_{3\times1}]^i\boldsymbol{M}\|, \\ \epsilon_{k+1} &= \textstyle\sum_i \|{}^i\boldsymbol{m}_{k+1} - K[\Delta R|\Delta \boldsymbol{t}]^i\boldsymbol{M}\|, \end{aligned} \tag{20}$$

where ${}^i\boldsymbol{m}_k$ represents the *i-th* 2D point in the image coordinate at frame k and ${}^i\boldsymbol{M}$ is the corresponding 3D point.

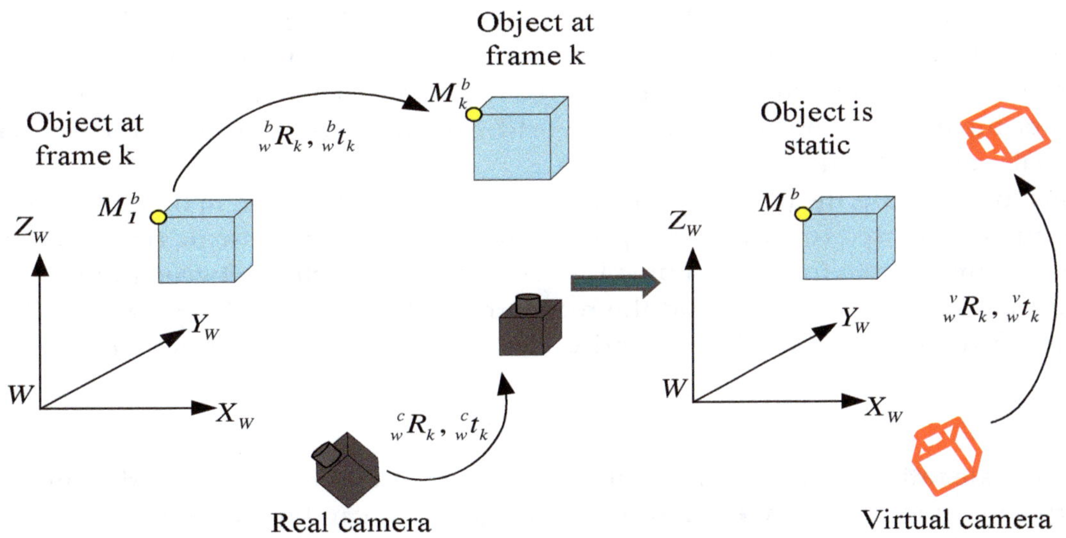

Figure 7. A concept of virtual camera.

4.2.2. Relative Motion Recovery for Virtual Camera

According to the pre-proposed concept of virtual camera, the motion of virtual camera is actually the combination motion of real camera and moving object. In addition, the intrinsic parameters of virtual camera is the same as those of real camera, but the motion of virtual camera is different from that of real camera with the presence of moving objects.

Meanwhile, the relative motion of virtual camera can be obtained by using the similar method as the real camera in Section 4.2.1. The only difference is that the relative rotation does not need to be recovered for the real camera because the real camera is rigidly attached with the IMU and the rotation of real camera can be pre-estimated from IMU-only.

4.2.3. Scale Adjustment

The baseline $\Delta \boldsymbol{t}$, recovered from E based on Label (19), can only have available direction because the camera motion is only estimated up to a scale. This is a so-called scale problem in monocular vision. Since there are multiple frames, the baseline estimated between each pair of consecutive frames is only determined up to an unknown and different scale factor as shown in Figure 8.

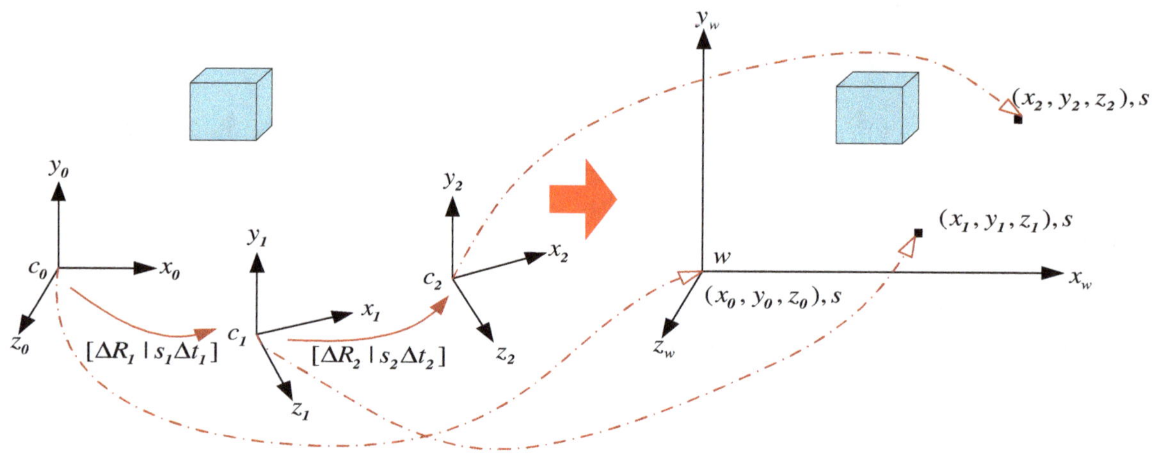

Figure 8. Unified scale recovery from videos.

In order to obtain a scale consistent trajectory estimation of the camera motion, the scale for each camera motion between two consecutive frames needs to be adjusted so that only one global scale parameter remains unknown. This global scale defines the true size of the reconstructed 3D structure and can be recovered if the information about the real world is introduced. In this subsection, an inertial measurement unit, which consists of three-axis accelerometer, gyroscope and magnetometer, is used to infer the information about the real world. Section 5 will introduce the estimation of this absolute global scale in details.

For adjusting the scale, the method proposed in [33] will be employed in this subsection, where the scale is computed in closed form with a 1-point algorithm. Given the scale free motion estimation ($[\Delta R|\Delta \boldsymbol{t}]$) of the camera from frame k to frame $k-1$, the feature matches between frame $k-1$ and frame k ($\boldsymbol{m} = (x, y, 1)^T = K^{-1} * (u, v, 1)^T$), and the reconstructed 3D points ($\boldsymbol{M} = (X, Y, Z, 1)^T$) obtained from three consecutive frames $k-2$, $k-1$ and k , the scale can be adjusted as follows:

$$\boldsymbol{m} = [\Delta R | s_k \Delta \boldsymbol{t}] \boldsymbol{M}, \tag{21}$$

where s_k is the scale ratio that relates the baseline between camera frame $k-2$ and frame $k-1$ and the baseline between camera frame $k-1$ and frame k. Label (21) can be rewritten as $\boldsymbol{A} s_k = \boldsymbol{b}$, where $\boldsymbol{A}$ and $\boldsymbol{b}$ are vectors. The vector $\boldsymbol{A}$ contains one constraint per row $\Delta t_x - \Delta t_z x$, defined by one 2D $\sim$ 3D correspondence. The vector $\boldsymbol{b}$ is defined as: $(\Delta \boldsymbol{r}_1 - \Delta \boldsymbol{r}_3 x) X$ where $\Delta \boldsymbol{r}_1$ is the first row of ΔR. Then, the scale s_k is solved by using SVD (Singular Value Decomposition) [10] for obtaining a solution in the least square sense as:

$$s_k = \frac{\boldsymbol{A}^T \boldsymbol{b}}{\boldsymbol{A}^T \boldsymbol{A}}. \tag{22}$$

Though only one 2D$\sim$3D correspondence is needed to solve the scale parameter, all available correspondences are used in this paper for robustness.

4.2.4. Camera Absolute Motion Recovery

Usually, the camera absolute poses, which are relative to the world coordinate, are essential to be obtained for motion estimation. However, from the 2D matched points, we can derive the relative rotation ΔR and translation $\Delta \boldsymbol{t}$ between two consecutive frames. If $(R_k, \boldsymbol{t}_k)$ and $(R_{k+1}, \boldsymbol{t}_{k+1})$ respectively represent the absolute rotation and translation of camera for frame k $(k = 1, 2, \cdots)$ and $k+1$, then a static 3D point $\boldsymbol{M}$ can be easily expressed between the camera frame and the world frame as shown in Labels (23) and (24):

$$\boldsymbol{M}_k^c = R_k \boldsymbol{M}_k^w + \boldsymbol{t}_k, \tag{23}$$

$$\boldsymbol{M}_{k+1}^c = R_{k+1} \boldsymbol{M}_{k+1}^w + \boldsymbol{t}_{k+1}. \tag{24}$$

The position of $\boldsymbol{M}$ will not be changed from frame k to frame $k+1$ because $\boldsymbol{M}$ is a static point and meanwhile the world frame does not move. In other words, we can easily define $\boldsymbol{M}_k^w = \boldsymbol{M}_{k+1}^w = \boldsymbol{M}^w$, then $\boldsymbol{M}^w$ can be derived from Label (23) as $\boldsymbol{M}^w = R_k^T(\boldsymbol{M}_k^c - \boldsymbol{t}_k)$. Thus, Label (25) is obtained by substituting $\boldsymbol{M}^w$ for $\boldsymbol{M}_{k+1}^w$ in Label (24):

$$\begin{aligned} \boldsymbol{M}_{k+1}^c &= R_{k+1} R_k^T \boldsymbol{M}_k^c - R_{k+1} R_k^T \boldsymbol{t}_k + \boldsymbol{t}_{k+1} \\ &= \Delta R \boldsymbol{M}_k^c + \Delta \boldsymbol{t}, \end{aligned} \tag{25}$$

with $\Delta R = R_{k+1} R_k^T$ and $\Delta \boldsymbol{t} = \boldsymbol{t}_{k+1} - R_{k+1} R_k^T \boldsymbol{t}_k$. Inversely, given $(\Delta R, \Delta \boldsymbol{t})$ and $(R_k, \boldsymbol{t}_k)$, the camera's absolute poses at frame $k+1$ cane be easily solved by using Label (26):

$$\begin{aligned} R_{k+1} &= \Delta R R_k, \\ \boldsymbol{t}_{k+1} &= \Delta \boldsymbol{t} + \Delta R \boldsymbol{t}_k. \end{aligned} \tag{26}$$

4.3. Motion Estimation for 3D Object

In this section, the motion of 3D objects in the world frame will be estimated from the motion of real camera and virtual camera. Assuming that a 3D point $\boldsymbol{M}_k^b$ is attached to a moving object as depicted in the left of Figure 7, $\boldsymbol{M}_k^b$ can be derived from the initial position $\boldsymbol{M}_1^b$ according to the motion of rigid object(${}_w^bR_k$ and ${}_w^b\boldsymbol{t}_k$) Label (27):

$$\boldsymbol{M}_k^b = {}_w^bR_k \boldsymbol{M}_1^b + {}_w^b\boldsymbol{t}_k, \tag{27}$$

where superscript b indicates the point $\boldsymbol{M}$ is attached to the moving object and subscript k denotes the point is viewed at frame k. It is clearly seen that the static rigid object is a special case where ${}_w^bR_k = \mathrm{I}$ and ${}_w^b\boldsymbol{t}_k = \boldsymbol{0}$.

Based on the motion of real camera ${}_w^cR_k$ and ${}_w^c\boldsymbol{t}_k$ at frame k, we can use Label (28) to obtain the 3D position of a point from the world frame to the current real camera frame:

$$\boldsymbol{M}_k^c = {}_w^cR_k \boldsymbol{M}_k^b + {}_w^c\boldsymbol{t}_k. \tag{28}$$

Combining Labels (27) and (28), the 3D position of point with respect to the *k-th* camera can be easily derived in Label (29):

$$\boldsymbol{M}_k^c = ({}_w^cR_k {}_w^bR_k)\boldsymbol{M}_1^b + ({}_w^cR_k {}_w^b\boldsymbol{t}_k + {}_w^c\boldsymbol{t}_k). \tag{29}$$

As aforementioned, the special case with ${}_w^bR_k = \mathrm{I}$ and ${}_w^b\boldsymbol{t}_k = \boldsymbol{0}$ can be thought as the static object observed by a moving camera, which can simplify Label (29) to be Label (8). Actually, the definition of the "virtual" camera originates from Label (29), which denotes a static object ($\boldsymbol{M}_1^b = \boldsymbol{M}_k^b$) viewed by a moving camera as shown in the right of Figure 7. Therefore, the motion of "virtual" camera $({}^{v}_{w}R_k, {}^{v}_{w}\boldsymbol{t}_k)$ at frame k can be denoted in Label (30):

$$\begin{aligned} {}^{v}_{w}R_k &= {}^{c}_{w}R_k {}^{b}_{w}R_k, \\ {}^{v}_{w}\boldsymbol{t}_k &= {}^{c}_{w}R_k {}^{b}_{w}\boldsymbol{t}_k + {}^{c}_{w}\boldsymbol{t}_k. \end{aligned} \tag{30}$$

It is clearly seen that the initial point has ${}^{b}_{w}R_k = \mathrm{I}$ and ${}^{b}_{w}\boldsymbol{t}_k = \mathbf{0}$ in frame 1, so the motion of virtual camera has the same motion as the real camera at frame 1: ${}^{v}_{w}R_1 = {}^{c}_{w}R_1 = \mathrm{I}$ and ${}^{v}_{w}\boldsymbol{t}_1 = {}^{c}_{w}\boldsymbol{t}_1 = \mathbf{0}$. During the following frames, the virtual camera's motion differs from the real camera's motion because of the motion of rigid objects.

As a result, the object pose $({}^{b}_{w}R_k, {}^{b}_{w}\boldsymbol{t}_k)$ can be derived by using Label (30) based on the real camera's motion $({}^{c}_{w}R_k, {}^{c}_{w}\boldsymbol{t}_k)$ and the virtual camera's motion $({}^{v}_{w}R_k, {}^{v}_{w}\boldsymbol{t}_k)$:

$$\begin{aligned} {}^{b}_{w}R_k &= ({}^{c}_{w}R_k)^{-1} {}^{v}_{w}R_k, \\ {}^{b}_{w}\boldsymbol{t}_k &= ({}^{c}_{w}R_k)^{-1}({}^{v}_{w}\boldsymbol{t}_k - {}^{c}_{w}\boldsymbol{t}_k). \end{aligned} \tag{31}$$

5. Multi-Rate Linear Kalman Filter

As we mentioned previously, the main problem of monocular vision is scale ambiguity. The inertial sensors can infer the position with absolute metric unit from the accelerometer, which suffers from the accumulated drift for long-term tracking. Therefore, the combination of monocular visual and inertial data is proposed in this paper to solve the scale ambiguity. In the state-of-the-art literature [8,17,24–26], the sensor fusion algorithm requires a nonlinear estimator to estimate both the orientation and the position in the same process, such as Extended Kalman Filter (EKF), Unscented Kalman Filter (UKF), etc. However, in this paper, a multi-rate linear estimator, called "AGOF/Linear Kalman Filter" as our previous work [30], was designed to integrate visual and inertial measurements together without updating orientation information, so that the model can be linear and only needs a small state vector. The following sections briefly review our proposed filter in [30].

5.1. State Vector Definition

The state vector $\boldsymbol{x}_k$ and the system process noise $\boldsymbol{n}$ can be expressed as follows

$$\begin{aligned} \boldsymbol{x}_k &= [{}^{c}_{e}\boldsymbol{p}_k; {}^{c}_{e}\boldsymbol{v}_k; {}^{c}_{e}\boldsymbol{a}_k; \lambda_k; \boldsymbol{b}_{a,k}], \\ \boldsymbol{n} &= [\boldsymbol{n}_a; n_\lambda; \boldsymbol{n}_{b_a}], \end{aligned} \tag{32}$$

where ${}^{c}_{e}\boldsymbol{p}_k$ is camera position without scale, ${}^{c}_{e}\boldsymbol{v}_k$ is camera velocity, ${}^{c}_{e}\boldsymbol{a}_k$ is camera acceleration expressed in metric unit (meter), $\lambda_k = 1/s_k$ is the reciprocal of the absolute scale factor, which leads to low-order polynomials and $\boldsymbol{b}_{a,k}$ is the accelerometer bias.

5.2. Dynamic Model

The system is assumed to have a uniformly accelerated linear translation at time k, so the translation of the camera can be modeled by an equation set. Thus, the dynamic model of the state is defined as follows:

$$\begin{aligned} {}^{c}_{e}\boldsymbol{p}_{k+1} &= {}^{c}_{e}\boldsymbol{p}_k + T\lambda_k {}^{c}_{e}\boldsymbol{v}_k + \tfrac{T^2\lambda_k}{2} {}^{c}_{e}\boldsymbol{a}_k + \tfrac{T^3\lambda_k}{6}\boldsymbol{n}_a, \\ {}^{c}_{e}\boldsymbol{v}_{k+1} &= {}^{c}_{e}\boldsymbol{v}_k + T {}^{c}_{e}\boldsymbol{a}_k + \tfrac{T^2}{2}\boldsymbol{n}_a, \\ {}^{c}_{e}\boldsymbol{a}_{k+1} &= {}^{c}_{e}\boldsymbol{a}_k + T\boldsymbol{n}_a, \\ \lambda_{k+1} &= \lambda_k + n_\lambda, \\ \boldsymbol{b}_{a,k+1} &= \boldsymbol{b}_{a,k} + T\boldsymbol{n}_{b_a}, \end{aligned} \tag{33}$$

where T represents the time span between k and $k+1$. λ_k is based on a random walk model and the bias $\boldsymbol{b}_{a,k}$ is based on the value and a white noise at time k.

5.3. Measurement Model

The involved sensors are with two different sampling rates, so two measurements are considered: one is ${}^{s}\boldsymbol{y}_k^m = \left[{}^{c}_{e}\boldsymbol{a}_k^m\right]$ when inertial measurements are available and the other is ${}^{c}\boldsymbol{y}_k^m = \left[{}^{c}_{e}\boldsymbol{p}_k^m\right]$ when visual measurements are available. Therefore, the updating equation of measurements for output states is:

$$\boldsymbol{y}_k = H\boldsymbol{x}_k + \boldsymbol{e}_k, \tag{34}$$

with $H_{s,k} = \begin{pmatrix} \mathbf{0}_{3\times3} & \mathbf{0}_{3\times3} & \boldsymbol{I}_{3\times3} & \mathbf{0}_{3\times4} \end{pmatrix}$ for available inertial measurements or $H_{c,k} = \begin{pmatrix} \boldsymbol{I}_{3\times3} & \mathbf{0}_{3\times3} & \mathbf{0}_{3\times4} & \mathbf{0}_{3\times3} \end{pmatrix}$ for available visual measurements.

In order to obtain reliable measurements from inertial sensors as the input of measurement model, the effect of the gravity ${}^{e}\boldsymbol{g} = [0 \quad 0 \quad -9.8]^T$ denoted in the earth coordinate system e should be firstly removed from the raw acceleration measurements ${}^{s}\boldsymbol{a}$ in sensor coordinate system s based on the preestimated robust orientation ${}^{s}_{e}\hat{\boldsymbol{q}}_f$ using the quaternion-based representation. The related equations are depicted in Label (35):

$$\begin{aligned} {}^{c}_{e}\boldsymbol{a}_k^m &= \mathcal{R}({}^{c}_{s}\boldsymbol{q}) * (\mathcal{R}({}^{s}_{e}\hat{\boldsymbol{q}}_{f,k}) * {}^{s}\boldsymbol{a}_k - {}^{e}\boldsymbol{g}) + {}^{c}_{s}\boldsymbol{t}, \\ {}^{s}\boldsymbol{a}_k &= {}^{s}\boldsymbol{a}_k^m - \boldsymbol{b}_{a,k} - \boldsymbol{e}_{a,k}, \end{aligned} \tag{35}$$

where the operator $\mathcal{R}$ denotes converting orientation from unit quaternion representation to rotation matrix representation; ${}^{c}_{s}\boldsymbol{q}$ and ${}^{c}_{s}\boldsymbol{b}$ can be obtained from the hand-eye calibration using the method in [34].

6. Experimental Results and Analysis

6.1. Experimental Setup

The performance of our proposed method was tested by a sunglass with wearable visual-inertial fusion system as shown in Figure 4c in different indoor environments. Firstly, three different experiments were performed in three different indoor environments, which are a hallway, an office room and a home-based environment. In order to test the accuracy of ego-motion estimation, the results from a Pioneer robot were as our ground truth shown in Figure 9. Moreover, the results were compared with those from EKF to verify our proposed MR-LKF more efficient. Secondly, a longer closed-loop path was performed, where a person was walking up and down the stairs with the visual-inertial system. Finally, an office-based dynamic environment was concerned, where a toy car was moving in a straight line.

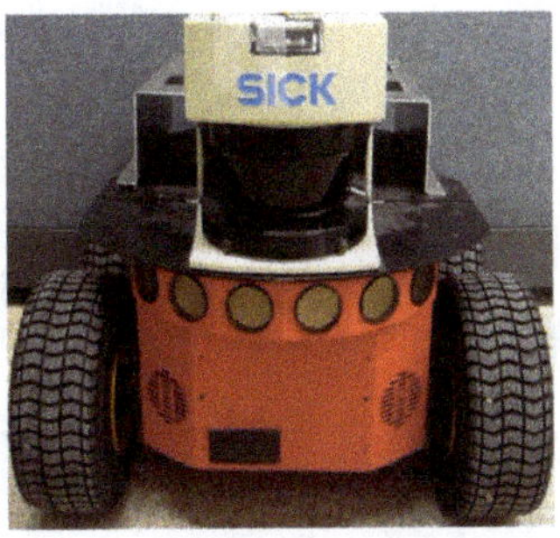

Figure 9. The Pioneer robot platform for experimental illustrations.

6.2. Experimental Results

6.2.1. Experiment I: Straight-Line Motion Estimation in a Hallway

The experiment was conducted to attach the proposed vIMU system on the Pioneer robot platform to follow a straight line in our office hallway. The tracked trajectory is shown in Figure 10g compared with the results from EKF and the Pioneer robot. It is clearly seen that the estimated trajectory is more accurate and closer to the ground truth. In addition, Figure 10h shows the inertrial measurements, which obviously shows the movement of the system as slow and smooth. Moreover, typical frames and 3D visualized tracked trajectory are clearly given in Figure 10a–f.

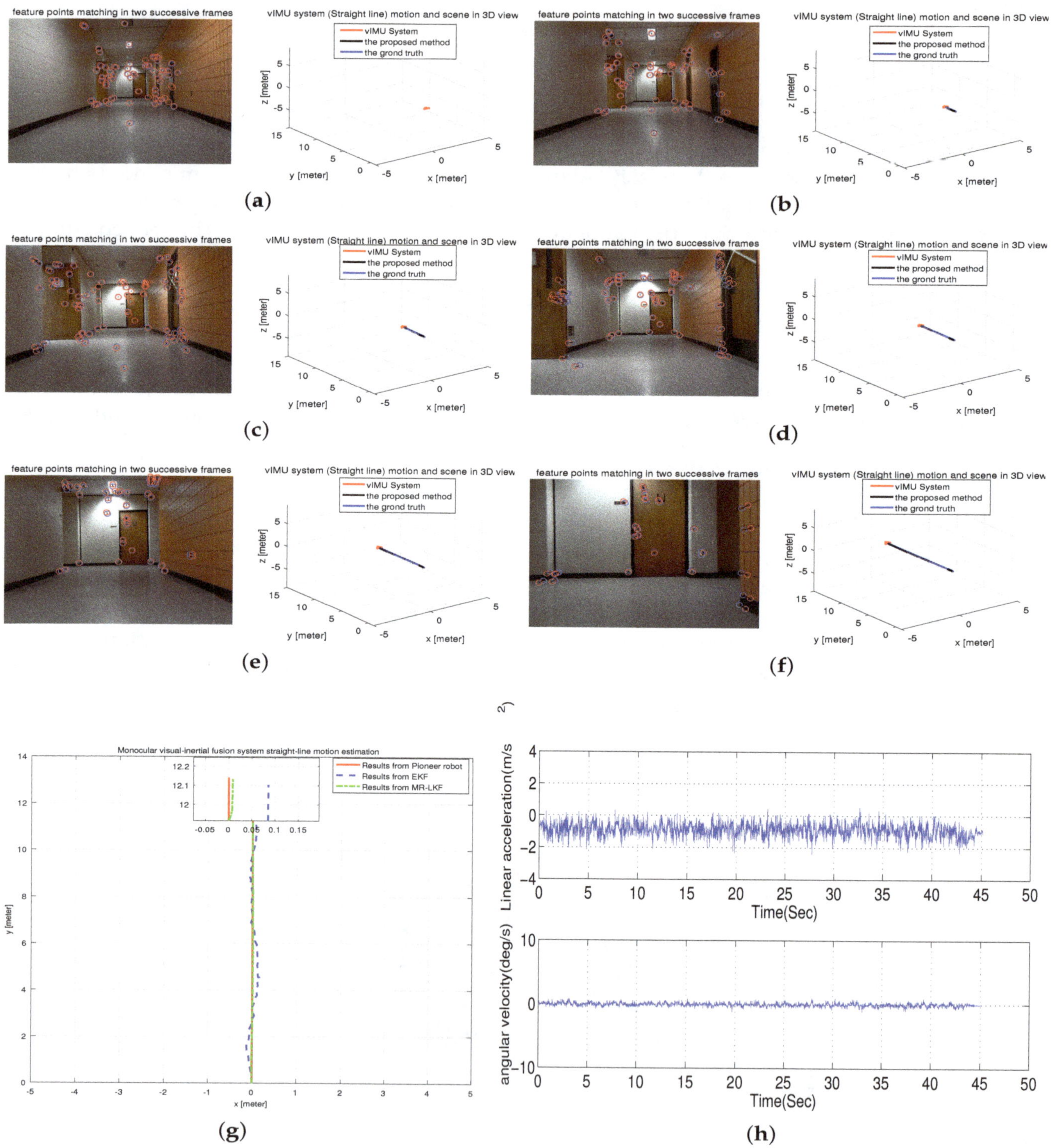

Figure 10. Straight-line Motion Estimation in a hallway. (**a**–**f**) typical frames; (**g**) estimated trajectory with a magnified final position; (**h**) inertial measurements.

6.2.2. Experiment II: Curve Motion Estimation in an Office Room

In this test scenario, the Pioneer robot attached the visual-inertial system to follow a curve in our office room. Figure 11h shows the inertial measurements, which obviously show that the system experienced fast rotational and translational motion. The tracked trajectory is shown in Figure 11g compared with the results from EKF and the Pioneer robot. It is clearly seen that the estimated trajectory is more accurate and closer to the ground truth. Moreover, typical frames and 3D visualized tracked trajectory are clearly given in Figure 11a–f.

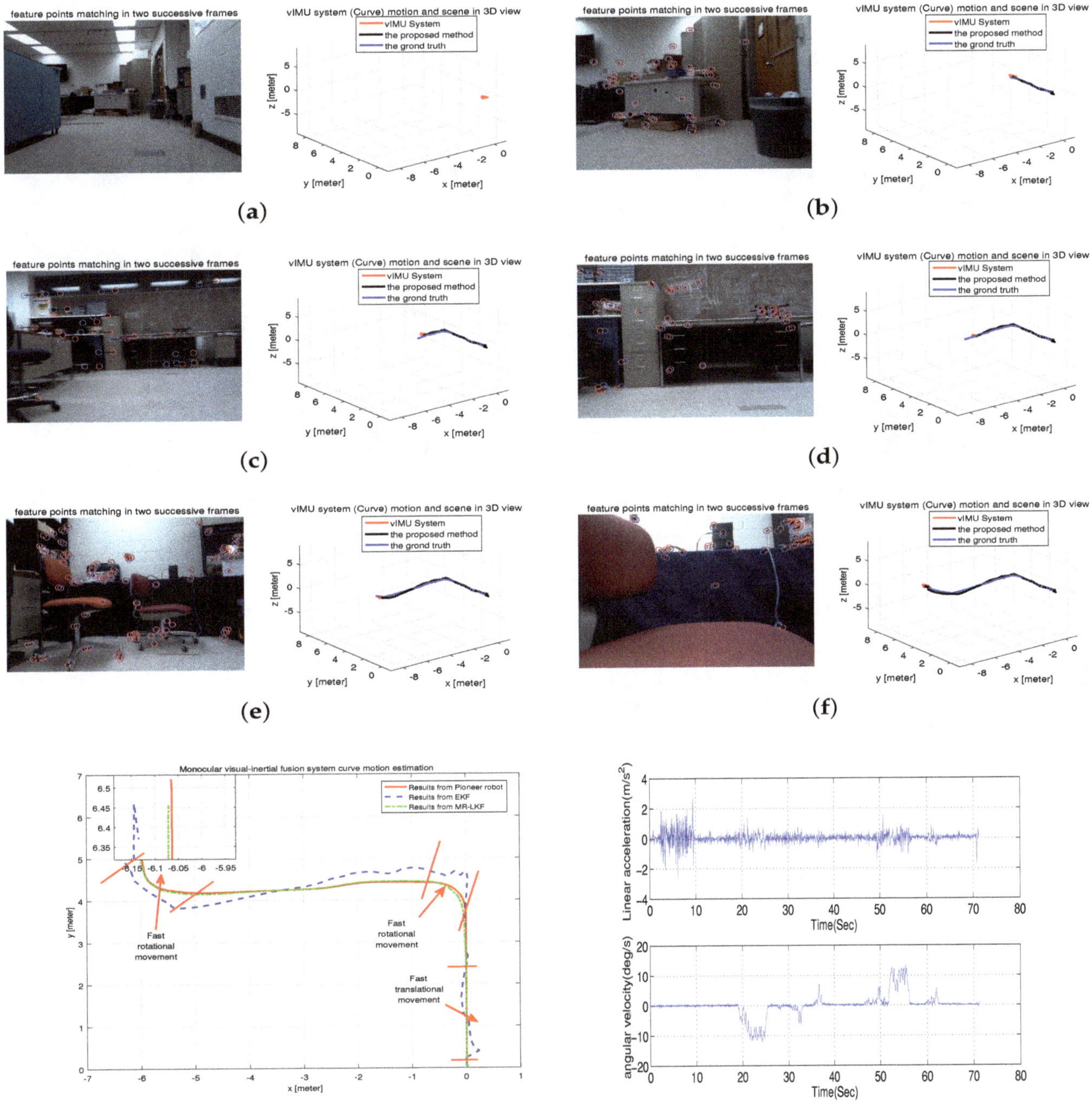

Figure 11. Curve Motion Estimation in an office room. (**a**–**f**) typical frames; (**g**) estimated trajectory with a magnified final position; (**h**) inertial measurements.

6.2.3. Experiment III: Semicircle Motion Estimation in A Home-Based Environment

This test was performed on a controllable robot arm to generate a semicircle movement in a home-based environment. Obviously, the radius of the semicircle is actually the length of the arm, so the accuracy of estimated results can be verified based on the known trajectory equation. The tracked trajectory is shown in Figure 12g compared with the results from EKF and the known trajectory. It is clearly seen that the estimated trajectory is more accurate and closer to the known trajectory. In addition, Figure 12h shows the orientation estimation from our AGOF orientation filter compared with the true orientation. Moreover, typical frames and 3D visualized tracked trajectory are clearly given in Figure 12a–f.

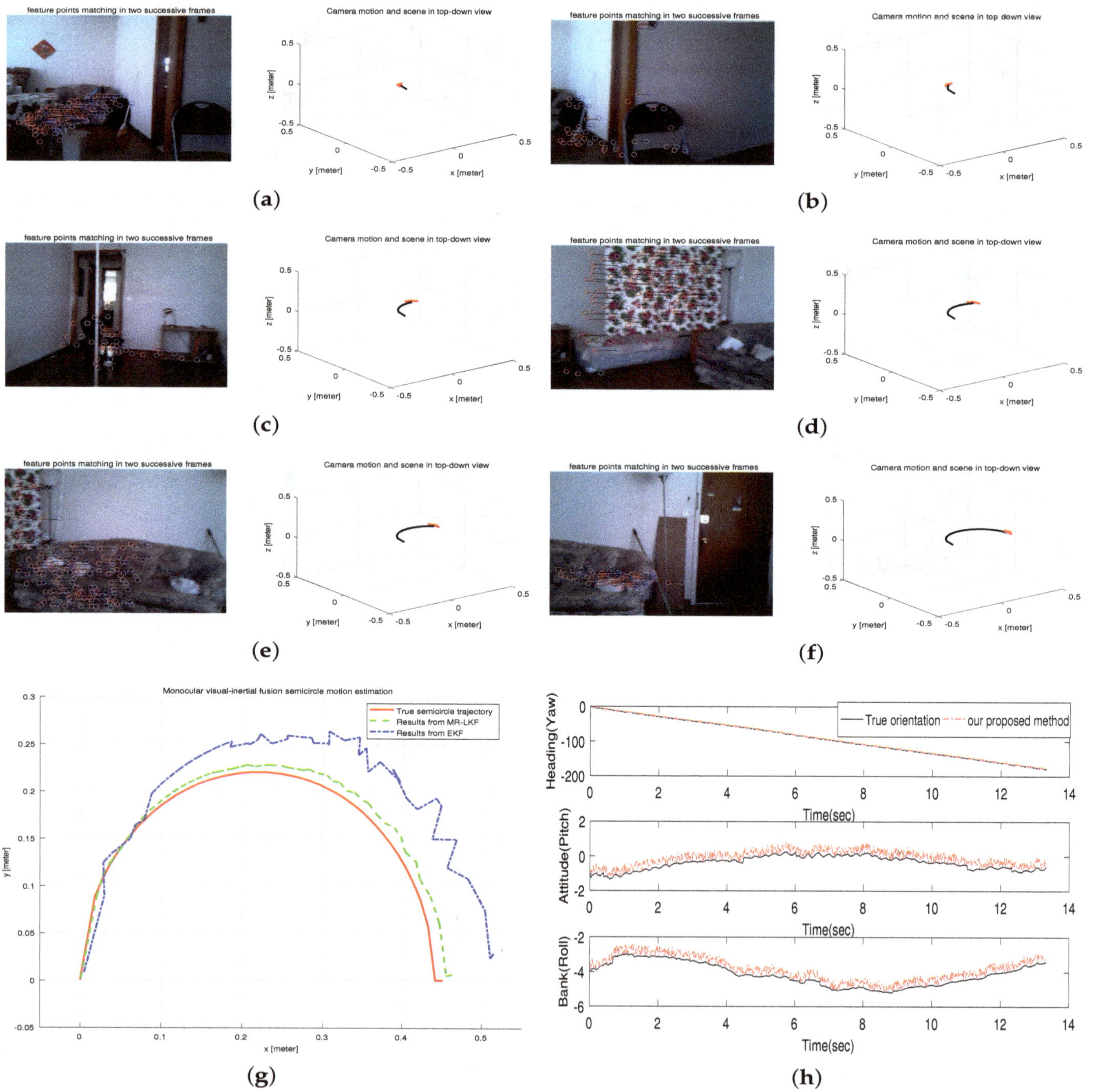

Figure 12. Semicircle Motion Estimation in a home-based environment. (**a**–**f**) typical frames; (**g**) estimated trajectory; (**h**) Orientation estimation.

6.2.4. Experiment IV: Closed-Loop Motion Estimation

In this test, a longer trial was performed to verify the efficiency of the proposed method in three-dimensional estimation, where a closed route was conducted by a person walking up and down stairs with the visual-inertial system. Figure 13a shows the estimated trajectory with a magnified final position. It is clearly seen that our proposed method can correct the drift and make the final position very close to the initial position. Moreover, the robust orientation estimation from our AGOF filter, shown in Figure 13b, plays an important role in reducing the drift.

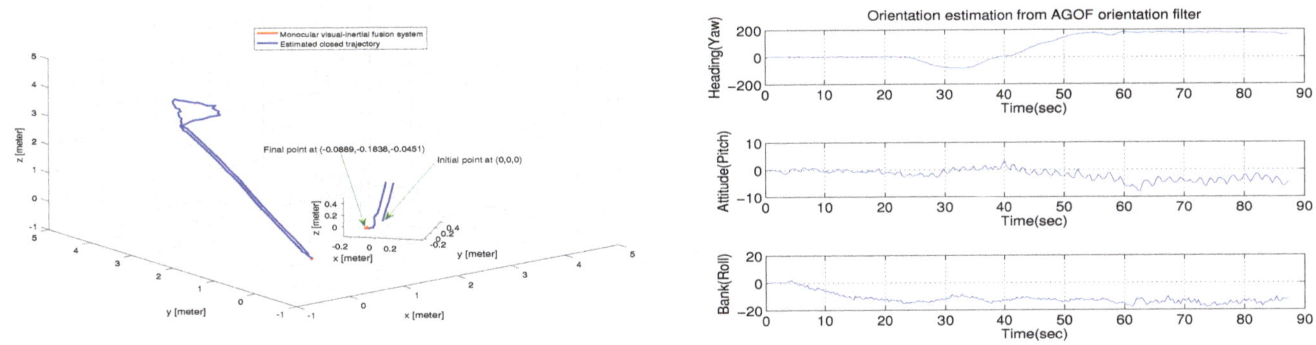

(a) (b)

Figure 13. Closed-loop Motion Estimation. (**a**) closed trajectory estimation; (**b**) orientation estimation from AGOF filter.

6.2.5. Experiment V: Motion Estimation with Moving Objects in an Office-Based Environment

During this test, a person wearing the visual-inertial system was walking in an office-based environment, where a moving toy car was viewed. In this test scenario, a straight line was performed by the moving toy car on a table. The detected moving toy car is labeled within a black bounding box and six key frames with this detected toy car are selected as denoted in Figure 14a–f. Figure 14g shows the motion of the real and virtual camera, which are labeled by using red and blue line, respectively. The motion of moving car is finally derived and labeled by green line in Figure 14g. In particular, the trajectory of a moving car is clearly seen by drawing the shadows of each motion on a 2D plane.

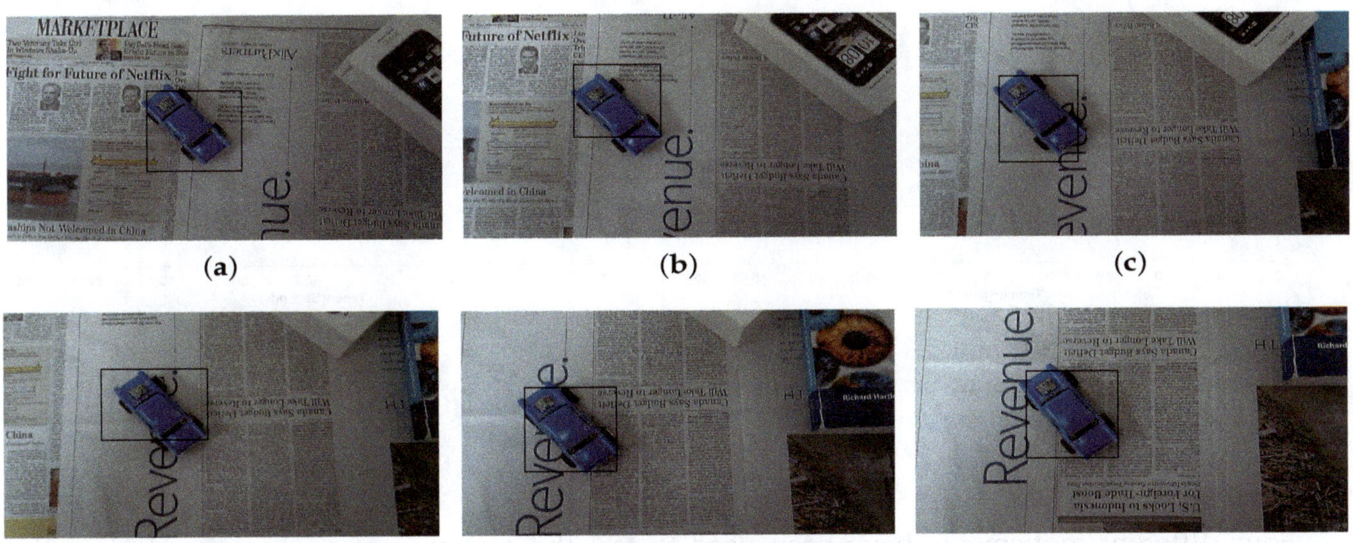

(a) (b) (c) (d) (e) (f)

Figure 14. *Cont.*

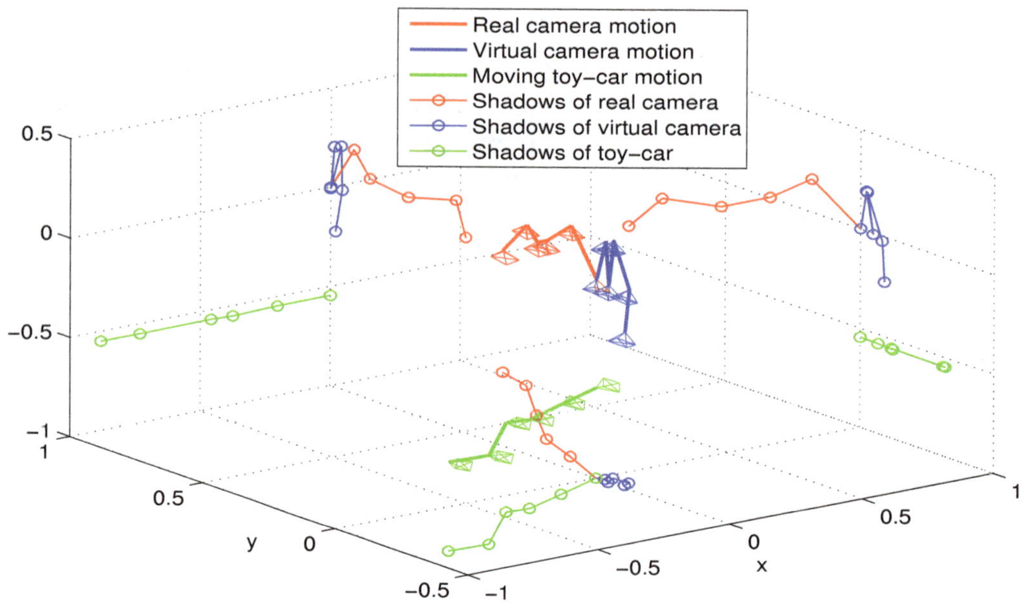

(g)

Figure 14. Motion estimation with moving objects in an office-based environment. (**a**–**f**) typical frames; (**g**) the 3D motion of real camera, virtual camera and moving toy car with 2D shadows.

6.3. Experimental Analysis

6.3.1. Scale Factor Analysis

Figure 15 shows the scale factor estimation for straight-line and curve movements. It is clearly illustrated that the scale factor *s* changes over time *t* and its converge time is about 10 s. Therefore, each experiment requires 10 s time calibration at the beginning.

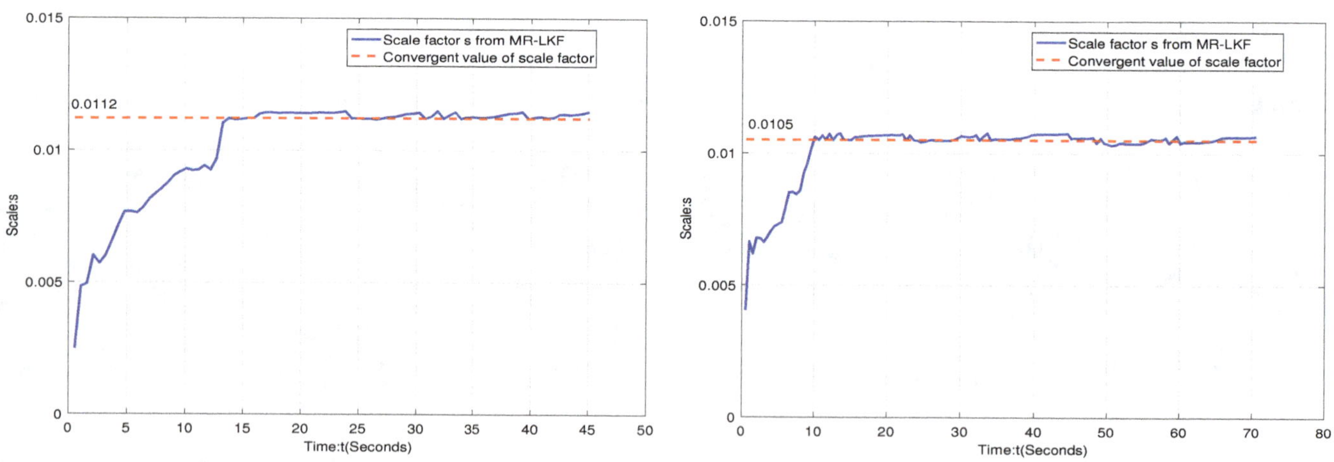

(a) (b)

Figure 15. Scale factor analysis. (**a**) scale factor estimation for straight-line motion; (**a**) scale factor estimation for curve motion.

6.3.2. Accuracy Analysis

Four different movements have been used to test the accuracy of our proposed algorithm. For Experiments I and II, the error of each camera position ${}^{c}_{e}\boldsymbol{p}_k$ in the reconstructed trajectory is calculated as the Euclidean distance between each point of the estimated camera trajectory and the trajectory $p_{robot,k}$ from Pioneer robot as shown in Label (36). Based on the known trajectory equation of the semicircle, the accuracy can be verified by Label (37), where $r = 0.221$ m is actually the length of robot arm. The accuracy of the fifth experiment is verified based on the known path of the moving toy car:

$$error_k = \sqrt{({}^c_e p_k - p_{robot,k})^T ({}^c_e p_k - p_{robot,k})}, \tag{36}$$

$$(x - r)^2 + y^2 = r^2. \tag{37}$$

Table 3 depicts the error accuracy analysis for four experiments. The true length of four different trajectories is respectively 12 m, 12.5 m, 0.69 m and 1 m. As clearly shown in Figures 10h and 11h, the robot platform experienced different motions with slow and smooth motion in Experiment I and fast rotational and translational motion in Experiment II. From Table 3, it is clearly seen that Experiment I has higher accuracy than Experiment II, but the estimated results from our proposed method in both of Experiments I and II are more accurate than those from the EKF as shown in Figures 10g and 11g.

Table 3. Error accuracy analysis in four experiments.

Trajectory Type and Length (m)	Mean Error (m)	Maximum Error (m)	Mean Error over the Trajectory
Experiment I: 12	0.17	0.28	1.42%
Experiment II: 12.5	0.3	0.55	2.4%
Experiment III: 0.69	0.015	0.03	2.2%
Experiment V: 1	0.035	0.12	3.5%

6.3.3. Dynamic Scene Segmentation Analysis

The experimental illustration was shown in Figure 16 to demonstrate our proposed AGOF-aided homography recovery constraint for dynamic scene segmentation. Figure 16a shows detected 2D feature points and matched in two consecutive frames (green circles in the first frame and red circles in the second frame). In Figure 16b, the feature points in the first frame are transformed and 2D motion paths are obtained based on homography recovery with the help of the AGOF orientation filter. It is clear seen from Figure 16c that the feature matches can be easily sorted out. Finally, the moving object can be detected and separated from the background as denoted in Figure 16d.

The experimental illustration for the proposed dynamic scene segmentation constrained by epipolar geometry is shown in Figure 17. Figure 17a depicts detected 2D feature points and matched in two consecutive frames. The distance errors between the points and their corresponding epipolar lines are shown in Figure 17b. As we described in Section 4.1.2, the larger the distance is, the more likely the 3D point belongs to an independently moving object. Therefore, the distance errors can be used to sort out the points belonging to the moving object. As a result, the moving object can be separated from the background and tracked in each frame as shown in Figure 17c,d.

6.3.4. Scale Adjustment and Estimation Analysis

Based on a set of scale inconsistent camera motions and 2D feature matches, the 3D structure could be reconstructed using a linear reconstruction method, such as singular value decomposition (SVD) [10]. While the reconstructed 3D structure could be very noisy and not consistent due to the frame-to-frame reconstruction and the inconsistent estimation of the camera motion. This also results in a duplicated structure as shown in Figure 18b. After adopting our proposed scale adjustment method, a refined 3D point cloud can be obtained with a unified scale. Figure 18c clearly shows that the reconstructed 3D structure is consistent and has no duplicated structure. Having obtained a set of scale consistent camera motions, an absolute global scale can be estimated with the help of the IMU sensor and the 3D reconstructed point cloud with metric scale is shown in Figure 18d.

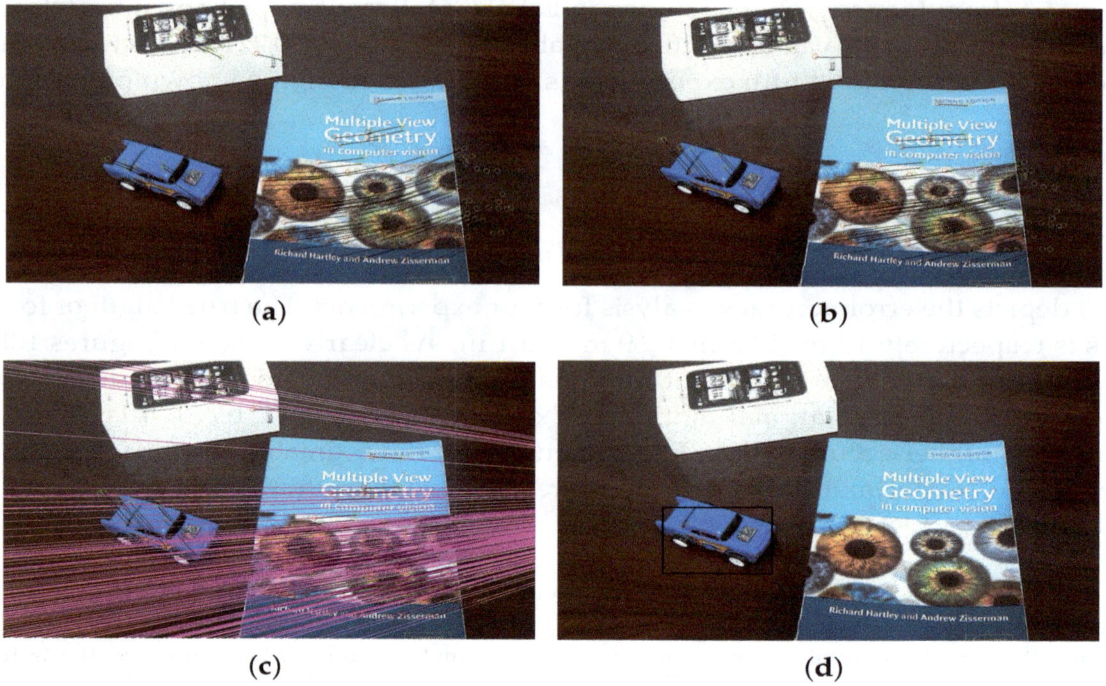

Figure 16. Experimental illustrations for homography recovery. (**a**) detected 2D feature points in first frame; (**b**) detected 2D feature points in second frame; (**c**) sorted feature matches; (**d**) detected toy car.

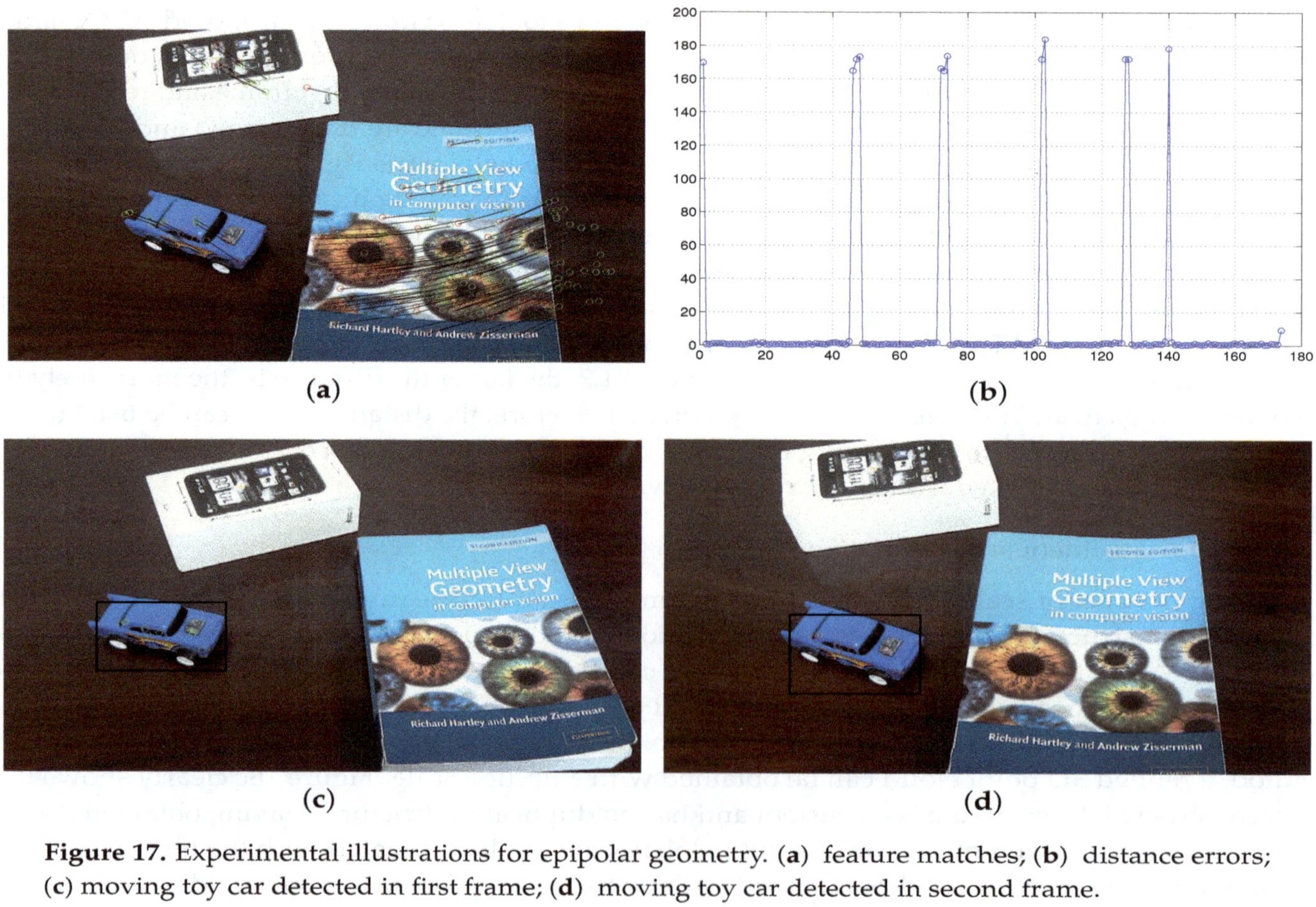

Figure 17. Experimental illustrations for epipolar geometry. (**a**) feature matches; (**b**) distance errors; (**c**) moving toy car detected in first frame; (**d**) moving toy car detected in second frame.

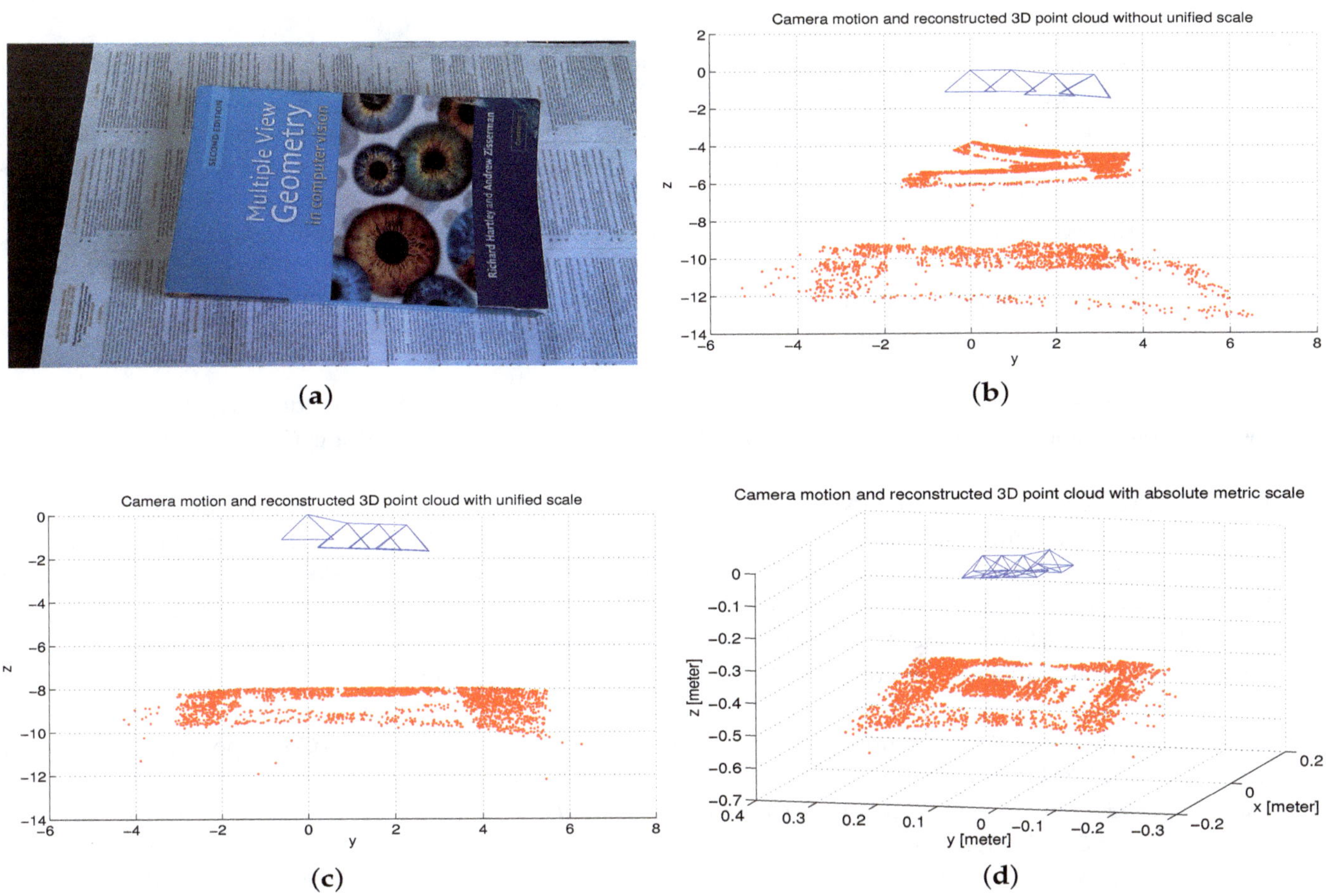

Figure 18. Experimental illustrations for scale adjustment and estimation. (**a**) original frame; (**b**) camera motion and 3D reconstructed point cloud without unified scale; (**c**) camera motion and 3D reconstructed point cloud with unified scale; (**d**) camera motion and 3D reconstructed point cloud with metric scale.

7. Conclusions

A novel wearable absolute ego-motion tracking system was proposed for indoor positioning. The use of pre-estimated orientation from inertial sensors can eliminate mismatched points based on geometry constraints. In addition, a novel concept of "virtual camera" was presented to represent the motion from the motion areas related to each moving object, which was actually the combined motion from the real camera and the moving object. Moreover, an adaptive multi-rare linear Kalman filter was adopted to solve not only scale ambiguity, but also the problem of different sampling rates. This proposed system has much potential to aid the visually impaired and blind people, so, in the future, the goal of our work will aim at several scenarios of real obstacles to test the robustness and effectiveness of the proposed system with motion alerts.

Acknowledgments: This work is partially supported by the National Science Foundation of China (NSFC) under Grant (No. 61403237 and No. 61573226) and Shandong Jianzhu University Doctoral Program Foundation under Grant (No. XNBS1330).

Author Contributions: Ya Tian and Zhe Chen designed the algorithm, performed the experiments, analyzed the data and wrote the paper. Shouyin Lu and Jindong Tan conceived of and designed the experiments. All authors contributed to the paper correction and improvments.

References

1. Aging Statistics from Administration on Aging. Available online: https://aoa.acl.gov/Aging-Statistics/index.aspx (accessed on 24 October 2017).
2. Tian, Y.; Wei, H.; Tan, J. An Adaptive-Gain Complementary Filter for Real-Time Human Motion Tracking With MARG Sensors in Free-Living Environments. *IEEE Trans. Neural Syst. Rehabilit. Eng.* **2013**, *21*, 254–264.
3. Davison, A. Real-time simultaneous localisation and mapping with a single camera. In Proceedings of the ICCV '03 Proceedings of the Ninth IEEE International Conference on Computer Vision, Washington, DC, USA, 13–16 October 2003; Volume 2, pp. 1403–1410.
4. Klein, G.; Murray, D. Parallel Tracking and Mapping for Small AR Workspaces. In Proceedings of the 6th IEEE and ACM International Symposium on Mixed and Augmented Reality, Nara, Japan, 13–16 November 2007; pp. 225–234.
5. Forster, C.; Pizzoli, M.; Scaramuzza, D. SVO: Fast Semi-Direct Monocular Visual Odometry. In Proceedings of the IEEE International Conference on Robotics and Automation (ICRA), Hong Kong, China, 31 May–7 June 2014; pp. 15–22.
6. Engel, J.; Cremers, D. Semi-dense Visual Odometry for a Monocular Camera. In Proceedings of the IEEE International Conference on Computer Vision, Sydney, Australia, 1–8 December 2014; pp. 1449–1456.
7. Randeniya, D.; Sarkar, S.; Gunaratne, M. Vision-IMU Integration Using a Slow-Frame-Rate Monocular Vision System in an Actual Roadway Setting. *IEEE Trans. Intell. Transp. Syst.* **2010**, *11*, 256–266.
8. Tardif, J.; George, M.; Laverne, M. A New Approach to Vision-Aided Inertial Navigation. In Proceedings of the IEEE/RSJ International Conference on Intelligent Robots and Systems, Taipei, Taiwan, 18–22 October 2010; pp. 4161–4168.
9. Scharstein, D.; Szeliski, R. A Taxonomy and Evaluation of Dense Two-Frame Stereo Correspondence Algorithms. *Int. J. Comput. Vis.* **2002**, *47*, 7–42.
10. Hartley, R.; Zisserman, A. *Multiple View Geometry in Computer Vision*; The Press Syndicate of the University of Cambridge: Cambridge, UK, 2003.
11. Pollefeys, M.; Van Gool, L.; Vergauwen, M.; Verbiest, F.; Cornelis, K.; Tops, J.; Koch, R. Visual Modeling with a Hand-Held Camera. *Int. J. Comput. Vis.* **2004**, *59*, 207–232.
12. Jebara, T.; Azarbayejani, A.; Pentland, A. 3D structure from 2D motion. *IEEE Signal Process. Mag.* **1999**, *16*, 66–84.
13. Chiuso, A.; Favaro, P.; Jin, H.; Soatto, S. Structure from motion causally integrated over time. *IEEE Trans. Pattern Anal. Mach. Intell.* **2002**, *24*, 523–535.
14. Esteban, I.; Dijk, J.; Groen, F. FIT3D toolbox: Multiple view geometry and 3D reconstruction for matlab. In *Electro-Optical Remote Sensing, Photonic Technologies, and Applications IV*; SPIE: Bellingham, WA, USA, 2010.
15. You, S.; Neumann, U.; Azuma, R. Hybrid Inertial and Vision Tracking for Augmented Reality Registration. In Proceedings of the IEEE Virtual Reality, Houston, TX, USA, 13–17 March 1999; pp. 260–267.
16. Huster, A.; Frew, E.; Rock, S. Relative position estimation for AUVs by fusing bearing and inertial rate sensor measurements. In Proceedings of the OCEANS '02 MTS/IEEE, Biloxi, MI, USA, 29–31 October 2002; Volume 3, pp. 1863–1870.
17. Bleser, G.; Stricker, D. Advanced Tracking Through Efficient Image Processing and Visual-Inertial Sensor Fusion. *Comput. Graph.* **2009**, *33*, 59–72.
18. Peter Corke, J.L.; Dias, J. An introduction to inertial and vision sensing. *Int. J. Robot. Res.* **2007**, *26*, 519–535.
19. Gemeiner, P.; Einramhof, P.; Vincze, M. Simultaneous motion and structure estimation by fusion of inertial and vision data. *Int. J. Robot. Res.* **2007**, *26*, 591–605.
20. Maes, K.; Lourens, E.; Nimmen, K.V.; Reynders, E.; Roeck, G.D.; Lombaert, G. Design of sensor networks for instantaneous inversion of modally reduced order models in structural dynamics. *Mech. Syst. Signal Process.* **2015**, *52–53*, 628–644.
21. Lourens, E.; Papadimitriou, C.; Gillijns, S.; Reynders, E.; Roeck, G.D.; Lombaert, G. Joint input-response estimation for structural systems based on reduced-order models and vibration data from a limited number of sensors. *Mech. Syst. Signal Process.* **2012**, *29*, 310–327.
22. Azam, S.E.; Chatzi, E.; Papadimitriou, C. A dual Kalman filter approach for state estimation via output-only acceleration measurements. *Mech. Syst. Signal Process.* **2015**, *60–61*, 866–886.

23. Azam, S.E.; Chatzi, E.; Papadimitriou, C.; Smyth, A. Experimental Validation of the Dual Kalman Filter for Online and Real-Time State and Input Estimation. In Proceedings of the IMAC XXXIII, Orlando, FL, USA, 2–5 February 2015; pp. 1–13.
24. Chen, J.; Pinz, A. Structure and Motion by Fusion of Inertial and Vision-Based Tracking. In Proceedings of the 28th OAGM/AAPR Conference, Hagenberg, Austria, 17–18 June 2004; Volume 179; pp. 55–62.
25. Li, M.; Mourikis, A.I. *High-Precision, Consistent EKF-Based Visual-Inertial Odometry*; Sage Publications, Inc.: Thousand Oaks, CA, USA, 2013.
26. Panahandeh, G.; Jansson, M. Vision-Aided Inertial Navigation Based on Ground Plane Feature Detection. *IEEE/ASME Trans. Mechatron.* **2014**, *19*, 1206–1215.
27. Diel, D.D.; DeBitetto, P.; Teller, S. Epipolar Constraints for Vision-Aided Inertial Navigation. In Proceedings of the IEEE Workshop on Motion and Video Computing, Breckenridge, CO, USA, 5–7 January 2005; Volume 2, pp. 221–228.
28. Liu, C.; Prior, S.D.; Teacy, W.L.; Warner, M. Computationally efficient visual-inertial sensor fusion for Global Positioning System-denied navigation on a small quadrotor. *Adv. Mech. Eng.* **2016**, *8*, doi:10.1177/1687814016640996.
29. Madgwick, S.O.H.; Harrison, A.J.L.; Vaidyanathan, R. Estimation of IMU and MARG orientation using a gradient descent algorithm. In Proceedings of the IEEE International Conference on Rehabilitation Robotics, Zurich, Switzerland, 29 June–1 July 2011; p. 5975346.
30. Tian, Y.; Hamel, W.R.; Tan, J. Accurate Human Navigation Using Wearable Monocular Visual and Inertial Sensors. *IEEE Trans. Instrum. Meas.* **2014**, *63*, 203–213.
31. Lowe, D. Distinctive image features from scale-invariant keypoints. *Int. J. Comput. Vis.* **2004**, *60*, 91–110.
32. Horn, B.K. Recovering Baseline and Orientaiton from Essential Matrix. *J. Opt. Soc. Am.* **1990**, *M*, 1–10.
33. Esteban, I.; Dorst, L.; Dijk, J. Closed form solution for the scale ambiguity problem in monocular visual odometry. In Proceedings of the Third International Conference on Intelligent Robotics and Applications, Shanghai, China, 10–12 November 2010; Part I; pp. 665–679.
34. Lobo, J.; Dias, J. Vision and Inertial Sensor Cooperation Using Gravity as a Vertical Reference. *IEEE Trans. Pattern Anal. Mach. Intell.* **2003**, *25*, 1597–1608.

Permissions

All chapters in this book were first published by MDPI; hereby published with permission under the Creative Commons Attribution License or equivalent. Every chapter published in this book has been scrutinized by our experts. Their significance has been extensively debated. The topics covered herein carry significant findings which will fuel the growth of the discipline. They may even be implemented as practical applications or may be referred to as a beginning point for another development.

The contributors of this book come from diverse backgrounds, making this book a truly international effort. This book will bring forth new frontiers with its revolutionizing research information and detailed analysis of the nascent developments around the world.

We would like to thank all the contributing authors for lending their expertise to make the book truly unique. They have played a crucial role in the development of this book. Without their invaluable contributions this book wouldn't have been possible. They have made vital efforts to compile up to date information on the varied aspects of this subject to make this book a valuable addition to the collection of many professionals and students.

This book was conceptualized with the vision of imparting up-to-date information and advanced data in this field. To ensure the same, a matchless editorial board was set up. Every individual on the board went through rigorous rounds of assessment to prove their worth. After which they invested a large part of their time researching and compiling the most relevant data for our readers.

The editorial board has been involved in producing this book since its inception. They have spent rigorous hours researching and exploring the diverse topics which have resulted in the successful publishing of this book. They have passed on their knowledge of decades through this book. To expedite this challenging task, the publisher supported the team at every step. A small team of assistant editors was also appointed to further simplify the editing procedure and attain best results for the readers.

Apart from the editorial board, the designing team has also invested a significant amount of their time in understanding the subject and creating the most relevant covers. They scrutinized every image to scout for the most suitable representation of the subject and create an appropriate cover for the book.

The publishing team has been an ardent support to the editorial, designing and production team. Their endless efforts to recruit the best for this project, has resulted in the accomplishment of this book. They are a veteran in the field of academics and their pool of knowledge is as vast as their experience in printing. Their expertise and guidance has proved useful at every step. Their uncompromising quality standards have made this book an exceptional effort. Their encouragement from time to time has been an inspiration for everyone.

The publisher and the editorial board hope that this book will prove to be a valuable piece of knowledge for researchers, students, practitioners and scholars across the globe.

List of Contributors

Mohiuddin Khan Shourav and Subin Kim
Department of Mechanical Engineering, Graduate School, Kookmin University, 77 Jeongneung-ro, Seongbuk-gu, Seoul 02707, Korea

Jung Kyung Kim
Department of Mechanical Engineering, Graduate School, Kookmin University, 77 Jeongneung-ro, Seongbuk-gu, Seoul 02707, Korea
School of Mechanical Systems Engineering, Kookmin University, 77 Jeongneung-ro, Seongbuk-gu, Seoul 02707, Korea

Kyunghoon Kim
School of Mechanical Systems Engineering, Kookmin University, 77 Jeongneung-ro, Seongbuk-gu, Seoul 02707, Korea
Department of Mechanical and Aerospace Engineering, North Carolina State University, Raleigh, NC 27695, USA

Jong Kang Park
Department of Biological Engineering, Massachusetts Institute of Technology, Cambridge, MA 02139, USA

Christopher J. Rowlands
Department of Chemical Engineering and Biotechnology, Cambridge University, Cambridge CB2 1TN, UK

Peter T. C. So
Department of Biological Engineering, Massachusetts Institute of Technology, Cambridge, MA 02139, USA
Laser Biomedical Research Center (LBRC), Massachusetts Institute of Technology, Cambridge, MA 02139, USA

Guangcan Zhou, Zi Heng Lim, Yi Qi and Guangya Zhou
Micro and Nano Systems Initiative, Department of Mechanical Engineering, National University of Singapore, Singapore 117575, Singapore

Chunlong Fei, Qidong Zhang, Yani Li and Yintang Yang
School of Microelectronics, Xidian University, Xi'an 710071, China

Di Li
School of Microelectronics, Xidian University, Xi'an 710071, China
Department of Ophthalmology and Biomedical Engineering, University of Southern California, Los Angeles, CA 90089-1111, USA

Chunlong Fei, Tianlong Zhao, Pengfei Lin, Di Li and Yintang Yang
School of Microelectronics, Xidian University, Xi'an 740071, China

Danfeng Wang
School of Microelectronics, Xidian University, Xi'an 740071, China
School of Electronic and Electrical Engineering, Wuhan Textile University, Wuhan 430200, China

Jianzheng Cheng
School of Electronic and Electrical Engineering, Wuhan Textile University, Wuhan 430200, China

Yi Quan
Electronic Materials Research Laboratory, Key Laboratory of the Ministry of Education & International Center for Dielectric Research, Xi'an Jiaotong University, Xi'an 740049, China

Chunlei Wang and Chunming Wang
School of Physics, State Key Laboratory of Crystal Materials, Shandong University, Jinan 250100, China

Yeong-Hyeon Seo, Kyungmin Hwang, Hyunwoo Kim and Ki-Hun Jeong
Department of Bio and Brain Engineering, KAIST, Daejeon 34141, Korea
KAIST Institute for Health Science and Technology, Daejeon 34141, Korea

Hui Yang and Sihui Chen
Laboratory of Biomedical Microsystems and Nano Devices, Bionic Sensing and Intelligence Center, Institute of Biomedical and Health Engineering, Shenzhen Institutes of Advanced Technology, Chinese Academy of Sciences, Shenzhen 518055, China

Yi Zhang
Institute of Biomedical Therapeutics, University of Southern California, Los Angeles, CA 90033, USA

Olutosin Charles Fawole
Livanova Inc., 100 Cyberonics Blvd, Houston, TX 77058, USA

Rui Hao
Laboratory of Biomedical Microsystems and Nano Devices, Bionic Sensing and Intelligence Center, Institute of Biomedical and Health Engineering, Shenzhen Institutes of Advanced Technology, Chinese Academy of Sciences, Shenzhen 518055, China
Pen-Tung Sah Institute of Micro-Nano Science and Technology, Xiamen University, Xiamen 361005, China

Subhashish Dolai
Electrical and Computer Engineering Department, University of Utah, Salt Lake City, UT 84112, USA

Hsuan-Yu Leu and Jules Magda
Chemical Engineering Department, University of Utah, Salt Lake City, UT 84112, USA

Massood Tabib-Azar
Electrical and Computer Engineering Department, University of Utah, Salt Lake City, UT 84112, USA
Bio Engineering Department, University of Utah, Salt Lake City, UT 84112, USA

Weizhi Qi, Qian Chen, Heng Guo and Lei Xi
Department of Biomedical Engineering, Southern University of Science and Technology, Shenzhen 518055, China
School of Physics, University of Electronic Science and Technology of China, Chengdu 610054, China

Huikai Xie
Department of Electrical and Computer Engineering, University of Florida, Gainesville, FL 32611, USA

Zhuoqing Yang, Jianhao Shi, Jinyuan Yao and Guifu Ding
National Key Laboratory of Science and Technology on Micro/Nano Fabrication, School of Electronics Information and Electrical Engineering, Shanghai Jiao Tong University, Shanghai 200240, China

Bin Sun
Institute of Biomedical and Health Engineering, Shenzhen Institute of Advanced Technology, Chinese Academy of Science, Shenzhen 518055, China

Renshi Sawada
Graduate School of Systems Life Science, Kyushu University, Fukuoka 819-0395, Japan

Zhen Qiu
Department of Biomedical Engineering, Institute for Quantitative Health Science and Engineering, Michigan State University, East Lansing, MI 48824, USA

Wibool Piyawattanametha
Department of Biomedical Engineering, Institute for Quantitative Health Science and Engineering, Michigan State University, East Lansing, MI 48824, USA
Departments of Biomedical Engineering, Faculty of Engineering King Mongkut's Institute of Technology Ladkrabang (KMITL), Bangkok 10520, Thailand

Kevin Brenner, Kamyar Firouzi, Morten Fischer Rasmussen, Quintin Stedman and Butrus (Pierre) Khuri-Yakub
E.L. Ginzton Lab., Stanford University, Stanford, CA 94305, USA

Arif Sanli Ergun
E.L. Ginzton Lab., Stanford University, Stanford, CA 94305, USA
Department of Electrical and Electronics Engineering, TOBB University of Economics and Technology, Ankara 06560, Turkey

Kebin Gu
Department of Mechanical Engineering, University of Washington, Seattle, WA 98185, USA

ChiLeung Tsui
Department of Electrical and Computer Engineering, University of Washington, Seattle, WA 98185, USA

Wei-Chih Wang
Department of Mechanical Engineering, University of Washington, Seattle, WA 98185, USA
Department of Electrical and Computer Engineering, University of Washington, Seattle, WA 98185,USA
Institute of Nanoengineering and Microsystems, National Tsinghua University, Hsinchu 300, Taiwan
Department of Power Mechanical Engineering, National Tsinghua University, Hsinchu 300, Taiwan

Changho Lee
Department of Nuclear Medicine, Chonnam National University Medical School & Hwasun Hospital, Hwasun 58128, Korea

Jin Young Kim
Departments of Mechanical Engineering, Pohang University of Science and Technology (POSTECH), Pohang 37673, Korea

Chulhong Kim
Departments of Mechanical Engineering, Pohang University of Science and Technology (POSTECH), Pohang 37673, Korea
Departments of Creative IT Engineering and Electrical Engineering, Pohang University of Science and Technology (POSTECH), Pohang 37673, Korea

Zeyu Chen
College of Mechanical & Electrical Engineering, Central South University, Changsha 410083, China
Department of Biomedical Engineering, University of Southern California, Los Angeles, CA 90089, USA

Xuejun Qian, Runze Li and Kirk Shung
Department of Biomedical Engineering, University of Southern California, Los Angeles, CA 90089, USA

Xuan Song
Department of Mechanical and Industrial Engineering, The University of Iowa, Iowa City, IA 52242, USA

Qiangguo Jiang and Rongji Huang
School of Electro-Mechanical Engineering, Guangdong University of Technology, Guangzhou 510006, China

Yang Yang and Yong Chen
Epstein Department of Industrial and Systems Engineering, University of Southern California, Los Angeles, CA 90089, USA

Qifa Zhou
Department of Biomedical Engineering, University of Southern California, Los Angeles, CA 90089, USA
Roski Eye Institute, University of Southern California, Los Angeles, CA 90089, USA

Zhe Chen
School of Information and Electrical Engineering, Shandong Jianzhu University, Jinan 250101, China

Ya Tian and Shouyin Lu
School of Information and Electrical Engineering, Shandong Jianzhu University, Jinan 250101, China
Shandong Provincial Key Laboratory of Intelligent Buildings Technology, Jinan 250101, China
Shandong Provincial Key Laboratory of Intelligent Technology for New Type Man-Machine Interaction and Robot System, Jinan 250101, China

Jindong Tan
Department of Mechanical, Aerospace, and Biomedical Engineering, The University of Tennessee, Knoxville, TN 37996, USA

Index

Printed in the USA
CPSIA information can be obtained
at www.ICGtesting.com
LVHW081322310823
756829LV00007B/324